Fundamentals of High-Resolution Lung CT

Common Findings, Common Patterns, Common Diseases, and Differential Diagnosis

Fundamentals of High-Resolution Lung CT

Common Findings, Common Patterns, Common Diseases, and Differential Diagnosis

BRETT M. ELICKER, M.D.

Associate Professor of Clinical Radiology and Biomedical Imaging
Chief, Cardiac and Pulmonary Imaging
University of California—San Francisco
San Francisco, California

W. RICHARD WEBB, M.D.

Professor Emeritus of Radiology and Biomedical Imaging
Emeritus Member, Haile T. Debas Academy of Medical Educators
University of California—San Francisco
San Francisco, California

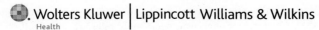

Wolters Kluwer | Lippincott Williams & Wilkins
Health

Philadelphia • Baltimore • New York • London
Buenos Aires • Hong Kong • Sydney • Tokyo

Executive Editor: Jonathan W. Pine, Jr.
Product Manager: Amy G. Dinkel
Senior Manufacturing Manager: Benjamin Rivera
Director of Marketing: Caroline Foote
Production Project Manager: David Orzechowski
Designer: Teresa Mallon
Production Service: Integra Software Services Pvt. Ltd.

Printed in China

Library of Congress Cataloging-in-Publication Data

Elicker, Brett M.
  Fundamentals of high-resolution lung CT : common findings, common patterns, common diseases, and differential diagnosis / Brett M. Elicker, W. Richard Webb.
     p. ; cm.
  Includes bibliographical references and index.
  ISBN 978-1-4511-8408-2 (alk. paper)
  I. Webb, W. Richard (Wayne Richard), 1945- II. Title.
  [DNLM: 1.   Lung—radiography. 2.   Tomography, X-Ray Computed. 3.   Diagnosis, Differential.
4.   Lung Diseases—radiography. WF 600]

  616.2'407572—dc23

                                        2012032695

Care has been taken to confirm the accuracy of the information presented and to describe generally accepted practices. However, the authors, editors, and publisher are not responsible for errors or omissions or for any consequences from application of the information in this book and make no warranty, expressed or implied, with respect to the currency, completeness, or accuracy of the contents of the publication. Application of the information in a particular situation remains the professional responsibility of the practitioner.

The authors, editors, and publisher have exerted every effort to ensure that drug selection and dosage set forth in this text are in accordance with current recommendations and practice at the time of publication. However, in view of ongoing research, changes in government regulations, and the constant flow of information relating to drug therapy and drug reactions, the reader is urged to check the package insert for each drug for any change in indications and dosage and for added warnings and precautions. This is particularly important when the recommended agent is a new or infrequently employed drug.

Some drugs and medical devices presented in the publication have Food and Drug Administration (FDA) clearance for limited use in restricted research settings. It is the responsibility of the health care provider to ascertain the FDA status of each drug or device planned for use in their clinical practice.

To purchase additional copies of this book, call our customer service department at (800) 638-3030 or fax orders to (301) 223-2320. International customers should call (301) 223-2300.

Visit Lippincott Williams & Wilkins on the Internet: at LWW.com. Lippincott Williams & Wilkins customer service representatives are available from 8:30 am to 6 pm, EST.

Dedication

To Emma, Cole, Jack, and
"The Old Salt"
from
B.M.E.

To E, C, and J
from
W.R.W. (i.e. "The Old Salt")

Preface

The accurate interpretation of high-resolution CT in patients with diffuse lung disease is fundamentally based on 1) the recognition of specific HRCT findings; 2) an understanding of what they mean and their relationship to differential diagnosis; 3) a basic knowledge of the lung diseases that most commonly result in diffuse lung disease; and 4) the typical constellation of findings associated with each of these diseases.

Although interpreting HRCT can seem to be a complicated task, an understanding of these four basic principles often leads to the recognition of a typical or classic "pattern" of lung disease and the correct diagnosis or a list of diagnostic possibilities. On the other hand, it is important to understand that some HRCT patterns are necessarily nonspecific and should lead to further evaluation and correlation with clinical findings or lung biopsy.

In some sense, this book is "HRCT Lite." It is intended to provide a simple and easily understandable approach to diagnosis and differential diagnosis. However, it is also important to emphasize that we do not consider this book to be an oversimplification of the HRCT principles and diagnosis of diffuse lung disease. The chapters and illustrations in this book are based upon, and demonstrate, the fundamental observations, rules, shortcuts, thought patterns, and differential diagnoses we use in everyday clinical practice and have built up over a period of years of HRCT-pathologic correlation. It also is intended to review our basic and practical understanding of the lung diseases commonly assessed using HRCT.

It is our intention that this book provides the fundamental insights and facts necessary to interpret HRCT in most clinical settings, in an easily understood and digestible format. Although it is not comprehensive, it is our hope that it provides a practical and useful understanding of HRCT and its use in the diagnosis of diffuse lung disease.

Brett M. Elicker
W. Richard Webb
San Francisco, California

Contents

Fundamentals of High-Resolution Lung CT

Common Findings, Common Patterns, Common Diseases, and Differential Diagnosis

1

HRCT FINDINGS

HRCT Indications, Technique, Radiation Dose, and Normal Anatomy

High-resolution computed tomography (HRCT) is widely used in the evaluation of a variety of diffuse lung diseases. The goal of this introductory chapter is to discuss the basics of HRCT, including indications, technique, and normal lung anatomy, as displayed using this modality.

INDICATIONS FOR HRCT

HRCT has several indications and uses in patients with, or suspected of having, diffuse lung disease (Table 1.1).

Detection of Diffuse Lung Disease

HRCT can be more sensitive and specific in the diagnosis of diffuse lung disease than other diagnostic tests (Fig. 1.1A, B), including plain radiographs and pulmonary function tests. For instance, HRCT may detect abnormalities in asymptomatic patients with connective tissue disease or other conditions, or with various exposures, before pulmonary function tests become abnormal. Detecting abnormalities at an early stage may allow for appropriate treatment, preventing progression of lung disease.

Table 1.1 Indications for HRCT
Detection of diffuse lung disease
• Detect abnormalities before other tests (e.g., chest x-ray) become abnormal
• Exclude certain diseases as a cause of symptoms
Characterization of diffuse lung disease
• Identification of specific abnormalities
• Formulation of a differential diagnosis
• Determine if reversible or irreversible abnormalities are likely present
• Help determine prognosis
Differential diagnosis and guidance for further testing
• HRCT findings (with clinical information) may be sufficiently diagnostic
• HRCT findings may suggest the appropriate study
• tree-in-bud: sputum analysis
• perilymphatic nodules or possible infection: transbronchial biopsy
• nonspecific diffuse lung disease: video-assisted thoracoscopic surgical lung biopsy
Sequential evaluation of abnormalities over time
• Response to treatment
• Assess patients with new symptoms

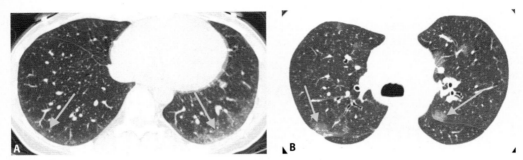

Figure 1.1

Detection of early lung disease. HRCT may be more sensitive than other tests in detecting diffuse lung disease. **A.** Mild subpleural ground glass opacity (*arrows*) is seen in a patient with nonspecific interstitial pneumonia associated with scleroderma. This patient has a normal chest x-ray and pulmonary function tests. **B.** In a patient with acquired immune deficiency syndrome and a normal chest x-ray, patchy ground glass opacity (*arrows*) is visible on HRCT. Bronchoscopy confirmed *Pneumocystis jiroveci* infection.

HRCT may also be used to exclude certain lung diseases as a cause of symptoms or abnormal pulmonary function test findings. For example, in patients with pulmonary hypertension, HRCT may be used to exclude emphysema and fibrotic lung disease as causative etiologies. As another example, in patients with acquired immune deficiency syndrome and a suspicion of *Pneumocystis jiroveci* infection, HRCT has a high negative predictive value, and further testing, such as bronchoscopy, is not generally required if the study is normal.

Characterization of Diffuse Lung Disease

The primary role of HRCT is in the identification of specific abnormalities that allow a characterization of diffuse lung disease and formulation of a differential diagnosis. The type and specific location of lung abnormalities may be determined using HRCT, and it may be suggested whether the disease present is primarily inflammatory or fibrotic or whether it is an airways disease (Fig. 1.2), interstitial disease, or alveolar (airspace) disease (Fig. 1.3).

HRCT findings may have important implications for treatment and prognosis. When findings of fibrosis are present on HRCT, patients are less likely to respond to various medications and, in general, have a poorer prognosis. Patients with HRCT findings suggestive of inflammation are generally treated more aggressively in the hope that the

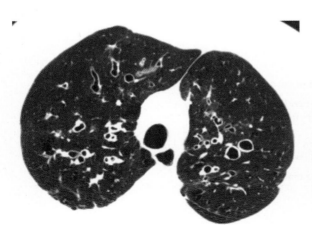

Figure 1.2

HRCT characterization of lung disease. HRCT allows the diagnosis of airways disease in this patient with chronic symptoms. It provides an accurate assessment of both acute and chronic abnormalities in patients with airways disease. Bronchiectasis, airway wall thickening, and luminal impaction are present in this patient with cystic fibrosis.

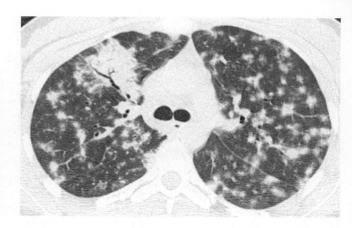

Figure 1.3

HRCT characterization of lung disease. HRCT provides an accurate diagnosis of diffuse alveolar or airspace disease in a patient with patchy consolidation and an air bronchogram. In this example, patchy nodular areas of peribronchovascular and subpleural consolidation are present in a patient with organizing pneumonia.

lung findings are reversible. HRCT is helpful in making this distinction.

Differential Diagnosis and Guidance for Further Diagnostic Testing

HRCT is more specific than chest radiography, physical examination, and pulmonary function tests in the diagnosis and characterization of lung abnormalities in patients with diffuse lung disease (Fig. 1.4A, B), and some HRCT findings may be highly suggestive of a specific disease. Nonetheless, most HRCT abnormalities are nonspecific and require a differential diagnosis.

The diagnosis of diffuse lung disease is generally based on a multidisciplinary approach, incorporating clinical information, HRCT findings, and sometimes pathology. Infrequently, one of these is sufficient to make a definitive diagnosis, and a combination of at least two is usually required to maintain a high degree of diagnostic accuracy and confidence. When HRCT is interpreted in conjunction with clinical information, the accuracy and specificity of diagnosis improve significantly (Table 1.2). Examples of clinical information useful in the diagnosis of diffuse lung abnormalities include patient age, duration of symptoms, a history of cigarette smoking, exposures (e.g., inhalational and environmental), immune status, drug treatment, and known systemic disorders such as connective tissue disease.

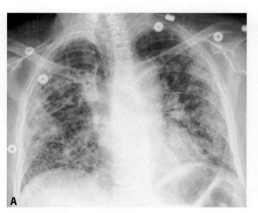

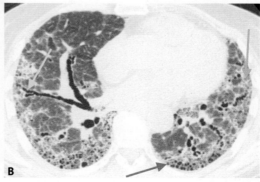

Figure 1.4

Specificity of HRCT. A. Frontal chest radiograph in a patient with idiopathic pulmonary fibrosis (IPF) shows diffuse nonspecific opacities. **B.** HRCT provides superior evaluation of lung abnormalities. Subpleural honeycombing (*red arrow*), traction bronchiectasis (*yellow arrow*), and irregular reticulation (*blue arrow*) are present. In the absence of known diseases or exposures, HRCT is considered diagnostic of IPF.

Table 1.2	Clinical information that may be useful in the interpretation of HRCT abnormalities

Age
Acute or chronic symptoms
Cigarette smoking
Exposures (drugs, dusts, and organic antigens)
Immune status
Connective tissue disease

In many cases, a combination of HRCT findings and clinical information may predict a single diagnosis with a high degree of accuracy (Fig. 1.5A, B). In such cases, further diagnostic testing may not be needed. For instance, when centrilobular nodules of ground glass opacity are present on HRCT in a patient with an exposure to birds, the diagnosis is very likely hypersensitivity pneumonitis. In such cases, biopsy is not usually required for diagnosis. Another example is an HRCT showing honeycombing in a subpleural and basilar distribution. This pattern is compatible with usual interstitial pneumonia (UIP) and a biopsy is not generally required for confirmation. In the absence of known diseases or exposures, the patient will be diagnosed as having idiopathic pulmonary fibrosis (IPF).

On the other hand, when the HRCT pattern is nonspecific, the suggested differential diagnosis may help to guide additional tests. For example, when tree-in-bud opacities are present on HRCT, a diagnosis is often obtained using sputum analysis, as this finding usually reflects an infectious cellular bronchiolitis with impaction of small airways. In patients with perilymphatic nodules visible on HRCT, there is a high likelihood of obtaining a histologic diagnosis on transbronchial biopsy, as this abnormality is often due to sarcoidosis or lymphangitic tumor spread (Fig. 1.6). Transbronchial biopsy is useful in the diagnosis of these two diseases, because they involve the airways or predominate in the peribronchovascular interstitium. It is also helpful in diagnosing some infections, when sputum analysis is not sufficient. Histologic samples obtained at transbronchial biopsy, however, have significant potential limitations, primarily because they represent small samples of lung, and the samples obtained may not be representative of the overall process that is present. HRCT, on the other hand, provides a global evaluation of the lung abnormalities present (Fig. 1.7).

Lung biopsy is obtained in cases in which the combination of clinical information and HRCT is not considered sufficient for diagnosis. Video-assisted thoracoscopic

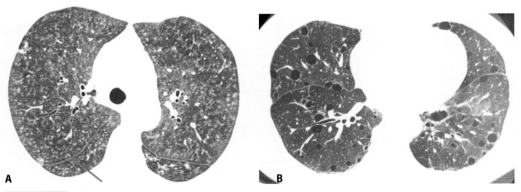

A   B

Figure 1.5

Correlation of HRCT findings with clinical information. A. HRCT shows diffuse indistinct centrilobular nodules (*arrows*). There are several possible diagnoses based upon the HRCT pattern. This patient has chronic symptoms and a history of recurrent exposure to birds. This combination of HRCT findings and clinical information is highly suggestive of hypersensitivity pneumonitis. **B.** HRCT in a patient with Sjögren's syndrome shows scattered lung cysts. While this finding is nonspecific, in a patient with a history of connective tissue disease, it is highly suggestive of lymphoid interstitial pneumonia.

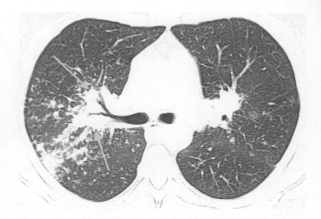

Figure 1.6

HRCT in sarcoidosis. HRCT shows clusters of nodules in the interstitium around the central bronchovascular bundles (*arrows*) suggestive of sarcoidosis. Given the proximity of these findings to the airways, bronchoscopy with transbronchial biopsy is the test of choice for confirmation of this diagnosis.

surgical (VATS) biopsies are most helpful as they obtain relatively large samples from multiple locations within the lung. In patients with nonspecific fibrosis on HRCT, a VATS biopsy is usually required for diagnosis. HRCT may help guide the surgeon to the most appropriate regions for biopsy. It is important to recognize, however, that even if a VATS biopsy is obtained, it is often important to consider it in association with the HRCT abnormalities.

Sequential Evaluation of Lung Abnormalities Over Time

HRCT may be used in the follow-up of patients after treatment or in those with new or progressive symptoms. Follow-up HRCT after treatment for diffuse lung disease (Fig. 1.8A, B) is particularly useful in determining the relative amounts of inflammation and fibrosis present. Improvement of findings on a repeat HRCT suggests that a reversible component was present on the initial examination. This is helpful

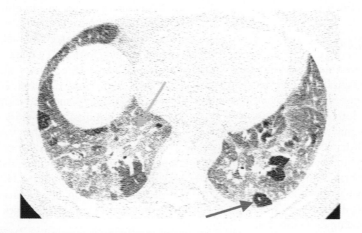

Figure 1.7

HRCT and biopsy in hypersensitivity pneumonitis. HRCT provides a global assessment of anatomic abnormalities, whereas biopsy represents a small sampling of lung abnormalities. In some cases, biopsy of small areas of lung may not be representative of the overall pattern present. HRCT in this case shows a combination of ground glass opacity (*yellow arrow*) and air trapping (*red arrow*), highly suggestive of hypersensitivity pneumonitis. Pathology showed nonspecific interstitial pneumonia. In this case, the imaging is more suggestive of the actual diagnosis, hypersensitivity pneumonitis.

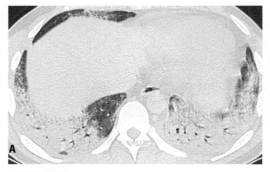 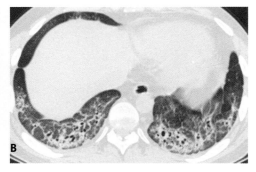

Figure 1.8

Sequential evaluation of HRCT abnormalities over time. A. HRCT shows subpleural and basilar predominant consolidation. **B.** After treatment, the consolidation has resolved, but there has been interval development of irregular reticulation and traction bronchiectasis, indicative of fibrosis. HRCT is able to distinguish the reversible and nonreversible components after treatment.

in patients presenting with ground glass opacity; this finding may represent inflammation, fibrosis, or a combination of both. Follow-up CT after treatment will help determine which of these abnormalities the ground glass opacity represented.

New symptoms in a patient with diffuse lung disease may be due to worsening of the patient's established lung disease or a superimposed process. HRCT may be helpful in making this distinction.

HRCT TECHNIQUES

Basic HRCT technique uses thin slices, scanning at full inspiration, and reconstruction with a sharp algorithm. To provide an accurate assessment of lung abnormalities, thin slices (0.625 to 1.25 mm) are required (Table 1.3). These are reconstructed using a sharp or edge-enhancing algorithm to improve characterization of abnormal findings. Rapid gantry rotation is optimal in reducing motion artifacts. Automatic milliampere (mA) adjustment is useful in reducing radiation dose.

There are many CT protocols that may be used in obtaining high-resolution images for the purpose of diagnosing diffuse lung disease. No one protocol is the "correct" one, although several specific techniques are helpful. In nearly all patients, images are routinely obtained in the supine position, at full inspiration.

Axial versus Volumetric Imaging

Traditionally, discontinuous images are acquired at 1 or 2 cm intervals using an axial (non-helical) technique (Table 1.3). This allows a sampling of lung abnormalities, which is usually sufficient for the diagnosis of diffuse lung diseases. This technique inherently results in a low radiation dose.

The current generation of multi-detector scanners also allows for volumetric acquisition of thin sections through the entire thorax using a short breath-hold. For this reason, many centers use volumetric thin-section imaging rather than axial imaging for HRCT (Table 1.3). Volumetric imaging allows detection of all abnormalities present (e.g., lung nodules) and reconstruction in different planes and is optimal if quantification of lung abnormalities is desired. It is not clear, however, whether volumetric imaging provides improved diagnostic accuracy in patients with diffuse interstitial lung disease. Disadvantages of volumetric HRCT include an increased radiation dose and images that are slightly fuzzier than axial images.

Prone Imaging

Prone imaging may be obtained as part of the initial HRCT examination or routinely in all patients. Many interstitial lung diseases first present in the posterior subpleural lung regions. This is particularly common with the interstitial pneumonias, namely

Table 1.3	HRCT scanning technique and examples of possible protocols

HRCT technique

Full inspiration
0.625–1.25 mm thick sections
Sharp (edge-enhancing) algorithm
Fast gantry rotation speed
Fixed mA or automatic mA adjustment

Axial (non-helical) protocol

Supine position
No table motion
Full inspiration
Sections acquired at 1 cm intervals
Prone scans at 1–2 cm intervals optional

Volumetric protocol

Supine position
Full inspiration
Contiguous images throughout the chest
Images reconstructed at 0.625-1.25 mm
Prone scans at selected levels or with
    volumetric acquisition optional

Post-expiratory imaging (static)

Supine position
Suspended full expiration
Levels of acquisition: aortic arch, tracheal
    carina, above diaphragm

Expiratory imaging (dynamic)

Sequential images acquired during forced
    expiration
Eight sequential images at 0.5 s intervals
No table motion
Levels of acquisition: aortic arch, tracheal
    carina, above diaphragm
Fast gantry rotation speed
mA = 100 or less

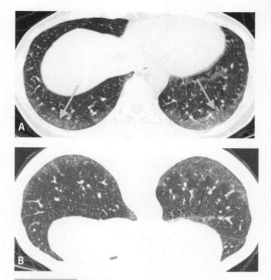

Figure 1.9

Use of prone HRCT. A. Supine HRCT shows subtle ground glass opacity involving the posterior lung (*yellow arrows*). This could represent normal dependent density or early interstitial lung disease. **B.** Prone HRCT shows persistence of these abnormalities (*red arrows*). The prone scan confirms that this finding is due to early interstitial lung disease.

UIP, nonspecific interstitial pneumonia, and desquamative interstitial pneumonia. In the supine position, normal patients may show increased opacity in the posterior subpleural region, reflecting dependent (gravitational) atelectasis. Prone imaging is useful in distinguishing early interstitial lung disease from normal dependent density (Fig. 1.9A, B). When the patient is placed in the prone position, normal dependent density should disappear, whereas early interstitial lung disease persists. Prone imaging may also help in the identification of specific abnormalities in the dependent lung such as honeycombing.

Expiratory Imaging

Expiratory images, obtained in order to detect air trapping, are important in the initial HRCT evaluation of most patients and in the follow-up of patients with suspected airways disease or chronic obstructive lung disease. As an example, chronic hypersensitivity pneumonitis may mimic the appearance of UIP and IPF on inspiratory images, but air trapping on expiratory images may allow these diseases to be distinguished.

Expiratory images may be acquired using a static post-expiratory technique or a dynamic technique during forced expiration (Table 1.3). Static post-expiratory images are produced by obtaining single scans at selected levels at end expiration (i.e., "take a big breath, blow it out, and hold your breath"). Dynamic expiratory imaging (Fig. 1.10A–H) involves obtaining

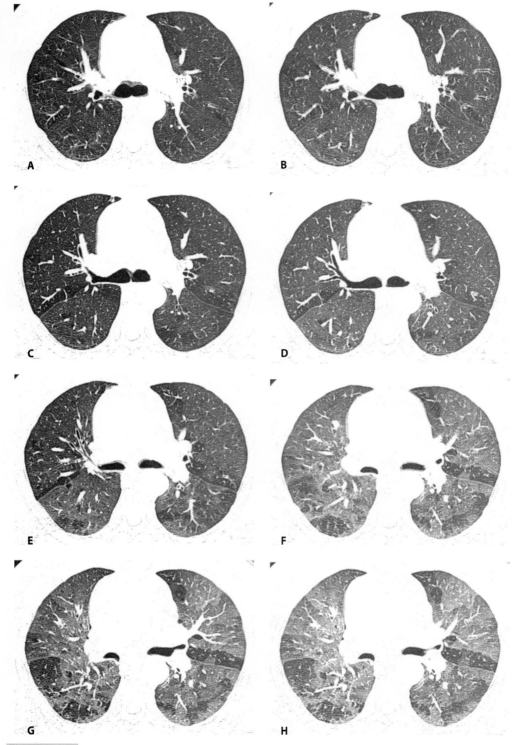

Figure 1.10

Dynamic expiratory imaging. Eight consecutive images were obtained at the level of the tracheal carina during forced expiration, using reduced mA. Image **(A)** is obtained at the beginning of expiration and image **(H)** at the end. During expiration there are several regions of lung that do not change in attenuation and remain lucent. This represents air trapping in a patient with hypersensitivity pneumonitis.

multiple (six to eight) sequential images (with a reduced mA setting) at the same anatomic location during forced expiration (i.e., "take a deep breath and blow it out as fast as you can"). The entire sequence may take 4 to 6 seconds. Dynamic imaging is more sensitive in the detection of air trapping.

Expiratory images are often acquired at three anatomic levels: aortic arch, tracheal carina, and above the diaphragm. Sometimes five levels are chosen. Volumetric post-expiratory imaging through the entire chest is another option, but it requires a much higher radiation dose.

HRCT AND RADIATION DOSE

People are exposed to nonmedical radiation on a routine basis, primarily in the form of cosmic radiation. The yearly dose that an individual receives from cosmic radiation varies, but on average, it is approximately 2.5 milliSieverts (mSv). For comparison, the dose from a posteroanterior chest radiograph is approximately 0.05 mSv.

CT dose (Table 1.4) varies significantly among different patients, CT scanners, and HRCT protocols. Radiation dose is directly related to the mA used, which may range from 100 to 400 mA for most chest CT. Varying mA in relation to body thickness and absorption can reduce dose. Decreased radiation dose is associated with increased image noise and decreased resolution, but images generally remain diagnostic.

HRCT using a variable mA of about 100, axial imaging, and 10 mm slice spacing results in a radiation dose of approximately 0.7 mSv. This dose is doubled if prone imaging is also used. Volumetric multi-detector HRCT imparts a dose in the range of 4 to 7 mSv if 300 mA is used, but volumetric HRCT with a reduced dose (100 mA) produces adequate images with a dose of 1 to 2 mSv. For a given dose, axial images are a little sharper than images obtained using helical technique.

Low-dose HRCT using spaced axial images may also be performed with 40 mA, although noise is increased and resolution is decreased. Dose using this technique may be as low as

Table 1.4	Comparison of radiation dose for chest imaging techniques	
		Effective radiation dose (mSv)
Annual background radiation		2.5
Posteroanterior chest radiograph		0.05
Spaced axial HRCT supine (10 mm spacing)		0.7
Spaced axial HRCT supine (20 mm spacing)		0.35
Low-dose spaced axial HRCT		0.02–0.2
Volumetric helical HRCT supine (300 mA)		4–7
Volumetric helical HRCT supine (100 mA)		1–2

Modified from Mayo JR, Aldrich J, Muller NL. Radiation exposure at chest CT: a statement of the Fleischner Society. Radiology 2003; 228: 15-21.

0.02 mSv (with widely spaced images) to 0.2 mSv (with images at 2 cm intervals, supine and prone, and with dynamic expiratory images).

NORMAL ANATOMY ON HRCT

The recognition of HRCT abnormalities is fundamentally based on an understanding of normal lung anatomy as demonstrated using this technique (Table 1.5). Understanding the *secondary pulmonary lobule* or simply *pulmonary lobule* (these two terms are synonyms) is fundamental in HRCT interpretation. The secondary lobule is described in detail below, but first things first.

Large Bronchi and Arteries
Within the central lung, bronchi and pulmonary artery branches are closely associated and branch in parallel. Central pulmonary arteries imaged in cross section normally appear as rounded or elliptical opacities on HRCT, accompanied by uniformly thin-walled bronchi of similar size and shape. When imaged along their axis, bronchi and vessels should appear roughly cylindrical or show slight tapering as they branch, depending on the length of the segment that is visible; tapering

of a vessel or bronchus is most easily seen when a long segment is visible.

The outer walls of pulmonary arteries form a smooth and sharply defined interface with the surrounding lung, whether they are seen in cross section or along their length. In normal subjects, the internal diameter of a bronchus (i.e., the bronchial lumen) averages about 0.7 of the diameter of the adjacent pulmonary artery. This measurement is termed the *bronchoarterial ratio*. A bronchoarterial ratio exceeding 1 generally indicates bronchial dilatation (i.e., bronchiectasis), although a ratio exceeding 1 may be seen in normal elderly patients or in people living at high altitudes (e.g., Denver).

The walls of large bronchi, outlined by lung on one side and air in the bronchial lumen on the other, should appear smooth and of uniform thickness. Generally speaking, the wall of a bronchus measures 1/5th to 1/10th of its outer diameter, and bronchial walls in different lung regions should appear similar in thickness. The lumen of a bronchus should be free of secretions.

Bronchi and pulmonary arteries are surrounded by the *peribronchovascular interstitium*, which extends from the pulmonary hila into the peripheral lung.

Table 1.5 Normal HRCT appearances

Large arteries and bronchi

Outer walls of arteries and bronchi smooth and sharply marginated
Bronchial walls 1/5th–1/10th of bronchial diameter
Ratio of bronchial lumen to adjacent artery (bronchoarterial ratio) averages 0.7
Bronchial walls similar in appearance in different lung regions

Secondary pulmonary lobule

Usually 1–2.5 cm in diameter
Interlobular septa uncommonly visible; very thin
Centrilobular artery visible about 5 mm from pleural surface (dot or branching)
Centrilobular bronchiole invisible

Pleural surfaces

Smooth and sharply marginated; fissures thin
A few linear or small nodular opacities are normal

The Peribronchovascular Interstitium

The peribronchovascular interstitium, also known as the axial interstitium, accompanies pulmonary artery, bronchial branches, and lymphatics from the hilar regions into the lung periphery. It is invisible in normals. The central or perihilar peribronchovascular interstitium is often affected by lymphatic diseases, such as sarcoidosis or lymphangitic spread of neoplasm, or infiltrative abnormalities, such as pulmonary edema. Such abnormalities may result in smooth, nodular, or irregular thickening of the peribronchovascular interstitium.

Pulmonary Lobule (Secondary Pulmonary Lobule)

The *secondary pulmonary lobule*, or simply *pulmonary lobule* (these are synonyms), is a key anatomic structure in understanding HRCT abnormalities (Fig. 1.11). The pulmonary lobule is the smallest unit of lung that is delineated by connective tissue septa, and many pathologic abnormalities occur in relation to specific components of the secondary lobule. Pulmonary lobules are generally polygonal in shape and measure from 1 to 2.5 cm.

Interlobular Septa

Pulmonary lobules are marginated by *interlobular septa* that contain pulmonary veins and lymphatics and form a web-like network throughout the lung. Only a few interlobular septa are seen on HRCT in normal subjects, and when visible, these tend to be inconspicuous (Figs. 1.11 and 1.12). Certain processes, such as pulmonary edema, may result in interlobular septal thickening easily seen on HRCT (Fig. 1.13). It may be smooth, nodular, or irregular.

Centrilobular Structures

A lobular artery and bronchiole are located in the center of pulmonary lobules or, in other words, in the *centrilobular region*. The *lobular artery* is normally visible as a dot-like or branching structure about 5 mm from the

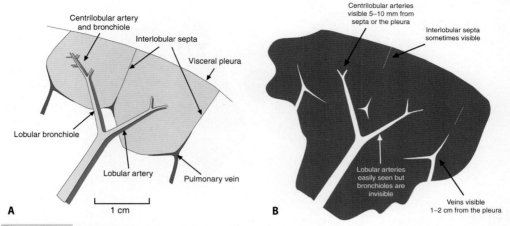

Figure 1.11

Normal (secondary pulmonary lobule). A. Two adjacent pulmonary lobules are depicted. The borders of the lobule are delineated by interlobular septa that are contiguous with the subpleural interstitium. The lobular bronchiole and artery are in the center of the pulmonary lobule, the centrilobular region. **B.** HRCT visibility of lobular structures.

pleural surface (in the lung periphery or adjacent to a fissure); the *lobular bronchiole* is not normally visible because its wall is too thin to be resolved using HRCT.

The bronchiole and pulmonary artery supplying a pulmonary lobule, and located in the centrilobular region, are also invested by the distal continuation of the peribronchovascular interstitium.

In the peripheral lung or adjacent to fissures, the centers of pulmonary lobules (i.e., the centrilobular region) are located approximately 0.5 cm from the pleural surface.

Small airways diseases and vascular diseases often are manifested by abnormalities affecting the centrilobular region (Fig. 1.14).

The Pleural Surfaces, Fissures, and Subpleural Interstitium

Interlobular septa are contiguous in the peripheral lung with the *subpleural interstitium* that lies directly beneath visceral pleural surfaces and adjacent to fissures. Fissures and the peripheral pleural surfaces should appear smooth in contour and sharply marginated, although a few linear

Figure 1.12

Normal interlobular septa. HRCT in normal subjects may show a few interlobular septa (*arrows*), but these are usually inconspicuous. Septa are easily seen only when they are thickened.

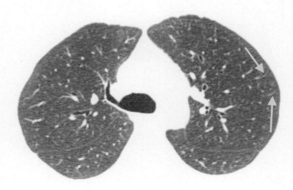

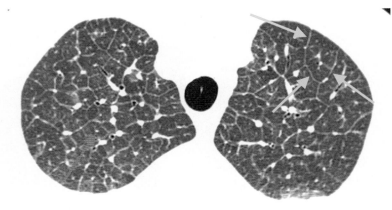

Figure 1.13

Interlobular septal thickening. Thickening of interlobular septa (*yellow arrows*) is present in a patient with pulmonary edema. There is a web-like network of interconnecting lines outlining polygonal structures 1–2.5 cm in size, representing the pulmonary lobules. Note small dots at the center of some lobules (*red arrow*), representing the centrilobular arteries.

opacities intersecting the pleura (interlobular septa) or nodular opacities (pulmonary veins or lymphoid aggregates) may be seen. Thickening of interlobular septa is typically associated with subpleural interstitial thickening (and thickening of fissures). Nodules may also be located in relation to the interlobular septa. Abnormalities of the subpleural interstitium may result in the pleural surfaces or fissures having an irregular or nodular appearance.

The Intralobular Interstitium

A fine network of interstitial connective tissue fibers extends throughout the lung, within pulmonary lobules, bridging the space between the interlobular septa and the centrilobular peribronchovascular interstitium. This interstitial network has been termed the *intralobular interstitium*. The intralobular interstitium is not normally visible, but it may become thickened in the presence of lung fibrosis or infiltration.

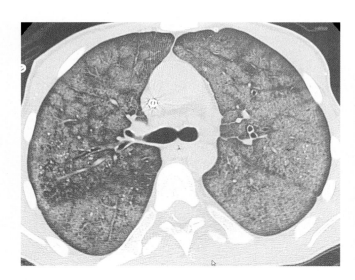

Figure 1.14

Disease affecting the centrilobular region. Areas of ground glass opacity are present that have shapes resembling pulmonary lobules. The periphery of the lobule and interlobular septa are spared in this case. Diseases that are centrilobular in location are generally related to the centrilobular artery or bronchiole. This patient has metastatic calcification associated with renal failure.

FURTHER READING

Arakawa H, Webb WR. Expiratory high-resolution CT scan. *Radiol Clin North Am*. 1998;36:189-209.

Austin JH, Müller NL, Friedman PJ, et al. Glossary of terms for CT of the lungs: recommendations of the Nomenclature Committee of the Fleischner Society. *Radiology*. 1996;200:327-331.

Elicker B, Pereira CA, Webb R, Leslie KO. High-resolution computed tomography patterns of diffuse interstitial lung disease with clinical and pathological correlation. *J Bras Pneumol*. 2008;34:715-744.

Gotway MB, Freemer MM, King TE Jr. Challenges in pulmonary fibrosis. 1: use of high resolution CT scanning of the lung for the evaluation of patients with idiopathic interstitial pneumonias. *Thorax*. 2007;62:546-553.

Gotway MB, Reddy GP, Webb WR, Elicker BM, Leung JW. High-resolution CT of the lung: patterns of disease and differential diagnoses. *Radiol Clin North Am*. 2005;43:513-542.

Griffin CB, Primack SL. High-resolution CT: normal anatomy, techniques, and pitfalls. *Radiol Clin North Am*. 2001;39:1073-1090.

Hansell DM, Bankier AA, MacMahon H, et al. Fleischner Society: glossary of terms for thoracic imaging. *Radiology*. 2008;246:697-722.

Klusmann M, Owens C. HRCT in paediatric diffuse interstitial lung disease—a review for 2009. *Pediatr Radiol*. 2009;39(suppl 3):471-481.

Mayo JR. CT evaluation of diffuse infiltrative lung disease: dose considerations and optimal technique. *J Thorac Imaging*. 2009;24:252-259.

Mayo JR, Aldrich J, Muller NL. Radiation exposure at chest CT: a statement of the Fleischner Society. *Radiology*. 2003;228:15-21.

Nishino M, Washko GR, Hatabu H. Volumetric expiratory HRCT of the lung: clinical applications. *Radiol Clin North Am*. 2010;48:177-183.

Quigley M, Hansell DM, Nicholson AG. Interstitial lung disease—the new synergy between radiology and pathology. *Histopathology*. 2006;49:334-342.

Sundaram B, Chughtai AR, Kazerooni EA. Multidetector high-resolution computed tomography of the lungs: protocols and applications. *J Thorac Imaging*. 2010; 25:125-141.

Webb WR. High resolution lung computed tomography: normal anatomic and pathologic findings. *Radiol Clin North Am*. 1991;29:1051-1063.

Webb WR. Thin-section CT of the secondary pulmonary lobule: anatomy and the image—the 2004 Fleischner lecture. *Radiology*. 2006;239:322-338.

Reticular Opacities

Reticular opacities seen on HRCT in patients with diffuse lung disease can indicate lung infiltration with interstitial thickening or fibrosis. Three principal patterns of reticulation may be seen. These are interlobular septal thickening, honeycombing, and irregular reticulation.

INTERLOBULAR SEPTAL THICKENING

Interlobular septal thickening is an uncommon manifestation of diffuse lung disease, but is easily recognized on HRCT.

HRCT Features

Interlobular septa variably marginate secondary pulmonary lobules (see Chapter 1). They comprise connective tissue and contain pulmonary veins and lymphatics. Interlobular septa are approximately 1 to 2 cm in length and 1/10th of a millimeter in thickness. Only a few interlobular septa are seen on HRCT in normal patients.

When interlobular septa are abnormally thickened, they are easily seen and form a web-like network of lines. These lines can usually be recognized as thickened interlobular septa because they outline what can be recognized as pulmonary lobules because of their characteristic size (1 to 2.5 cm) and polygonal shape and because a centrilobular artery is usually visible in its center as a dot-like or branching opacity (Fig. 2.1).

Interlobular septal thickening can be associated with thickening of the intralobular interstitium (see Chapter 1), which results in a fine network of lines within lobules (Fig. 2.2).

Intralobular interstitial thickening results in an irregular reticular pattern smaller in scale than the reticular pattern of interlobular septal thickening.

Significance of Interlobular Septal Thickening

The presence of a few thickened interlobular septa can be seen in a wide variety of diffuse lung diseases and is, in general, a nonspecific finding. For the purposes of differential diagnosis, thickened septa should be ignored unless they represent a predominant abnormality (Fig. 2.3A, B).

When significant interlobular septal thickening is present, the abnormal septa may appear smooth in contour (this is most common), nodular, or irregular. The morphologic pattern primarily determines the differential diagnosis (Fig. 2.4A–C, Table 2.1).

Smooth Interlobular Septal Thickening

Smooth interlobular septal thickening is present when the septa are easily seen and appear thicker than normal, but otherwise have a normal appearance (Fig. 2.4A, Table 2.1). It is usually a manifestation of pulmonary edema or lymphangitic spread of tumor. This appearance is due to fluid or tumor infiltration of the lymphatics located within the septa. Septal thickening in lymphangitic spread of tumor may be either smooth or nodular, but smooth thickening is more common. Symmetric involvement of both lungs favors edema, while asymmetric involvement favors lymphangitic tumor. Most patients with lymphangitic

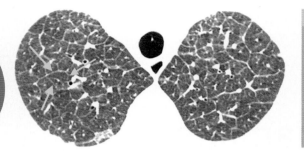

Figure 2.1

Interlobular septal thickening. Smooth interlobular septal thickening is present in a patient with pulmonary edema. Note the thin, 1–2 cm long lines that form an interconnecting network and outline polygonal structures (*arrows*). These are the secondary pulmonary lobules. An artery is visible in the center of the lobules.

spread of tumor have a known malignancy or other evidence of malignancy on HRCT.

Nodular Interlobular Septal Thickening

Nodular interlobular septal thickening is most commonly seen in patients with sarcoidosis or lymphangitic spread of tumor. This appearance reflects involvement of lymphatics within the septa, with the nodules representing clusters of granulomas or tumor nodules (Fig. 2.4B, Table 2.1). In sarcoidosis, nodules are almost always seen in other locations as well, including the peribronchovascular regions and the centrilobular and/or subpleural regions. This

appearance reflects a perilymphatic distribution of nodules, described in Chapter 3.

Irregular Interlobular Septal Thickening

Irregular interlobular septal thickening usually reflects lung fibrosis and is similar in significance to irregular reticulation, which is described later. The architectural distortion associated with fibrosis causes the septa to become jagged or angulated in appearance (Fig. 2.4C, Table 2.1). Irregular septal thickening may be seen with any cause of fibrotic lung disease, and other findings, such as honeycombing and traction bronchiectasis, are more helpful in the formulation of a differential diagnosis.

HONEYCOMBING

Honeycombing is easily recognized and indicates the presence of lung fibrosis. It is relatively common.

HRCT Features

Pathologically honeycombing represents interstitial fibrosis with lung destruction and dilatation of peripheral airspaces. On HRCT, honeycombing results in air-filled cystic spaces (black holes) with easily seen walls, usually 3 to 10 mm in diameter, but sometimes smaller or larger.

Honeycombing is the most specific HRCT sign of fibrosis. When honeycombing is present, one can be confident that the patient has fibrotic lung disease. To make a confident diagnosis of honeycombing, several HRCT findings must be present (Table 2.2, Figs. 2.5 to 2.8):

1. *Honeycombing always involves the subpleural lung.* Unless lucencies are visible in the

Figure 2.2

Intralobular interstitial thickening. HRCT in a patient with pulmonary edema. The interconnecting lines (*arrow*) are on a smaller scale than interlobular septa.

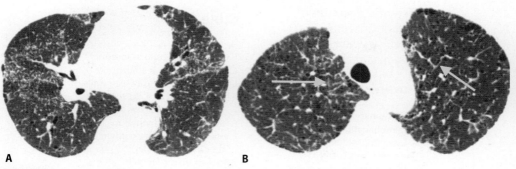

2

A   B

Figure 2.3

Interlobular septal thickening as an insignificant finding. A. HRCT shows perilymphatic nodules with a patchy distribution and predominance along the fissures (*red arrow*) in a patient with amyloidosis. **B.** At a higher level, HRCT shows interlobular septal thickening (*yellow arrows*). Septal thickening should be ignored in terms of differential diagnosis unless it is the predominant finding.

immediate subpleural region, honeycombing cannot be diagnosed with certainty.
2. *Most cysts are 3 to 10 mm in diameter.* Some may be larger or smaller.
3. *The cysts have a thick wall.* The wall of honeycombing cysts should be easily seen. This finding helps in distinguishing honeycombing from emphysema or areas of subpleural air trapping.

4. *A layer or cluster of subpleural cysts should be visible.* Early honeycombing may be seen in only one layer beneath the pleural surface (Fig. 2.6) or an isolated cluster of subpleural cysts may be visible. A single subpleural cyst is not sufficient to call it honeycombing. Adjacent cysts share walls.

As honeycombing becomes more severe, it extends inward to involve more central

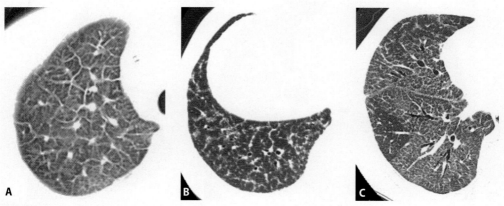

A   B   C

Figure 2.4

Differential diagnosis of smooth, nodular, and irregular interlobular septal thickening (ILS). When ILS is the predominant abnormality seen on HRCT, the differential diagnosis depends upon the morphology of the thickening. **A. Smooth ILS.** The diagnosis is most likely pulmonary edema or lymphangitic carcinomatosis. This represents pulmonary edema. **B. Nodular ILS.** The diagnosis is most likely sarcoidosis or lymphangitic carcinomatosis. This represents sarcoidosis. **C. Irregular ILS.** This usually represents fibrotic lung disease. The differential diagnosis is the same as that of irregular reticulation. This represents nonspecific interstitial pneumonia in a patient with connective tissue disease.

Table 2.1	Differential diagnosis of interlobular septal thickening when it is the predominant abnormality
Morphology of septal thickening	**Differential diagnosis**
Smooth	Pulmonary edema
	Lymphangitic carcinomatosis
	Lymphoproliferative disease
	Amyloidosis (rare)
	Pulmonary veno-occlusive disease (rare)
	Lymphangiomatosis (rare)
	Erdheim-Chester disease (rare)
Nodular	Sarcoidosis
	Lymphangitic carcinomatosis
	Lymphoproliferative disease
	Amyloidosis (rare)
Irregular	Fibrotic lung disease

Table 2.2	HRCT features of honeycombing

Cysts are subpleural in location
Cysts are usually 3–10 mm
Cysts have thick, easily seen walls
The cysts occur in a cluster or layer and share walls (multiple layers are seen in late disease)
Cysts are of air attenuation (i.e., black)
Cysts are empty; they contain no "anatomy"; they are black holes
The cysts do not branch
They are associated with other signs of fibrosis (traction bronchiectasis and irregular reticulation)

lung regions, and honeycomb cysts appear in multiple layers and clusters. In patients with extensive disease, the stacked appearance of cysts, sharing walls with one another, is what gives this finding its resemblance to a

honeycomb. Remember that the interstitium adjacent to the fissures is also subpleural, and subpleural honeycombing may be seen in this location.

5. *The cysts of honeycombing should be of air attenuation* (i.e., they should be black), having the same density as air in the bronchi.

6. *There should be no "anatomy" within the cysts.* Vessels, bronchi, or septations are not visible within honeycomb cysts. The cysts are empty black holes.

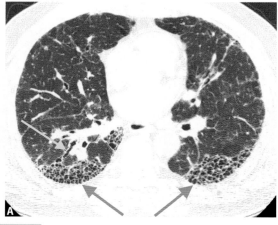 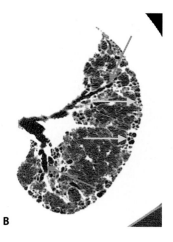

Figure 2.5

Features of honeycombing in two patients with usual interstitial pneumonia and idiopathic pulmonary fibrosis. A. HRCT shows advanced honeycombing. Note that cysts range from about 3 mm to less than 1 cm in diameter, are of air attenuation (i.e., black), have relatively thick walls, involve the subpleural lung, share walls, and are stacked in multiple layers (*red arrows*). There is associated traction bronchiectasis in the right lower lobe (*yellow arrow*). **B.** HRCT of a patient with idiopathic pulmonary fibrosis shows honeycombing (*yellow arrows*) and traction bronchiectasis (*red arrows*). The honeycomb cysts appear in clusters and layers in the subpleural lung.

2

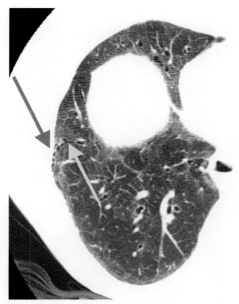

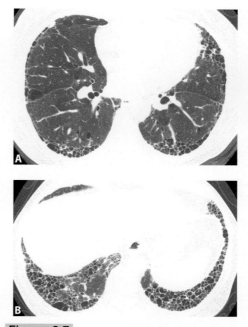

Figure 2.6

Early honeycombing in a single layer. Early honeycombing is seen in a patient with mixed connective tissue disease. Note at least three adjacent subpleural, air-attenuation cysts with well-defined walls (*red arrow*) associated with mild traction bronchiectasis (*yellow arrow*).

Figure 2.7

HRCT of a definite usual interstitial pneumonia pattern. Images through the mid-lung **(A)** and lung bases **(B)** show subpleural and basilar fibrosis with significant honeycombing. No ground glass opacity, mosaic perfusion, or diffuse nodules are seen.

7. *The cysts of honeycombing do not branch.* Branching cystic structures, even in the subpleural lung, likely represent traction bronchiectasis (described below).

8. *Associated signs of fibrosis are present in the same lung regions.* These findings include traction bronchiectasis, irregular reticulation, and volume loss. If cysts are not associated with other findings of fibrosis, they may represent emphysema or cystic lung disease.

Significance of Honeycombing and the "UIP Pattern"

Honeycombing is often associated with the histologic pattern termed *usual interstitial pneumonia (UIP)*, and in some cases, honeycombing may be diagnostic of that pattern. However, there are a number of diseases that can show honeycombing on HRCT (Table 2.3).

The presence of honeycombing, by itself, is not sufficient to confidently diagnose what is termed a *UIP pattern* (the combination of HRCT abnormalities predicting the presence of UIP). In UIP, findings of fibrosis, including honeycombing, typically have a subpleural, posterior, and lower lobe predominance, and the posterior costophrenic angles are almost always involved (Fig. 2.8, Table 2.4). Also, features that would suggest an alternative diagnosis, such as isolated regions of ground glass opacity (seen in areas not showing findings of fibrosis), mosaic perfusion, air trapping, segmental or lobar consolidation, and small nodules, must be absent. The accurate HRCT diagnosis of UIP is particularly important in the diagnosis of patients with idiopathic pulmonary fibrosis (IPF; see Chapter 9). For a detailed review of this topic, refer to the paper by Raghu et al., listed at the end of this chapter.

When all of the features listed in Table 2.4 are present, a diagnosis of UIP can be made with a high degree of confidence (Figs. 2.7 and 2.8).

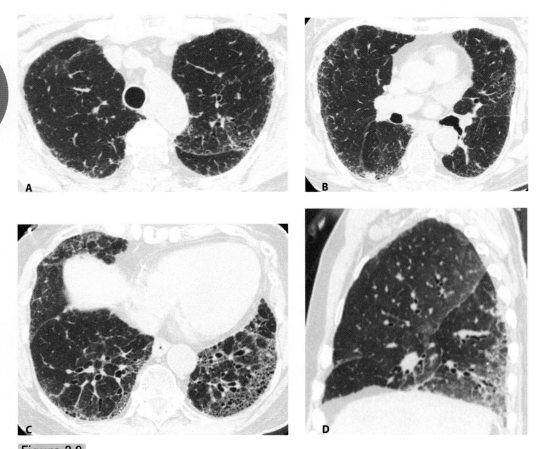

Figure 2.8

HRCT of a definite usual interstitial pneumonia pattern in a patient with idiopathic pulmonary fibrosis. HRCT through the upper lungs **(A)** and mid-lung **(B)** shows irregular reticulation as the predominant abnormality. Scan through the lung bases **(C)** shows subpleural and basilar fibrosis with significant honeycombing. The abnormalities predominate at the lung bases. **D.** Sagittal reformation shows predominance of abnormalities at the bases and in the posterior lung, including the costophrenic angles.

In these classic cases, there is a close correlation between the HRCT and pathologic patterns, and lung biopsy is uncommonly performed. Remember that UIP is not a disease, but a histologic pattern with an HRCT correlate (i.e., the UIP pattern).

When a definite UIP pattern is present, the differential diagnosis of honeycombing is limited (Table 2.5) and generally includes four diseases or conditions: IPF, connective tissue disease, drug-related fibrosis, and asbestosis.

Think of IPF as idiopathic UIP. UIP associated with connective tissue disease, drug-related fibrosis, and asbestosis may be indis-

Table 2.3	Differential diagnosis of honeycombing on HRCT

Idiopathic pulmonary fibrosis
Connective tissue disease
Drug-related fibrosis
Asbestosis
Hypersensitivity pneumonitis
Sarcoidosis
Nonspecific interstitial pneumonia
    (mild honeycombing)
Pneumoconioses other than asbestosis
Post–acute respiratory distress syndrome fibrosis

Table 2.4	HRCT findings confidently predicting a usual interstitial pneumonia pattern (all are necessary)

Honeycombing (in significant amounts)
Supportive signs of fibrosis (irregular reticulation and traction bronchiectasis)
Subpleural and basilar predominant distribution
Absence of upper or mid-lung or peribronchovascular predominance
Absence of extensive ground glass opacity
Absence of segmental or lobar consolidation
Absence of discrete bilateral cysts (away from honeycombing)
Absence of significant mosaic perfusion or air trapping (bilateral ≥ 3 lobes)
Absence of profuse micronodules

tinguishable from IPF on HRCT (Fig. 2.9A–C), but there are often clinical clues that suggest the appropriate diagnosis. Patients with connective tissue disease may have joint symptoms, muscle weakness, rashes, or abnormal blood tests. Patients with drug fibrosis have a history of treatment with a drug that is a known offender such as cyclophosphamide, chlorambucil, nitrofurantoin, and pindolol. Patients with asbestosis usually have a clear exposure history and 90% or more have associated pleural thickening or plaques visible on HRCT.

If the patient has a classic HRCT appearance of a UIP pattern, and no appropriate history or clinical manifestations to suggest the later three diagnoses, a presumptive diagnosis of IPF will be made. As this diagnosis is based primarily upon the HRCT appearance, it is very important to be conservative in labeling a patient as having a UIP pattern.

Table 2.5	Differential diagnosis of common causes of a UIP pattern on HRCT

Idiopathic pulmonary fibrosis
Connective tissue disease (rheumatoid arthritis most common)
Drug fibrosis
Asbestosis

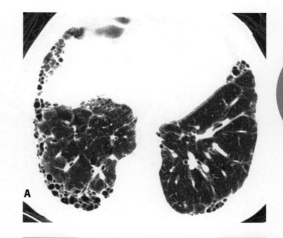
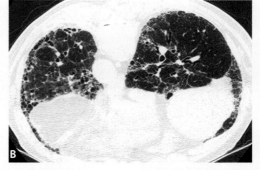
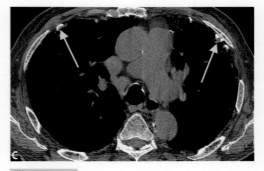

Figure 2.9

Differential diagnosis of a usual interstitial pneumonia pattern. A. A patient with rheumatoid arthritis–related interstitial lung disease shows a classic usual interstitial pneumonia pattern of subpleural and basilar predominant fibrosis with honeycombing. **B and C.** A patient with asbestosis shows a usual interstitial pneumonia pattern of lung disease that is indistinguishable from idiopathic pulmonary fibrosis. Note pleural plaques (**C**, *arrows*) in the patient with asbestosis.

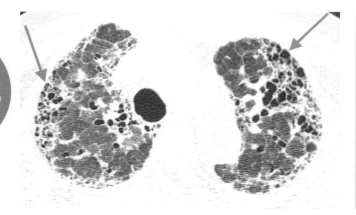

Figure 2.10

Honeycombing with patchy fibrosis in hypersensitivity pneumonitis. While honeycombing is present (*red arrows*), the distribution of fibrosis is patchy and involves the central lung. It does not predominate in the subpleural lung, as would be typical of usual interstitial pneumonia, and involves the upper lobes, which is also atypical. This patient was diagnosed with hypersensitivity pneumonitis on lung biopsy.

Significance of Honeycombing: Alternate Diagnoses

In patients with honeycombing visible on HRCT, the clinical history, the distribution of findings of fibrosis, and additional findings present may suggest that the diagnosis is not UIP.

Chronic hypersensitivity pneumonitis is often associated with a history of exposure to organic antigens. Hypersensitivity pneumonitis is classically mid- to lower lung predominant, with sparing of the inferior costophrenic angles, and may predominate in the upper lobes. It often shows abnormalities that are diffuse or central in the axial plane, without the subpleural predominance of UIP (Fig. 2.10). In other words, it may predominate in the peribronchovascular regions or involve the entire cross section of lung as seen on HRCT. The presence of ground glass opacity or centrilobular nodules outside of areas of fibrosis or mosaic perfusion or air trapping (Fig. 2.11)

also suggests hypersensitivity pneumonitis. It is rare for UIP to present with ground glass opacity as an isolated abnormality, but ground glass opacity is often visible in areas of lung that also show findings of fibrosis (i.e., honeycombing, irregular reticulation, and traction bronchiectasis). Additionally, nonspecific interstitial pneumonia (NSIP) may demonstrate significant ground glass opacity and subpleural sparing that should not be present with IPF.

Sarcoidosis typically has an upper lobe and central peribronchovascular predominant distribution.

Pneumoconioses, such as silicosis, may show a distribution similar to sarcoidosis, being upper lobe and peribronchovascular predominant. Large mass-like areas of fibrosis, progressive massive fibrosis, are common in pneumoconioses, but not typical of UIP.

Post–acute respiratory distress syndrome (ARDS) fibrosis involves the subpleural lung,

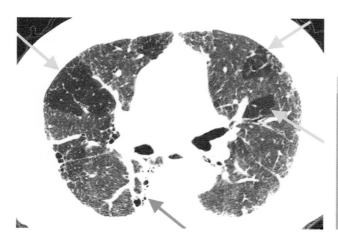

Figure 2.11

Honeycombing associated with mosaic perfusion in hypersensitivity pneumonitis. Mild honeycombing is present in the right lower lobe (*red arrow*), but with significant associated mosaic perfusion (*yellow arrows*). This combination of findings is strongly suggestive of hypersensitivity pneumonitis.

Figure 2.12

Severe fibrosis in nonspecific interstitial pneumonia. Extensive irregular reticulation and traction bronchiectasis are present at the lung bases, with only minimal honeycombing. While it is possible that this represents idiopathic pulmonary fibrosis, the relative lack of honeycombing and relative sparing of the subpleural lung favor nonspecific interstitial pneumonia.

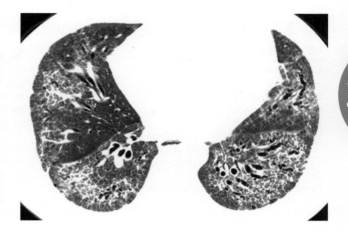

but usually has a strong anterior and mid-lung predominance.

Another situation in which a confident diagnosis of UIP cannot be made is when there is significant fibrosis, but only minimal honeycombing (Fig. 2.12). When the severity of fibrosis is out of proportion to the amount of honeycombing that is present, other etiologies should be entertained. *NSIP* may have a similar distribution to UIP (subpleural and basilar) and may show honeycombing. In most cases, however, the honeycombing is mild, and other findings of fibrosis, such as reticulation and traction bronchiectasis, predominate (Fig. 2.12). Relative sparing of the subpleural lung may also be seen with NSIP. This finding is uncommon in UIP.

Keep in mind that IPF may present with atypical findings, so even if the HRCT does not meet strict criteria for a definite UIP pattern, IPF is still often included in the differential diagnosis (Fig. 2.13A, B).

Diseases other than UIP may, in some cases, demonstrate a UIP pattern on histology. This is particularly problematic when areas of severe fibrosis are sampled at lung biopsy. The HRCT in such patients usually shows features atypical for UIP (Table 2.6).

Honeycombing Pitfalls

Paraseptal emphysema may resemble honeycombing because it occurs in a subpleural location, but there are several distinguishing features (Table 2.7, Fig. 2.14A, B). Paraseptal emphysema

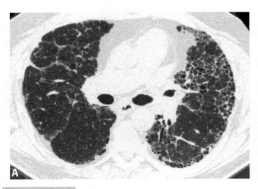
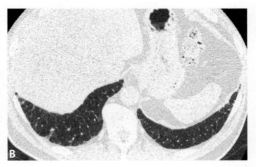

Figure 2.13

Atypical distribution of usual interstitial pneumonia (UIP) in idiopathic pulmonary fibrosis (IPF). HRCT of a patient with IPF presenting with atypical HRCT findings not diagnostic of a UIP pattern. **A.** Honeycombing is present but the disease is patchy, asymmetrical, and not strongly subpleural predominant. **B.** Sparing of the posterior costophrenic angles, present in this case, is also atypical for IPF. Even with an atypical HRCT appearance, IPF is often still included in the differential diagnosis.

Table 2.6   Features atypical for UIP in patients with honeycombing

HRCT feature	Likely alternative diagnoses
Ground glass opacity outside areas of fibrosis	Nonspecific interstitial pneumonia (NSIP), hypersensitivity pneumonitis
Mosaic perfusion/air trapping	Hypersensitivity pneumonitis
Centrilobular nodules	Hypersensitivity pneumonitis
Perilymphatic nodules	Sarcoidosis, pneumoconioses
Subpleural fibrosis with only minimal honeycombing, subpleural sparing	NSIP
Upper lobe distribution of abnormalities	Sarcoidosis, pneumoconioses, hypersensitivity pneumonitis
Parahilar peribronchovascular predominance	NSIP, hypersensitivity pneumonitis, sarcoidosis, pneumoconioses
Lower lobe distribution of findings, not subpleural predominant	Hypersensitivity pneumonitis

Table 2.7   Comparison of the features of paraseptal emphysema and honeycombing

	Paraseptal emphysema	Honeycombing
Layers	Always one layer	One or more layers
Wall thickness	Very thin	Thick
Associated findings	± centrilobular emphysema	Traction bronchiectasis, irregular reticulation
Distribution	Upper lobes	Lower lobes
Size	Large	Small
Overall lung volume	Increased	Decreased
Associated reticulation or traction bronchiectasis	Absent	Present

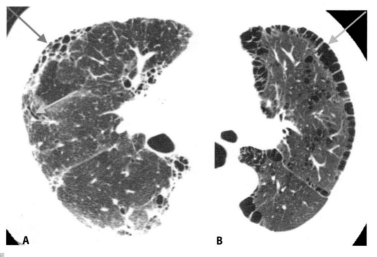

A   B

Figure 2.14

Paraseptal emphysema versus honeycombing. Comparison of honeycombing **(A)** and paraseptal emphysema **(B).** Both abnormalities are subpleural. Honeycomb cysts **(A,** *yellow arrow)* are clustered and stacked in multiple layers, have relatively thick walls, and are associated with reticulation and traction bronchiectasis **(A,** *red arrow).* Paraseptal emphysema **(B,** *blue arrow)* occurs in one layer, results in larger cysts, has very thin walls, and is associated with centrilobular emphysema, rather than signs of fibrosis.

2

Figure 2.15

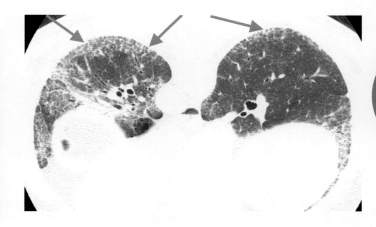

Subpleural reticulation mimicking honeycombing. Irregular reticulation is present in the subpleural lung in a patient with nonspecific interstitial pneumonia. The areas of reticulation seem to outline several rounded structures (*arrows*). However, these are distinguished from honeycombing by the fact that they are not of air attenuation (i.e., they are not black).

always occurs in one layer and is often associated with centrilobular emphysema; honeycombing may occur in multiple layers. Lucencies in paraseptal emphysema are usually larger than honeycomb cysts, ranging up to several centimeters in diameter. Honeycombing is typically associated with other signs of fibrosis such as traction bronchiectasis, irregular reticulation, and volume loss, while paraseptal emphysema is not. Honeycombing is usually lower lobe predominant, whereas paraseptal emphysema is usually seen in the upper lobes. Keep in mind, however, that paraseptal emphysema and honeycombing may coexist. In such cases, bubbly lucencies may be seen from the lung apex to the base.

Irregular reticulation in the subpleural lung may appear to outline rounded cysts that resemble honeycombing; however, the density of the central portion of these areas is not of air attenuation and may contain visible vessels (Fig. 2.15).

Honeycombing must involve the subpleural lung if a confident diagnosis is to be made. If a cystic abnormality does not involve the subpleural lung, it likely represents another finding such as emphysema, bronchiectasis, traction bronchiectasis (Fig. 2.16), or cystic lung disease.

Rarely primary cystic lung diseases, specifically lymphoid interstitial pneumonia (LIP), have a subpleural predominance (Fig. 2.17). In these cases, the cysts closely resemble honeycombing. Patients with LIP usually have a known history of connective tissue disease or immunosuppression (e.g., common variable immunodeficiency). Also, the lack of other signs of fibrosis in the same regions as the cysts may be a clue that honeycombing is not present.

IRREGULAR RETICULATION

Irregular reticulation is nonspecific. Simply stated, irregular reticulation is said to be present

Figure 2.16

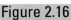

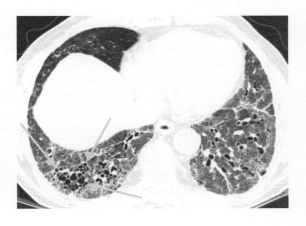

Traction bronchiectasis mimicking honeycombing. Clusters of rounded air-density structures are seen at the lung bases (*arrows*), resembling honeycombing. However, they do not involve the subpleural lung. These represent areas of traction bronchiectasis in a patient with nonspecific interstitial pneumonia.

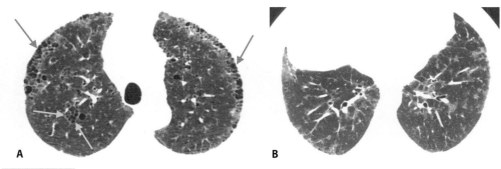

Figure 2.17

Subpleural cystic lung disease mimicking honeycombing. A. HRCT of a patient with rheumatoid arthritis and lymphoid interstitial pneumonia shows subpleural cysts (*red arrows*) that closely resemble honeycombing. These are distinguished from honeycombing by the lack of other signs of fibrosis and by the presence of cysts in the more central lung regions (*yellow arrows*). **B.** Image through the lung bases shows ground glass opacity without evidence of fibrosis.

when abnormal reticular opacities do not clearly represent one of the other two patterns, namely interlobular septal thickening and honeycombing. Irregular reticulation may be seen in combination with the other two reticular patterns.

Although some appearances of irregular reticulation have specific names (e.g., intralobular interstitial thickening, parenchymal bands, and subpleural lines), knowing them does not help much in diagnosis.

Irregular reticulation is moderately specific for fibrosis, although it also may be seen with infiltrative diseases such a pulmonary edema or inflammatory diseases that cause interstitial thickening.

HRCT Features

The lines of irregular reticulation can be thick or thin, fine or coarse, straight or curved, and may or may not be associated with distortion of the underlying lung architecture.

If irregular reticulation is associated with honeycombing, it can be assumed to reflect fibrosis. In this case, it is the presence of honeycombing that is most important in the differential diagnosis.

Another finding termed *traction bronchiectasis* is also helpful in suggesting that fibrosis is present when irregular reticulation is visible. On the other hand, if irregular reticulation

is associated with ground glass opacity, and traction bronchiectasis is absent, consider an infiltrative or inflammatory disease as most likely.

Irregular Reticulation with Traction Bronchiectasis

Traction bronchiectasis is a finding that is highly specific for fibrosis. The bronchi themselves are not intrinsically diseased, but are dilated secondary to traction on their walls from adjacent lung fibrosis. In traction bronchiectasis, bronchi appear irregular and distorted and are cork-screwed in shape (Figs. 2.12 and 2.16). Traction bronchiectasis may be distinguished from inflammatory bronchiectasis by a lack of mucous impaction and wall thickening and by its association with irregular reticulation (Fig. 2.18A, B). When traction bronchiectasis is visible, a close inspection for the presence of honeycombing should be undertaken. If honeycombing is also present, then that finding should be used to formulate the differential diagnosis.

Traction bronchiectasis may be seen in association with any fibrotic lung disease and is less specific than honeycombing with respect to the differential diagnosis. When significant traction bronchiectasis is unassociated with honeycombing, UIP is less likely as a diagnosis than when honeycombing is

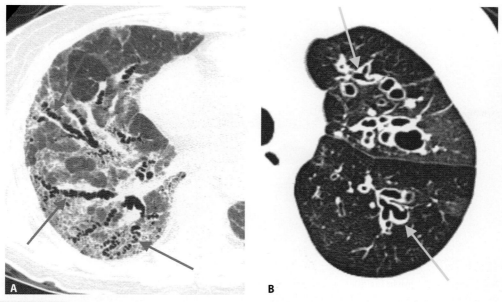

Figure 2.18

Traction versus inflammatory bronchiectasis. A. The bronchi in traction bronchiectasis are irregular and cork-screw shaped (*red arrows*) without evidence of bronchial inflammation. Associated lung disease is present. **B.** Inflammatory bronchiectasis (i.e., airways disease) shows extensive airway wall thickening, dilatation (*yellow arrows*), and mucoid impaction without signs of fibrosis.

present, and other abnormalities, such as sarcoidosis, hypersensitivity pneumonitis, and NSIP, should be considered (Figs. 2.12, 2.16, and 2.19). If irregular reticulation with traction bronchiectasis is the predominant abnormality in a patient with known connective tissue disease, a diagnosis of NSIP will generally be made. Otherwise, a biopsy is usually performed for diagnosis.

Irregular Reticulation with Ground Glass Opacity

Often it is best to approach the differential diagnosis of this pattern by considering the differential diagnosis of ground glass opacity and associated symptoms (see Chapter 4). Acute symptoms in the presence of ground glass opacity and reticulation suggest pulmonary edema, infection, diffuse alveolar damage,

Figure 2.19

Traction bronchiectasis in nonspecific interstitial pneumonia. In this patient with scleroderma, HRCT shows a peripheral distribution of irregular reticulation and traction bronchiectasis (*arrow*), without honeycombing. While usual interstitial pneumonia may occasionally present without honeycombing, the HRCT is more typical of nonspecific interstitial pneumonia.

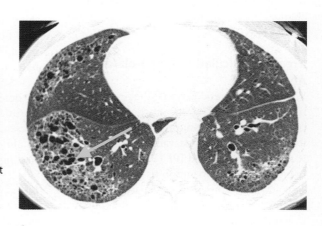

2

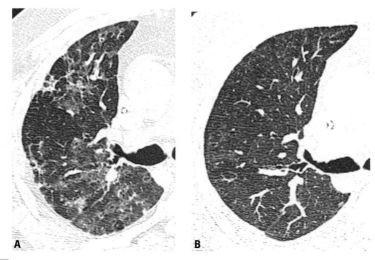

A   B

Figure 2.20

Irregular reticulation associated with ground glass opacity. HRCT at the same anatomic level is shown, performed 3 months apart. **A.** The initial HRCT shows irregular reticulation and ground glass opacity in a patient with bleomycin-induced pulmonary toxicity. **B.** Follow-up HRCT after treatment shows near-complete resolution of the previous abnormalities. While irregular reticulation often represents fibrosis, it may in some cases represent inflammation particularly when associated honeycombing and traction bronchiectasis are absent.

or hemorrhage. Chronic symptoms are most suggestive of hypersensitivity pneumonitis or NSIP. A biopsy is usually required for diagnosis in patients with chronic symptoms, unless the patient has a history of connective tissue disease. Patients with irregular reticulation and ground glass opacity may occasionally show improvement or resolution of abnormalities with appropriate treatment (Fig. 2.20A, B).

Rarely UIP presents with irregular reticulation and ground glass opacity as the predominant finding, without honeycombing or traction bronchiectasis. In this setting, these changes represent fibrosis below the resolution of HRCT.

Irregular Reticulation as an Isolated Abnormality

When irregular reticulation is the predominant finding, and no significant honeycombing, traction bronchiectasis, or ground glass opacity is present, the appearance is nonspecific. It may reflect UIP and IPF (Fig. 2.21A), NSIP, hypersensitivity pneumonitis (Fig. 2.21B), sarcoidosis, or other fibrotic, infiltrative, or inflammatory diseases. Biopsy is often pursued in these cases.

A GENERAL APPROACH TO THE DIAGNOSIS OF POSSIBLE FIBROTIC LUNG DISEASE

In the evaluation of HRCT in a patient with diffuse lung disease, a close inspection for the presence of fibrosis is an important step. This has significant implications in terms of diagnosis, prognosis, and potential response to treatment. Certain diseases, such as IPF, tend to be predominantly fibrotic, whereas others, such as desquamative interstitial pneumonia (DIP), typically have little to no fibrosis. Regardless of their specific diagnosis, patients with significant fibrosis on HRCT tend to have a poorer prognosis than those who do not and are less likely to show improvement with treatment.

Several considerations are important in determining the differential diagnosis of fibrotic lung disease on HRCT, including the presence of honeycombing, the distribution of abnormalities, and presence of associated findings such as air trapping.

HRCT Findings of Fibrosis

There are several HRCT findings that may indicate the presence of fibrosis. The most

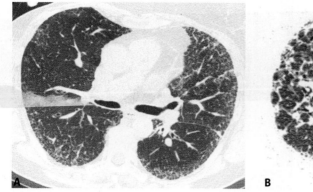
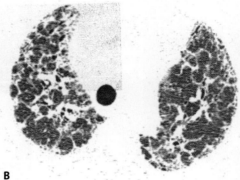

Figure 2.21

Irregular reticulation as the predominant finding. A. Mild subpleural reticulation is present without other signs of fibrosis. This abnormality is nonspecific with respect to diagnosis, but the subpleural distribution suggests one of the interstitial pneumonias. Lung biopsy yielded a diagnosis of usual interstitial pneumonia due to idiopathic pulmonary fibrosis. **B.** The irregular reticulation in this case is much more extensive and associated with mild traction bronchiectasis. It would be unusual for usual interstitial pneumonia to have such extensive abnormalities without honeycombing. This patient was diagnosed with hypersensitivity pneumonitis.

important of these are honeycombing, traction bronchiectasis, and irregular reticulation (Fig. 2.22A–C). Honeycombing is the most specific finding, and if present, one can be very confident about the presence of fibrosis (Fig. 2.7A). Traction bronchiectasis almost always indicates that fibrosis is present, particularly when associated with irregular reticulation. However, in some patients with ground glass opacity, traction bronchiectasis may be transient, resolving with treatment. Irregular reticulation is moderately specific for the presence of fibrosis, but in some cases may represent infiltration or inflammation, and can improve or resolve with treatment. Ground glass opacity is a nonspecific finding that reflects the presence of abnormalities below the resolution of HRCT and may occasionally be a manifestation of fibrotic lung disease (Fig. 2.7B).

Step-by-Step Analysis

Step 1: Is Fibrosis Present?

First, ask yourself this question. The presence of fibrosis is important in terms of diagnosis, prognosis, and possible response to treatment. Carefully search for any signs of fibrosis,

specifically honeycombing, traction bronchiectasis, and irregular reticulation (Fig. 2.23A, B).

Step 2: Is Honeycombing Present?

Honeycombing is arguably the most important sign on HRCT, thus a careful inspection for honeycombing should be undertaken (Fig. 2.24). It is highly specific for fibrosis and is often associated with a pattern of UIP and IPF.

Step 3: What Is the Craniocaudal Distribution of Abnormalities?

There are many ways to classify the distribution of a diffuse lung disease. Certain diseases tend to affect the upper lobes and others predominate in the mid- or lower lung (Table 2.8). An upper lobe predominance of disease is typical of sarcoidosis, prior granulomatous infection such as tuberculosis, pneumoconioses, radiation fibrosis, and ankylosing spondylitis. A lower lobe predominance of disease is typical of IPF, connective tissue disease, drug fibrosis, asbestosis, hypersensitivity pneumonitis, and chronic aspiration.

Pay particular attention to the costophrenic angles. In general, the idiopathic interstitial pneumonias, including UIP, NSIP, and DIP,

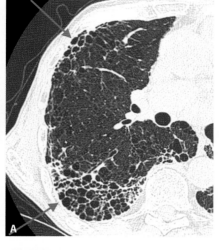

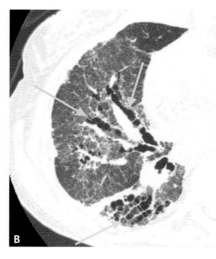

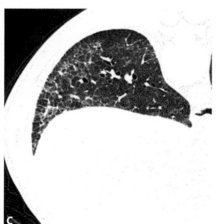

Figure 2.22

HRCT signs of fibrosis. A. Honeycombing. This is manifested by stacked subpleural cysts with relatively thick walls (*red arrows*). This finding is highly specific for fibrosis and is often seen in association with other findings such as traction bronchiectasis. **B. Traction bronchiectasis.** Bronchial dilatation associated with fibrosis is irregular, cork-screw shaped (*yellow arrows*), and unassociated with findings of airway inflammation such as bronchial wall thickening. This finding is also highly specific for fibrosis. **C. Irregular reticulation.** This finding is manifested by irregular lines associated with architectural distortion. It often represents fibrosis, but occasionally is a manifestation of inflammation, particularly in the setting of nonspecific interstitial pneumonia.

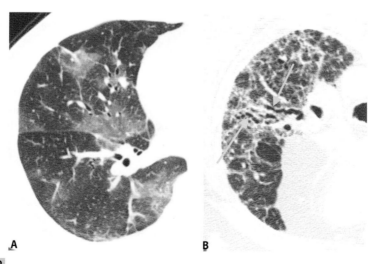

Figure 2.23

Approach to fibrosis, step 1: Is fibrosis present? A. Ground glass opacity only, no fibrosis present. HRCT in a patient with subacute hypersensitivity pneumonitis shows ground glass opacity and no evidence of fibrosis. These changes represented inflammation and resolved after treatment. **B. Severe fibrosis present.** Prone HRCT in a patient with chronic hypersensitivity pneumonitis shows traction bronchiectasis (arrows) and irregular reticulation. These findings represent fibrosis and were unresponsive to treatment.

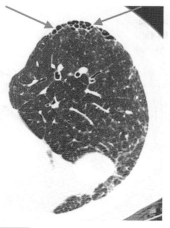

Figure 2.24

Approach to fibrosis, step 2: Is honeycombing present? Prone HRCT shows subpleural honeycombing (*arrows*) in a patient with idiopathic pulmonary fibrosis. While this finding may be found with several different diseases, its presence favors a pattern of usual interstitial pneumonia and represents irreversible fibrosis.

Table 2.8	Differential diagnosis of fibrosis based upon craniocaudal distribution of findings on HRCT
Upper lobe predominant	**Lower lobe predominant**
Sarcoidosis	Idiopathic pulmonary fibrosis
Prior tuberculosis	Connective tissue disease
Prior fungal infection	Drug fibrosis
Radiation fibrosis (e.g., head & neck cancer treatment)	Asbestosis
Pneumoconioses (silicosis, coal worker's, beryllium, talc)	Hypersensitivity pneumonitis
Ankylosing spondylitis	Chronic aspiration

involve the posterior costophrenic angles. Fibrosis resulting from ARDS is often subpleural and anterior in distribution. Most other diseases will show sparing of the inferior-most costophrenic angles (Fig. 2.25A–C). This is

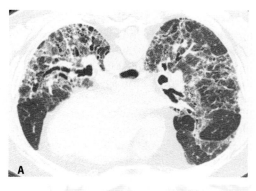

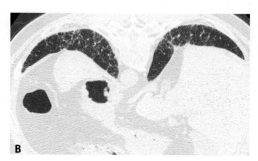

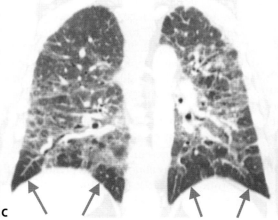

Figure 2.25

Approach to fibrosis, step 3: What is the craniocaudal distribution? Prone HRCT through the mid–lower lung **(A)**, inferior costophrenic angles **(B)**, and a coronal reformation **(C)** in a patient with hypersensitivity pneumonitis shows a mid–lower lung predominance with sparing of the costophrenic angles (**C**, *arrows*). This sparing of the costophrenic angle is very usual for usual and nonspecific interstitial pneumonia and suggests an alternative cause of fibrosis.

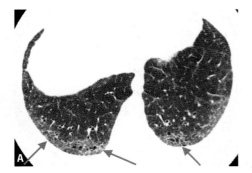

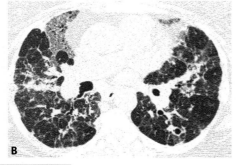

Figure 2.26

Approach to fibrosis, step 4: What is the axial distribution? A. Peripheral distribution in nonspecific interstitial pneumonia. HRCT shows a strong peripheral distribution (*arrows*) of ground glass opacity, irregular reticulation, and traction bronchiectasis. This distribution of findings strongly suggests an interstitial pneumonia, namely usual interstitial pneumonia, nonspecific interstitial pneumonia, or desquamative interstitial pneumonia. **B. Diffuse distribution of hypersensitivity pneumonitis.** In contrast to usual interstitial, nonspecific, and desquamative interstitial pneumonia, other fibrotic lung diseases tend to show a central or diffuse distribution of findings. This patient with hypersensitivity pneumonitis shows both peripheral and central areas of fibrosis.

particularly helpful in distinguishing chronic hypersensitivity pneumonitis from the interstitial pneumonias, as hypersensitivity pneumonitis is typically mid–lower lung predominant and yet spares the costophrenic angles.

Step 4: What Is the Axial (Cross-Sectional) Distribution of Abnormalities?

The cross-sectional distribution of abnormalities (Fig. 2.26A, B) may also be helpful (Table 2.9). Whether a disease is strongly

Table 2.9	Differential diagnosis based upon axial distribution of findings	
Subpleural predominant	**Diffuse or central distribution**
Idiopathic pulmonary fibrosis	Sarcoidosis
Connective tissue disease	Pneumoconioses
Drug fibrosis	Hypersensitivity pneumonitis
Asbestosis	Chronic aspiration
Post–acute respiratory distress syndrome fibrosis	Prior tuberculosis or fungal infection

peripheral or involves the more central or peribronchovascular lung regions can serve to focus the differential diagnosis. The interstitial pneumonias tend to be strongly peripheral in distribution. Keep in mind that the subpleural region includes the interstitium just deep to the fissures. Other diseases tend to show a central or diffuse distribution.

Step 5: Are There Significant Associated Findings That Help in Diagnosis?

Findings that accompany those of fibrosis are important in determining the cause. The most important of these include mosaic perfusion, air trapping, and nodules. The combination of fibrosis and mosaic perfusion and/or air trapping is strongly suggestive of hypersensitivity pneumonitis (Fig. 2.27A, B). A patient with perilymphatic nodules and fibrosis likely has sarcoidosis. Note that these additional findings need to be significant in extent to be used for diagnosis. For instance, it is not uncommon for someone with IPF to have a small amount of air trapping (Fig. 2.28A, B). It is only when the presence of air trapping is moderate to severe that it should be considered helpful in diagnosing hypersensitivity pneumonitis.

Step 6: If Fibrosis Is Present, Is It the Predominant Abnormality?

If fibrosis is present, it is important to determine if the lung abnormality is predominantly fibrotic (Fig. 2.29). For example, IPF is predominantly a fibrotic disease. If there are areas of isolated ground glass opacity, consolidation, or nodules, findings that generally do

2

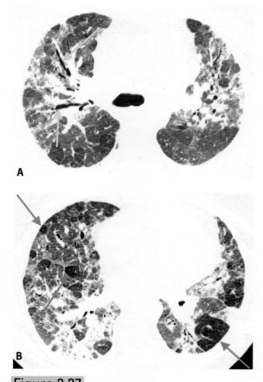

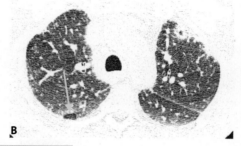

Figure 2.27

Approach to fibrosis, step 5: Are there associated findings? Other findings associated with fibrosis may be useful in diagnosis. The combination of fibrosis and significant mosaic perfusion/air trapping is very suggestive of hypersensitivity pneumonitis. Note the patchy irregular reticulation and traction bronchiectasis (**A**, *yellow arrows*) associated with significant areas of air trapping on expiratory images (**B**, *red arrows*).

Figure 2.28

Approach to fibrosis, step 5: Are there associated findings? A patient with idiopathic pulmonary fibrosis shows minimal air trapping. In order to be useful in diagnosis, additional findings associated with fibrosis need to be a significant part of the picture. This patient with idiopathic pulmonary fibrosis shows peripheral fibrosis with honeycombing in the lower lobes typical for a usual interstitial pneumonia pattern. The minimal air trapping in the right upper lobe (**B**, *arrow*) should be ignored as it is not a significant abnormality.

not indicate fibrosis, then there may be active inflammation present and the patient likely warrants more aggressive treatment.

Step 7: Is Useful Clinical Information Available?

Basic clinical information is vital in placing HRCT findings in context (Table 2.10). Age has an impact on which disease is most likely. For instance, IPF is rare in patients under 50 years of age, but in patients older than 50 years, it is one of the most common causes of lung fibrosis. Drug toxicity, asbestosis, and other pneumoconioses are also most common in patients older than 50 years. Sarcoidosis and

collagen vascular disease typically present in patients under 40 years. Hypersensitivity pneumonitis has a wide age range at presentation.

Fibrosis in a cigarette smoker is most commonly due to UIP or DIP. Exposures to dust or organic antigens are associated with pneumoconiosis or hypersensitivity pneumonitis, respectively. Connective tissue disease is most commonly associated with NSIP, but a UIP pattern may also be seen in these patients. Drug-induced fibrosis will be seen in patients with an appropriate medication history. The most common categories of drugs to produce fibrosis are the chemotherapeutic agents, cardiac medications, and antibiotics.

2

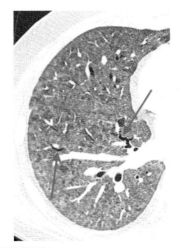

Figure 2.29

Approach to fibrosis, step 6: Is fibrosis the predominant abnormality? HRCT showing extensive ground glass opacity and minimal traction bronchiectasis (*red arrows*). While fibrosis is present, it is a very small component to the disease. Most of the abnormality is likely inflammatory and reversible.

Table 2.10	Clinical information and the most likely associated diagnoses presenting with fibrosis
Age > 50 y	Idiopathic pulmonary fibrosis, drug toxicity, asbestosis, pneumoconioses, hypersensitivity pneumonitis
Age < 50 y	Sarcoidosis, collagen vascular disease, hypersensitivity pneumonitis
Cigarette smoking	Idiopathic pulmonary fibrosis, desquamative interstitial pneumonia
Exposures to dust	Silicosis, coal worker's pneumoconiosis, talcosis, and other pneumoconioses
Exposures to organic antigens	Hypersensitivity pneumonitis
Connective tissue disease	Nonspecific interstitial pneumonia and usual interstitial pneumonia

FURTHER READING

Andreu J, Hidalgo A, Pallisa E, Majo J, Martinez-Rodriguez M, Caceres J. Septal thickening: HRCT findings and differential diagnosis. *Curr Probl Diagn Radiol.* 2004;33:226-237.

Austin JH, Müller NL, Friedman PJ, et al. Glossary of terms for CT of the lungs: recommendations of the Nomenclature Committee of the Fleischner Society. *Radiology.* 1996;200:327-331.

Collins J. CT signs and patterns of lung disease. *Radiol Clin North Am.* 2001;39:1115-1135.

Elicker B, Pereira CA, Webb R, Leslie KO. High-resolution computed tomography patterns of diffuse interstitial lung disease with clinical and pathological correlation. *J Bras Pneumol.* 2008;34:715-744.

Gotway MB, Freemer MM, King TE Jr. Challenges in pulmonary fibrosis. 1: use of high resolution CT scanning of the lung for the evaluation of patients with idiopathic interstitial pneumonias. *Thorax.* 2007;62:546-553.

Gotway MB, Reddy GP, Webb WR, Elicker BM, Leung JW. High-resolution CT of the lung: patterns of disease and differential diagnoses. *Radiol Clin North Am.* 2005;43:513-542.

Hansell DM, Bankier AA, MacMahon H, et al. Fleischner Society: glossary of terms for thoracic imaging. *Radiology.* 2008;246:697-722.

Kang EY, Grenier P, Laurent F, Müller NL. Interlobular septal thickening: patterns at high-resolution computed tomography. *J Thorac Imaging.* 1996;11:260-264.

Lynch DA, Travis WD, Muller NL, et al. Idiopathic interstitial pneumonias: CT features. *Radiology.* 2005;236:10-21.

Müller NL, Miller RR. Computed tomography of chronic diffuse infiltrative lung disease: part 1. *Am Rev Respir Dis.* 1990;142:1206-1215.

Müller NL, Miller RR. Computed tomography of chronic diffuse infiltrative lung disease: part 2. *Am Rev Respir Dis.* 1990;142:1440-1448.

Primack SL, Hartman TE, Hansell DM, Müller NL. End-stage lung disease: CT findings in 61 patients. *Radiology.* 1993;189:681-686.

Raghu G, Collard HR, Egan JJ, et al. An official ATS/ERS/JRS/ALAT statement: idiopathic pulmonary fibrosis: evidence-based guidelines for diagnosis and management. *Am J Respir Crit Care Med.* 2011;183:788-824.

Souza CA, Müller NL, Flint J, Wright JL, Churg A. Idiopathic pulmonary fibrosis: spectrum of high-resolution CT findings. *AJR Am J Roentgenol.* 2005;185:1531-1539.

Suh RD, Goldin JG. High-resolution computed tomography of interstitial pulmonary fibrosis. *Semin Respir Crit Care Med.* 2006;27:623-633.

Webb WR. High resolution lung computed tomography: normal anatomic and pathologic findings. *Radiol Clin North Am.* 1991;29:1051-1063.

Webb WR. Thin-section CT of the secondary pulmonary lobule: anatomy and the image—the 2004 Fleischner lecture. *Radiology.* 2006;239:322-338.

Woodhead F, Wells AU, Desai SR. Pulmonary complications of connective tissue diseases. *Clin Chest Med.* 2008;29:149-164.

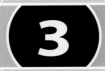

Nodular Lung Disease

Diffuse lung diseases presenting with small nodules (less than 1 cm in diameter) represent a wide variety of entities in many different disease categories. HRCT is generally used to suggest a focused differential diagnosis and guide further diagnostic evaluation. In some cases, HRCT may be diagnostic of a single disease.

The HRCT evaluation of a patient with nodular lung disease is based on several findings and patterns. These include (a) the craniocaudal distribution of nodules, (b) the appearance and attenuation of the nodules, and (c) the specific distribution of the nodules relative to lung structures.

CRANIOCAUDAL DISTRIBUTION OF NODULES

The craniocaudal distribution of nodules is helpful in the differential diagnosis of nodular

lung disease (Table 3.1). Certain diseases, such as sarcoidosis and other granulomatous diseases, tend to predominate in the upper lobes (Fig. 3.1A–C), whereas others, such as hematogenous metastases, tend to be lower lobe predominant (Fig. 3.2A, B). However, on its own, the craniocaudal distribution of nodules is insufficient for diagnosis and should be used in combination with other findings. There is overlap between the distributions of different diseases and variability among patients with the same disease.

APPEARANCE AND ATTENUATION OF NODULES

The appearance of nodules may help to determine whether they are interstitial or alveolar (airspace) in origin (Table 3.2, Fig. 3.3A, B). *Interstitial nodules* commonly have well-defined borders and are of soft tissue attenuation. Hematogenous metastases are a good example;

Table 3.1	Differential diagnosis of nodules based upon craniocaudal distribution	
Upper lobe predominant nodules	**Lower lobe predominant nodules**	**Variable (upper or lower lobe predominant nodules)**
Sarcoidosis	Hematogenous metastases	Lymphangitic carcinomatosis
Pneumoconioses (e.g., silicosis, coal worker's pneumoconiosis, berylliosis)		Hypersensitivity pneumonitis
Langerhans cell histiocytosis		Endobronchial spread of infection
Respiratory bronchiolitis		Invasive mucinous adenocarcinoma
		Miliary tuberculosis
		Miliary fungal infection
		Follicular bronchiolitis

3

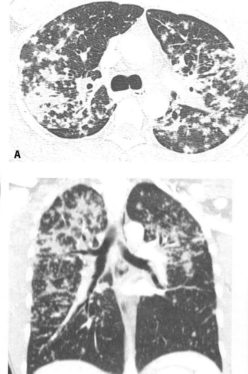

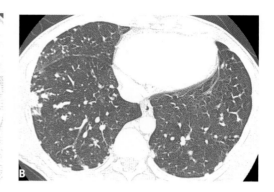

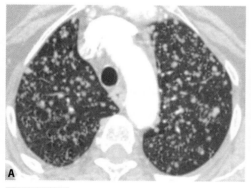

Figure 3.1

Upper lobe predominance of nodules in sarcoidosis.
A and **B.** HRCT in a patient with sarcoidosis shows
nodules to be more numerous and larger in the upper
(**A**) rather than in the lower (**B**) lungs. **C.** The marked
upper lobe predominance of sarcoidosis is clearly
demonstrated on a coronal reformation.

even small nodules in patients with metastases tend to be sharply marginated. *Alveolar
(or airspace) nodules* typically have ill-defined
borders. For instance, endobronchial spread of
infection (bronchopneumonia) results from

airway infection, and as the infection spreads
outward to involve the adjacent alveoli, the
leading edge of the resulting nodular opacity
will be indistinct because of heterogeneous
alveolar involvement. Alveolar nodules may

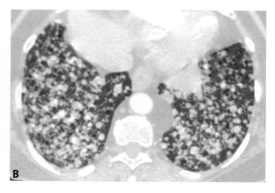

Figure 3.2

Lower lobe predominance of nodules in metastatic neoplasm. A and **B.** HRCT in a patient with
hematogenous spread of thyroid cancer to the lungs. Note the marked lower lobe predominance in the size
and number of nodules (**B**), as compared with a scan through the upper lobes (**A**). This reflects the differences
in blood flow to the lower and upper lobes.

Table 3.2 Differential diagnosis of nodules based upon appearance

Well-defined borders	Ill-defined borders	Either well-defined or ill-defined borders
Sarcoidosis	Hypersensitivity pneumonitis	Langerhans cell histiocytosis
Metastases	Respiratory bronchiolitis	Lymphoid interstitial pneumonia
Miliary infections	Follicular bronchiolitis	Pneumoconioses
Amyloidosis	Infections	
	Invasive mucinous adenocarcinoma (bronchioloalveolar carcinoma)	
	Aspiration	
	Pulmonary edema	
	Pulmonary hemorrhage	
	Pulmonary arterial hypertension	
	Metastatic calcification	

be of soft tissue attenuation or of ground glass opacity (GGO). Soft tissue airspace nodules are typical of bacterial infection, while GGO nodules may be due to atypical infections or inflammatory disease.

Using the appearance of nodules to determine their differential diagnosis, without considering other findings, is of limited accuracy; there are many exceptions to the rule. For instance, hypersensitivity pneumonitis (HP) is predominantly an interstitial lung disease (ILD), but is characterized by very indistinct nodules. Also, many diseases have both interstitial and alveolar components.

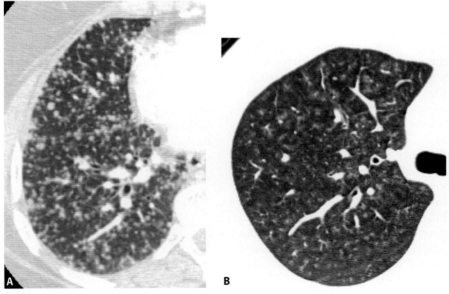

Figure 3.3

Appearances of different types of nodules. Different HRCT appearances of interstitial and airspace nodules. **A.** Hematogenous metastases involving the lung interstitium are sharply defined. **B.** Ground glass opacity nodules associated with viral pneumonia, with variable involvement of alveoli, are indistinct with poorly marginated borders.

DISTRIBUTION OF NODULES RELATIVE TO LUNG STRUCTURES

The preferred method by which to evaluate diffuse nodular lung disease on HRCT is to determine the specific distribution of nodules with respect to lung structures. This approach allows a limited differential diagnosis and also gives some insight into the pathophysiology of disease spread. When used in conjunction with clinical information, the craniocaudal distribution of nodules, and their appearance, it may be diagnostic of a single disease. When it is not diagnostic, HRCT can be helpful in guiding further tests.

There are three specific distributions of small nodules that can be distinguished on HRCT: (a) perilymphatic; (b) random; and (c) centrilobular. Recognizing one of these three distributions is fundamental to HRCT interpretation in patients with nodular lung disease. HRCT is 90% to 95% accurate in determining the pattern present and the correct differential diagnosis.

Perilymphatic Nodules

Diseases with a perilymphatic distribution of nodules are characterized by involvement of, or spread through, pulmonary lymphatics. For example, sarcoidosis is characterized by clusters of granulomas occurring in relation to lymphatics. Also, silicosis and coal worker's pneumoconiosis (CWP) result from inhalation of dusts, which are cleared via lymphatic channels.

Pulmonary lymphatics predominate in four specific locations: (1) the parahilar peribronchovascular interstitium, (2) the subpleural interstitium, (3) the interlobular septa, and (4) the centrilobular peribronchovascular interstitium. On HRCT, perilymphatic diseases typically show nodules predominating in, or limited to, one or more of these four locations (Fig. 3.4).

Peribronchovascular nodules are seen adjacent to large bronchi and vessels in the central lung regions (Fig. 3.4A, green nodules). They can give the walls of bronchi and arteries a nodular appearance, or clusters of nodules may be seen. *Subpleural nodules*, or clusters

of nodules forming "plaques" or masses, are seen immediately beneath the pleural surfaces and adjacent to the interlobar fissures (Fig. 3.4A, yellow nodules). *Interlobular septal nodules* give the septa a "beaded" appearance (Fig. 3.4A, red nodules). *Centrilobular peribronchovascular nodules* are seen in relation to small airways and vessels in the centers of pulmonary lobules. They give the centrilobular artery a knobby or beaded appearance or result in a centrilobular cluster of small nodules (Fig. 3.4A, blue nodules). Each of these regions need not be involved, or need not be involved to a similar degree, in patients having a perilymphatic pattern. At the level of individual pulmonary lobules, perilymphatic diseases may show centrilobular and interlobular septal nodules.

The combination of two of the four possible sites is usually sufficient for diagnosis. Globally, because the nodules occur only in relation to these specific locations, a perilymphatic distribution of nodules usually appears patchy, with some lung regions appearing abnormal and some lung regions appearing normal (Fig. 3.4A).

The most common diseases that result in a perilymphatic distribution of nodules are (a) sarcoidosis (Figs. 3.4B, C and 3.5A–D), (b) lymphangitic spread of neoplasm, and (c) several pneumoconioses, such as silicosis, CWP, berylliosis, talcosis, and rare earth pneumoconiosis (Table 3.3). Rare causes include lymphoid interstitial pneumonia (LIP) and amyloidosis.

There is some variation in the specific distribution of nodules, and the

Table 3.3	Differential diagnosis of perilymphatic nodules

Sarcoidosis (common)
Lymphangitic carcinomatosis or lymphoma/
   leukemia
Some pneumoconioses (e.g., silicosis, coal worker's
   pneumoconiosis, berylliosis, talc, rare earths)
Lymphoid interstitial pneumonia (rare)
Amyloidosis (rare)

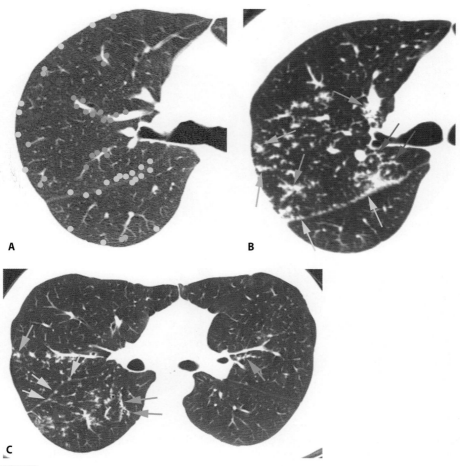

Figure 3.4

Perilymphatic nodules. A. In a perilymphatic pattern, the nodules predominate in relation to the peribronchovascular interstitium (*green dots*), subpleural interstitium (*yellow dots*), centrilobular regions (*blue dots*), and interlobular septa (*red dots*). In patients with a perilymphatic pattern, the distribution of nodules is often patchy. The specific distribution of perilymphatic nodules varies in different diseases and in different patients. **B** and **C.** Perilymphatic nodules in two patients with sarcoidosis. As in **(A)**, nodules are seen involving peribronchovascular (*green arrows*), subpleural (*yellow arrows*), centrilobular (*blue arrows*), and interlobular septal (*red arrows*) interstitium. The overall appearance is that of patchy lung involvement, with some lung regions appearing abnormal and some appearing normal.

predominant regions involved, among the different diseases associated with this pattern and in different patients with the same disease. These variations are discussed below.

HRCT findings, considered in conjunction with clinical information, may help distinguish among the several causes of perilymphatic nodules.

Sarcoidosis

Sarcoidosis is, by far, the most common disease in this category (see Chapter 12). On HRCT, nodules tend to predominate in the parahilar peribronchovascular and subpleural regions (Figs. 3.4B, C and 3.5A–D). Individual nodules are usually sharply marginated and of soft tissue attenuation and are easily seen when only a few millimeters in diameter. Peribronchovascular

3

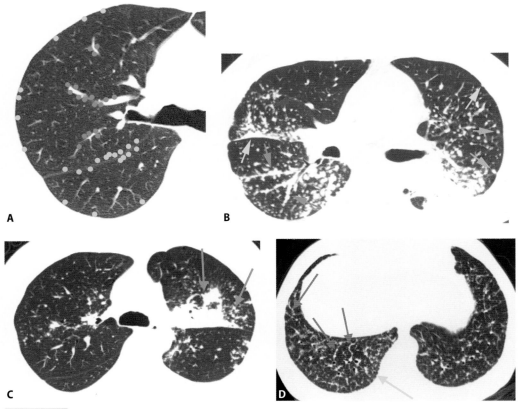

A

B

C

D

Figure 3.5

Perilymphatic nodules in sarcoidosis. A. A typical perilymphatic distribution in sarcoidosis. In sarcoidosis, nodules typically predominate in relation to the peribronchovascular interstitium (*green dots*) and the subpleural interstitium (*yellow dots*), but centrilobular and septal nodules may also be seen. **B.** A classic perilymphatic pattern in a patient with sarcoidosis shows patchy, clustered nodules that predominate in relation to the central bronchovascular bundles (*green arrows*) and subpleural regions (*yellow arrows*). Note that some centrilobular peribronchovascular nodules (*blue arrows*) and septal nodules (*red arrow*) are also present. Conglomeration of nodules is visible in the left lung. **C.** CT "galaxy sign" in sarcoidosis. In a different patient, HRCT shows a parahilar mass-like conglomerate of confluent nodules in the left upper lobe. The mass reflects profuse peribronchovascular nodules. Smaller "satellite" nodules are visible at the periphery (*arrows*) of the confluent mass. This appearance is most common in the parahilar regions and has been termed the "galaxy sign." The galaxy sign may be seen in other diseases, such as silicosis and talcosis. Asymmetry, as seen in this case, may be seen in sarcoidosis. **D.** Interlobular septal nodules in sarcoidosis. A patient with sarcoidosis shows numerous nodules in relation to interlobular septa (*yellow arrow*). Numerous subpleural nodules (*red arrows*) are also present.

nodules may be few in number or numerous and confluent. HRCT may show a few peribronchovascular nodules, clusters of nodules, or large parahilar masses made up of multiple confluent nodules (Fig. 3.5C). Air-filled bronchi (air bronchograms) may be visible within large masses. Individual small nodules are usually visible adjacent to large masses; these are termed *satellite nodules*, and the appearance of a large mass with satellite nodules has been termed *the galaxy sign* of sarcoidosis (Fig. 3.5C). Subpleural nodules are also common in the lung periphery or adjacent to fissures. They may be seen as individual nodules or as clusters or subpleural plaques or masses.

Interlobular sepal nodules and centrilobular peribronchovascular nodules are less common (Fig. 3.5B, D), but occasionally are a predominant feature (Fig. 3.5D). Mediastinal and hilar lymph node enlargement may be associated, but need not be present to suggest the diagnosis.

Sarcoidosis typically shows an upper lobe predominance of nodules, but this is not always the case. Bilateral abnormalities are typical, but asymmetry is common.

Sarcoidosis is more frequently seen in younger patients than the other causes of perilymphatic nodules. Often, patients with extensive nodules are relatively asymptomatic, so there may be a discrepancy between the HRCT appearance and the severity of the patient's symptoms. There is a geographic variability in the incidence of sarcoidosis; sarcoidosis is much less common in countries close to the equator and in Asia than in the United States.

If sarcoidosis is suspected on HRCT, transbronchial biopsy is often the next diagnostic test. As the nodules are often located within the peribronchovascular interstitium, transbronchial biopsy has a high yield.

Lymphatic Spread of Neoplasm

On HRCT, lymphangitic spread of neoplasm, either carcinoma or lymphoma, most frequently results in smooth thickening of the interstitium, including the interlobular septa, peribronchovascular interstitium, and the subpleural interstitium (see Chapter 17). When nodules are present, which occurs in a minority of cases, they also tend to predominate in relation to the interlobular septa (Fig. 3.6A–E), the parahilar peribronchovascular interstitium, and the subpleural regions. A combination of smooth interstitial thickening and nodules may be seen; this appearance is not common in sarcoidosis. Mediastinal and hilar lymph node enlargement may be associated. Pleural effusion, rare in sarcoidosis, may be seen.

In lymphangitic spread of neoplasm, nodules are sharply marginated and of soft tissue attenuation. The overall distribution is variable. An upper or lower lobe predominance may be present, and nodules may be unilateral or bilateral.

Patients with lymphangitic spread of tumor usually have a history of malignancy and are older and more symptomatic (i.e., dyspneic) than patients with sarcoidosis. As with sarcoidosis, lymphangitic spread of neoplasm can often be diagnosed using transbronchial biopsy.

Silicosis and CWP

History is important in suggesting silicosis or CWP in a patient with nodules (see Chapter 16). Patients with silicosis or CWP have a significant history of long-term exposure in professions such as mining, quarrying, stone cutting, or sand blasting. On HRCT, silicosis and CWP have a similar appearance despite the fact that different dusts are involved, and the histology is different.

Silicosis and CWP are frequently associated with centrilobular nodules (reflecting deposition of dust and fibrosis around small airways and involving lymphatics) and interlobular septal or subpleural nodules because of lymphatic clearance of the dust (Fig. 3.7A, B). Centrilobular nodules are more frequent in these pneumoconioses than with the other causes of perilymphatic nodules.

Large masses in the parahilar regions may be seen, usually representing central conglomerations of nodules in CWP or masses made up of confluent nodules and fibrosis (*progressive massive fibrosis*) in silicosis (Fig. 3.7B). As these masses develop, the number of lung nodules often appears to decrease. Satellite nodules are common, and areas of emphysema may be seen in the peripheral lung.

A distinct upper lobe predominance is typical in both silicosis and CWP, and nodules are often most numerous in the posterior lung. Abnormalities are usually symmetrical. Nodules are usually a few millimeters in diameter, of soft tissue attenuation, and more sharply margined in silicosis than in CWP.

Rare Diseases

LIP should be considered in patients with connective tissue disease or immunosuppression (e.g., human immunodeficiency virus and common variable immunodeficiency) (see Chapters 9 and 17). The HRCT

3

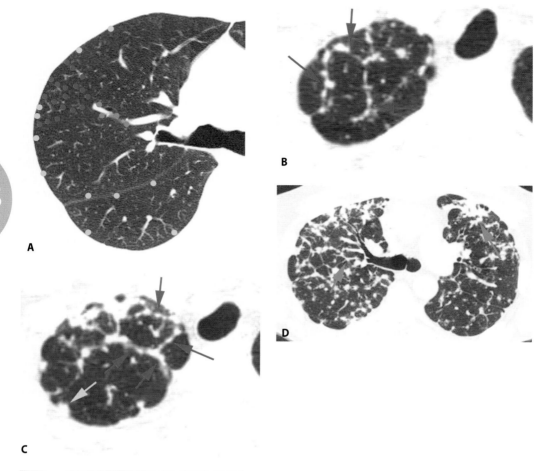

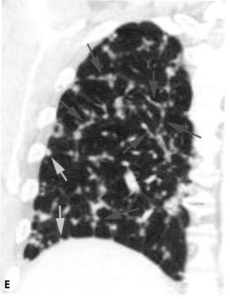

Figure 3.6

Perilymphatic nodules in lymphangitic spread of neoplasm. A. In lymphangitic spread of neoplasm, perilymphatic nodules tend to predominate in relation to the interlobular septa (*red dots*), the parahilar peribronchovascular interstitium (*green dots*), and the subpleural regions (*yellow dots*). The abnormality may be diffuse or patchy. **B–D.** Colon cancer with lymphangitic carcinomatosis. Extensive nodular interlobular septal thickening (*red arrows*) is seen throughout both lungs. A few subpleural nodules are also present (*yellow arrow*, **C**). Although lymphangitic carcinomatosis often predominates in relation to interlobular septa, it also may involve the peribronchovascular lymphatics (*green arrows*, **D**). **E.** Coronal reconstruction in the same patient as in **(B)–(D)** shows nodular interlobular septal thickening (*red arrows*) and subpleural nodules (*yellow arrows*).

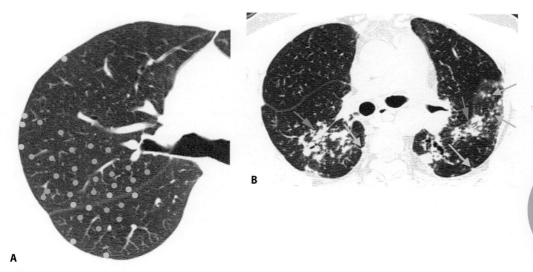

A

B

3

Figure 3.7

Perilymphatic nodules in silicosis. A. In silicosis, nodules usually predominate in the centrilobular (*blue dots*) and subpleural regions (*yellow dots*). A posterior lung predominance is common. **B.** HRCT in a patient with silicosis shows nodules in the subpleural regions (*yellow arrows*) and centrilobular regions (*blue arrows*). Peribronchovascular nodules are also visible (*green arrows*).

appearance of LIP is variable, but some combination of subpleural, interlobular septal, and centrilobular nodules is usually seen (Fig. 3.8). *Amyloidosis* may be seen in patients with multiple myeloma or may be idiopathic (see Chapter 18). Subpleural and septal nodules are most typical.

Random Nodules

Random nodules have no particular distribution with respect to the lung structures or the pulmonary lobule (Fig. 3.9). They typically show a diffuse and homogeneous distribution; they occur anywhere and everywhere. Subpleural nodules are present in patients with a random pattern, but there is no predominance of nodules in this location, as there often is with a perilymphatic distribution. Overall, random nodules are diffuse and uniform in distribution, while perilymphatic nodules usually appear patchy. Random nodules are usually of soft tissue attenuation, sharply marginated, and easily visible when only a few millimeters in size. At diagnosis, they are often smaller (1 to 2 mm) than nodules in patients with sarcoidosis.

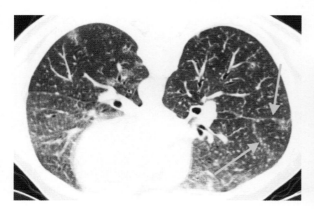

Figure 3.8

Perilymphatic nodules in lymphoid interstitial pneumonia. Prone HRCT of a patient with human immunodeficiency virus infection shows small nodules with a patchy distribution. Note the predominance of nodules in the subpleural interstitium (*arrows*) reflecting a perilymphatic distribution of disease.

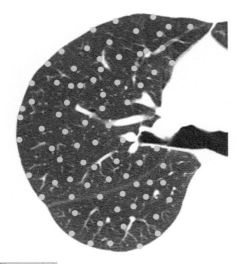

Figure 3.9

Random nodules. Nodules are diffuse and show a homogeneous distribution. Note that subpleural nodules are present, but there is no preponderance of nodules in this location.

Table 3.4	Differential diagnosis of random nodules

Miliary tuberculosis
Miliary fungal infection
Hematogenous metastases
Perilymphatic processes (occasionally
  appear random)

A random pattern is most common with processes that spread hematogenously (Fig. 3.10A, B). As blood flow is relatively homogeneous, it stands to reason that processes that spread in this manner are also diffuse in distribution. As there is proportionally more blood flow to the lung bases, random nodules may show a basilar predominance in size and number. On the other hand, miliary tuberculosis may show an upper lobe predominance because the organism grows best in the presence of high oxygen tension (which is present in the upper lobes).

The differential diagnosis (Table 3.4) of random nodules primarily includes miliary tuberculosis and other mycobacteria, miliary fungal infection (e.g., histoplasmosis and coccidioidomycosis) (see Chapter 14), and hematogenous spread of malignancy.

Occasionally, diseases that typically produce a perilymphatic pattern (e.g., sarcoidosis) appear random in distribution when the nodules are very numerous. However, there are usually clues to the correct diagnosis. For example, close inspection may show proportionally too many nodules along the fissures or within the peribronchovascular interstitium (Fig. 3.11). Also, in some patients with metastases, HRCT may show features of both random and perilymphatic patterns, likely because both types of spread are actually present.

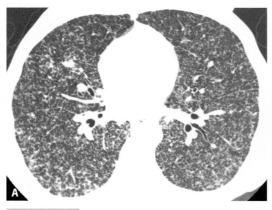
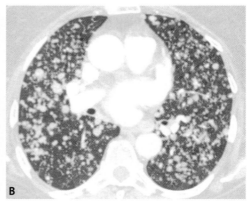

Figure 3.10

Random nodules. A and **B.** Two examples of a random distribution of pulmonary nodules in patients with miliary tuberculosis **(A)** and hematogenous spread of metastases **(B).** Notice the diffuse and uniform distribution of nodules with involvement of the pleural surfaces.

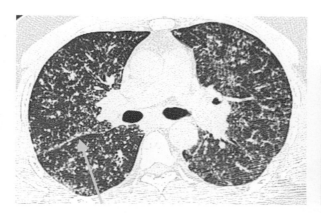

Figure 3.11

Perilymphatic nodules simulating a random distribution in sarcoidosis. Upon initial inspection, the nodules in this case appear to have a diffuse random distribution. However, note the predominance of nodules along the major fissure (*arrow*), a finding that suggests a perilymphatic distribution in this patient.

3

The size of nodules may be helpful in determining the most likely diagnosis. Tiny nodules, a few millimeters in diameter, are most commonly due to miliary tuberculosis, whereas larger nodules are more commonly due to malignancy. However, there is considerable overlap in the size of nodules that each of these diseases produces. Miliary tuberculosis can result in nodules larger than 5 mm.

History may be important in the differential diagnosis of this pattern. If the patient has a known diagnosis of malignancy, this pattern is usually diagnostic of hematogenous spread of tumor. If signs of infection are present (fever and increased white blood cell count), miliary tuberculosis or fungal infection is likely. One caveat: miliary tuberculosis may be associated with very few symptoms in elderly or debilitated patients. Transbronchial biopsy is often positive in patients with miliary infection or neoplasm.

Centrilobular Nodules

Centrilobular nodules occur in diseases that primarily involve the centrilobular bronchiole, artery, or lymphatics. The differential diagnosis of centrilobular nodules is quite broad and encompasses a wide variety of different etiologies and categories of disease. However, small airways disease is the most common cause of centrilobular nodules.

Centrilobular nodules demonstrate several HRCT findings that distinguish them from the other patterns. These include (1) sparing of the subpleural interstitium and (2) a similar spacing between adjacent nodules (Fig. 3.12).

As the centers of the most peripheral pulmonary lobules are about 5 to 10 mm from

pleural surfaces, the most peripheral nodules seen with this pattern are generally 5 mm from the pleural surface or fissures. Subpleural nodules are characteristically absent with a centrilobular distribution (Fig. 3.13), although a large centrilobular nodule may reach the pleural surface, or involve the entire lobule (Fig. 3.14). At a lobular level, centrilobular nodules (or a cluster of nodules) may be seen to surround the centrilobular artery, but do not involve the interlobular septa.

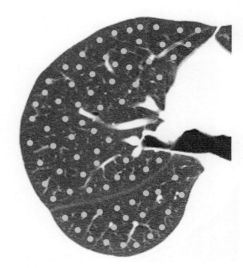

Figure 3.12

Centrilobular nodules. Nodules involve the centrilobular regions, and the most peripheral nodules are separated from the pleural surfaces by 5 to 10 mm; no subpleural nodules are present. Nodules also appear evenly spaced. In patients with centrilobular nodules, the overall distribution may be diffuse (as in this illustration) or patchy.

3

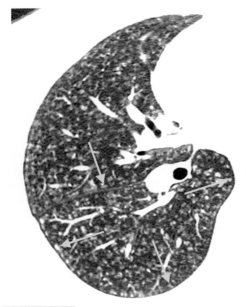

Figure 3.13

Centrilobular nodules in hypersensitivity pneumonitis. Diffuse nodules are present. Note sparing of the subpleural interstitium in the peripheral lung and along the fissure; the most peripheral nodules are about 5 mm from the pleural surface (*arrows*). No nodules arise at the pleural surface. The nodules appear evenly spaced.

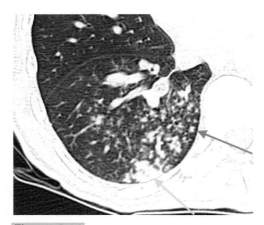

Figure 3.14

Centrilobular nodules in bacterial bronchopneumonia. Centrilobular nodules are visible in the right lower lobe. Their centers are about 5 mm from the pleural surface (*red arrow*). In areas that are more severely affected, the entire pulmonary lobule is involved (*yellow arrow*).

As pulmonary lobules are all about the same size, the centers of the pulmonary lobules (and any centrilobular nodules present) are about the same distance from one another. In other words, centrilobular nodules appear evenly spaced on HRCT.

The differential diagnosis of centrilobular nodules varies depending on several additional findings, including (1) their attenuation (whether they are of GGO or homogeneous soft tissue attenuation), (2) their overall distribution (i.e., diffuse, symmetrical, or patchy), and (3) their association with the finding of tree-in-bud (TIB).

GGO Centrilobular Nodules

Centrilobular nodules of GGO may be the result of airways disease or vascular disease (Table 3.5). Airways disease is more likely. Centrilobular nodules with this appearance typically reflect processes that produce peribronchiolar inflammation, infiltration, or fibrosis without dense consolidation or obliteration of alveoli.

HP represents a reaction to inhaled organic antigens that produces peribronchiolar inflammation with ill-defined granulomas (see Chapter 13). HP is one of the most common diseases to produce centrilobular nodules of GGO (Fig. 3.15). Clinical history is extremely important in the diagnosis of a patient with diffuse

Table 3.5	Differential diagnosis of ground glass opacity centrilobular nodules
Airways diseases	Hypersensitivity pneumonitis
	Respiratory bronchiolitis (RB or RB-ILD)
	Follicular bronchiolitis
	Langerhans cell histiocytosis
	Pneumoconioses (e.g., coal worker's pneumoconiosis, siderosis)
	Infection (most commonly atypical/viral pneumonia)
Vascular diseases	Pulmonary edema
	Pulmonary hemorrhage
	Pulmonary arterial hypertension
	Metastatic calcification

RB-ILD, respiratory bronchiolitis interstitial lung disease.

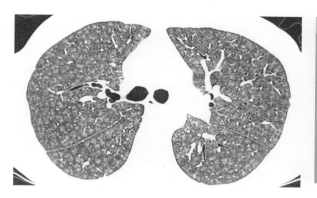

Figure 3.15

Subacute hypersensitivity pneumonitis (HP) with ground glass opacity centrilobular nodules. Diffuse centrilobular nodules of ground glass opacity are visible. There is sparing of the subpleural interstitium in the lung periphery and adjacent to the fissures. In the presence of an identifiable exposure, such as birds kept as pets, this pattern is diagnostic of HP. Otherwise lung biopsy is typically required for diagnosis.

GGO nodules. The combination of an identifiable exposure to an organic antigen and a HRCT showing diffuse centrilobular GGO nodules is usually considered diagnostic of HP and biopsy is not typically necessary. In the absence of such an exposure, additional diagnostic workup is likely indicated. In patients with HP, symptoms are usually subacute or chronic.

Respiratory bronchiolitis (RB) or *RB-ILD* is the most likely diagnosis when diffuse GGO nodules are visible in a patient with a history of cigarette smoking (Fig. 3.16) (see Chapter 11).

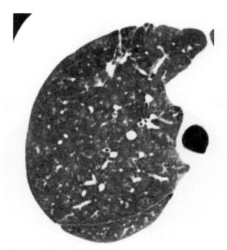

Figure 3.16

Respiratory bronchiolitis interstitial lung disease with ground glass opacity centrilobular nodules. HRCT shows very indistinct centrilobular nodules of ground glass opacity with sparing of the subpleural interstitium. This patient was a smoker with mild dyspnea.

RB represents an inflammatory bronchiolitis lesion present histologically in almost all smokers. RB-ILD is said to be present when RB is associated with symptoms, such as dyspnea. Langerhans cell histiocytosis in a smoker may occasionally present with GGO nodules. Symptoms in each of these smoking-related diseases are usually subacute or chronic.

Follicular bronchiolitis, an inflammatory bronchiolitis associated with lymphoid follicles, may present with diffuse GGO nodules (Fig. 3.17) (see Chapters 10 and 17). Patients usually have a history of connective tissue disease or immunosuppression. Follicular bronchiolitis is the sole manifestation of LIP in some patients.

Pneumoconioses can show centrilobular GGO nodules that indicate peribronchiolar deposition of the inhaled dust or mild peribronchiolar fibrosis (see Chapter 16). The pneumoconioses typically showing ground glass nodules as the predominant abnormality tend to be those that are not highly fibrogenic, such as CWP and siderosis. Obviously, in these cases, an exposure history is important.

Vascular abnormalities and diseases that may produce centrilobular GGO nodules include pulmonary edema (Fig. 3.18), pulmonary hemorrhage, metastatic calcification (calcification occurring in relation to small vessels in patients with abnormal serum calcium and phosphate), and pulmonary arterial hypertension (see Chapter 7). The cause of nodules in pulmonary hypertension is not clear, but is most likely due to perivascular edema or hemorrhage or their residua. These

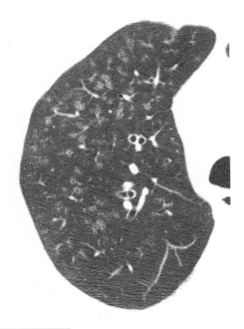

Figure 3.17

Follicular bronchiolitis with centrilobular nodules. HRCT shows centrilobular nodules of ground glass opacity. Many of the nodules are associated with abnormal airways. Biopsy showed follicular bronchiolitis.

vascular causes should be considered when an abnormality is diffuse or symmetric.

Several other diseases may present with GGO centrilobular nodules including bacterial, mycobacterial, or fungal infections and invasive mucinous adenocarcinoma of the lung (formerly termed diffuse bronchioloalveolar carcinoma; see Chapter 17), but the nodules in these cases are more commonly of soft tissue attenuation. In these diseases, nodules are often patchy rather than diffuse.

In a patient with chronic symptoms and diffuse GGO nodules, the most likely causes include HP, RB, and follicular bronchiolitis.

In a patient with acute symptoms and diffuse GGO nodules, atypical (viral or pneumocystis) pneumonia, pulmonary edema, and pulmonary hemorrhage are considerations (see Chapters 8 and 14). HP may occasionally present with acute symptoms.

Soft Tissue Attenuation Centrilobular Nodules

Centrilobular nodules of homogeneous soft tissue attenuation are characterized by inflammation or infiltration with consolidation of peribronchiolar alveoli or dense peribronchiolar fibrosis (Fig. 3.19). Bronchiolar filling or impaction may be present. As the

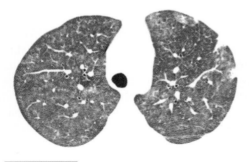

Figure 3.18

Pulmonary hemorrhage in a patient with systemic lupus erythematosus and hemoptysis. HRCT shows symmetric, diffuse centrilobular nodules of ground glass opacity. While this pattern is nonspecific, it may be seen with vascular diseases resulting in hemorrhage or edema.

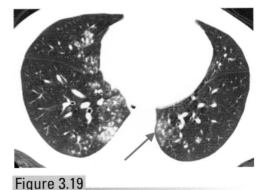

Figure 3.19

Endobronchial spread of infection in bacterial bronchopneumonia. HRCT shows patchy, asymmetric soft tissue attenuation centrilobular nodules. Note that the nodules all spare the subpleural regions (*arrow*).

Table 3.6	Differential diagnosis of soft tissue attenuation centrilobular nodules

Endobronchial spread of infection (bacterial, mycobacterial, fungal, viral)
Endobronchial spread of tumor (invasive mucinous adenocarcinoma)
Aspiration
Langerhans cell histiocytosis
Pulmonary edema
Pulmonary hemorrhage

disease progresses, the entire lobule may be involved.

The differential diagnosis of centrilobular nodules of soft tissue attenuation includes processes that are associated with endobronchial spread, such as bronchopneumonia, aspiration, and tumor (invasive mucinous adenocarcinoma) (Table 3.6, Fig. 3.20).

Bronchopneumonia resulting from bacterial, mycobacterial (tuberculosis and atypical organisms), fungal, or sometimes viral organisms is the most common cause of this abnormality (see Chapter 14). Symptoms are

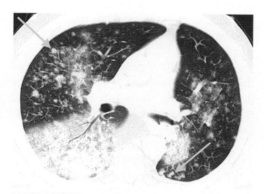

Figure 3.20

Invasive mucinous pulmonary adenocarcinoma.
Extensive patchy consolidation and soft tissue attenuation centrilobular nodules (*arrows*) are present. The nodules are evenly spaced and show striking sparing of the subpleural interstitium. This reflects endobronchial spread of tumor. Some ground glass opacity centrilobular nodules are also visible.

generally acute, and the nodules are focal, multifocal, or patchy in distribution, rather than diffuse.

Invasive mucinous adenocarcinoma may result in multifocal or patchy nodules, sometimes associated with larger areas of consolidation or GGO. Multiple lobes and both lungs may be involved.

Langerhans cell histiocytosis may be associated with centrilobular nodules early in the course of the disease. The nodules represent peribronchiolar accumulation of Langerhans cells and other inflammatory cells or peribronchiolar fibrosis (see Chapter 11).

Vascular diseases may produce either GGO or soft tissue attenuation centrilobular nodules depending upon the severity and confluence of alveolar involvement. Pulmonary edema and pulmonary hemorrhage are the most common vascular diseases to appear as soft tissue attenuation nodules.

Distribution in Differential Diagnosis: Diffuse, Symmetrical, and Patchy

The overall distribution of centrilobular nodules should be used in conjunction with nodule attenuation in formulating a differential diagnosis (Table 3.7).

In general, a diffuse and symmetrical distribution of centrilobular nodules is seen in patients with HP, RB or RB-ILD, follicular bronchiolitis, atypical infections, pneumoconioses, pulmonary edema, and other vascular abnormalities.

A symmetrical distribution of nodules with an upper or mid-lung predominance may be seen in HP, RB, Langerhans histiocytosis, pneumoconioses (e.g., CWP, silicosis, and siderosis), and metastatic calcification.

Patchy or multifocal nodules are most frequent with endobronchial spread of infection (bacteria, mycobacteria, and fungal), invasive mucinous adenocarcinoma, aspiration, and Langerhans cell histiocytosis. Such nodules are often asymmetric.

Tree-in-Bud

TIB opacities, when present, are seen in a centrilobular location. They may be associated

Table 3.7	Differential diagnosis of centrilobular nodules based upon overall distribution
Diffuse distribution	Hypersensitivity pneumonitis
	Respiratory bronchiolitis (RB or RB-ILD)
	Follicular bronchiolitis
	Atypical/viral infections
	Pneumoconioses
	Pulmonary edema
	Pulmonary hemorrhage
	Pulmonary arterial hypertension
Upper or mid-lung predominance	Hypersensitivity pneumonitis
	Respiratory bronchiolitis (RB or RB-ILD)
	Langerhans histiocytosis
	Pneumoconioses
	Metastatic calcification
Patchy distribution	Endobronchial infection (bacterial, mycobacterial, fungal)
	Invasive mucinous adenocarcinoma
	Aspiration
	Langerhans cell histiocytosis

RB-ILD, respiratory bronchiolitis interstitial lung disease.

Table 3.8	Differential diagnosis of the tree-in-bud pattern and its mimics
Infections	Bacterial infection
	Mycobacterial infection
	Fungal infection
	Viral infection
Infectious variants	Cystic fibrosis
	Ciliary disorders
	Immunodeficiency
	Panbronchiolitis
	Allergic bronchopulmonary aspergillosis
Noninfectious bronchiolar diseases	Invasive mucinous adenocarcinoma
	Follicular bronchiolitis
	Aspiration
Vascular abnormalities	Talcosis
	Intravascular metastases
Perilymphatic disease	Sarcoidosis

with centrilobular nodules (see Chapter 14). On HRCT, TIB is characterized by the presence of branching opacities, 1 to 2 mm in thickness and 1 to 2 cm in length, often associated with small nodules at the tips of the branches or along their length. The HRCT finding of TIB is usually due to dilatation and impaction of centrilobular bronchioles by pus or mucus (the branches), associated with small regions of peribronchiolar inflammation or fibrosis (the buds). TIB resembles a budding tree; its appearance is characteristic (Fig. 3.21A–E).

TIB is important because of its specificity; it is almost always due to infection with involvement of the small peripheral airways (Table 3.8). In fact, in a patient with lung disease, it is only necessary to visualize one good example of TIB to be confident that infection is present. TIB is not specific with regard to the type of infection, but bacterial and mycobacterial infections are most frequent. Depending on the cause or duration of infection, bronchiectasis or bronchial wall thickening may also be present (Figs. 3.21C–E and 3.22).

Because TIB is generally taken to mean that infection is present, it is vital to describe this finding only when you are sure that it is present. Your goal should be not to overcall TIB.

There are several noninfectious causes of TIB associated with bronchiolar abnormalities, but these are relatively rare and findings are often atypical. These include endobronchial spread of invasive mucinous adenocarcinoma, follicular bronchiolitis (usually in patients with connective tissue disease), mucoid impaction in asthma and allergic bronchopulmonary aspergillosis, and aspiration.

On occasion, a centrilobular vascular abnormality can mimic the appearance of TIB. Examples include talcosis due to injection of crushed pills (Fig. 3.23) in which fibrosis

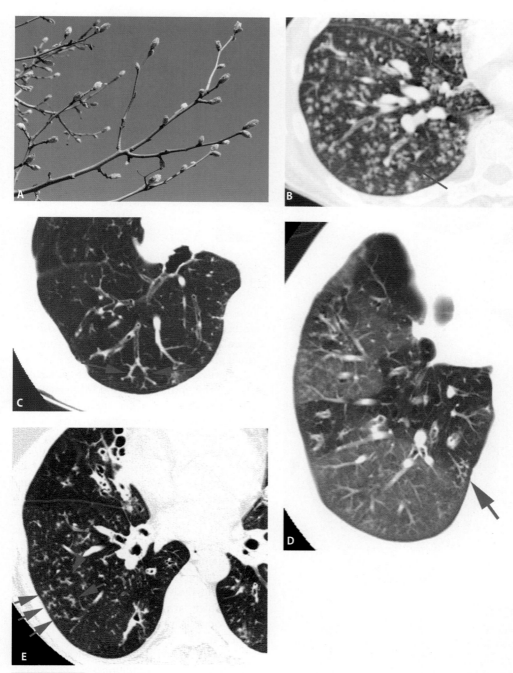

Figure 3.21

Tree-in-bud pattern. A. Tree-in-bud resembles the branches of a tree as its buds begin to swell prior to opening. **B.** On CT, tree-in-bud results in the appearance of a centrilobular branching opacity with nodules at the tips of the branches. This appearance reflects the presence of dilatation and impaction of small distal airways (*arrows*) and is highly specific for endobronchial infection. As in this patient with pneumonia, it may be associated with centrilobular nodules. **C.** Tree-in bud (*arrows*) in a patient with chronic airway infection. Note associated bronchial wall thickening. **D.** Tree-in bud (*arrow*) in a patient with cystic fibrosis. **E.** Tree-in bud (*arrows*) associated with bronchiectasis and chronic infection.

3

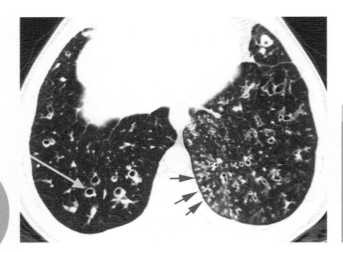

Figure 3.22

Primary ciliary dyskinesia with tree-in-bud. Extensive large airways inflammation is present, manifested by bronchiectasis and bronchial wall thickening (*yellow arrow*). Chronic infection and mucostasis in the distal airways is manifested primarily by tree-in-bud opacities (*red arrows*).

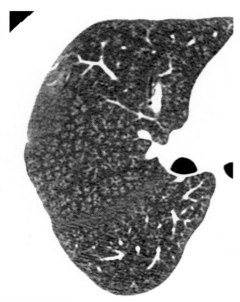

Figure 3.23

Talcosis, a vascular cause of centrilobular nodules. HRCT of the right lung in a body builder who injected crushed steroid tablets shows branching opacities that resemble the tree-in-bud sign. The process is diffuse. This distribution would be very unusual for endobronchial infection. Note the sparing of the fissures and peripheral subpleural interstitium. Talcosis results in deposition of mineral and fibrosis in relation to small centrilobular arteries.

occurs in relation to small vessels and intravascular metastases with nodules of tumor in small vessels.

Perilymphatic processes such as sarcoidosis are sometimes associated with small clusters of nodules in a centrilobular location. As the nodules are visible adjacent to the branching centrilobular artery, the appearance can mimic a TIB pattern. However, nodules in other locations, such as the parahilar peribronchovascular and subpleural regions, are often present, allowing a correct diagnosis to be made (Fig. 3.24).

HRCT may guide the next diagnostic test in patients with centrilobular nodules. In patients with patchy, soft tissue attenuation centrilobular nodules or the TIB pattern, sputum analysis or bronchoscopy with bronchoalveolar lavage often yields a diagnosis; infection is a very common cause of these appearances.

In patients with GGO nodules and acute symptoms, further evaluation is usually clinical. On occasion, bronchoscopy may be performed to diagnose a suspected infection. Sputum analysis in a patient with centrilobular nodules of GGO is not usually helpful. In patients with chronic symptoms and GGO nodules, a video-assisted thoracoscopic

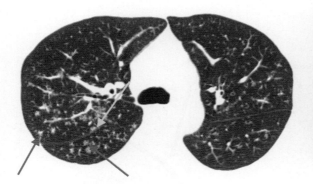

Figure 3.24

Perilymphatic nodules mimicking a centrilobular pattern. Clusters of centrilobular peribronchovascular nodules (*red arrows*) in a patient with sarcoidosis resemble the tree-in-bud sign. However, perilymphatic diseases such as sarcoidosis also show nodules in other locations such as the subpleural (*yellow arrow*) and parahilar peribronchovascular interstitium.

3

surgical biopsy is typically required for definitive diagnosis.

AN APPROACH TO DIAGNOSIS OF NODULAR LUNG DISEASE

Being able to differentiate the three patterns of nodules on HRCT will enable the formulation of an appropriate and focused differential diagnosis. A comparison of the characteristics of the three different distributions of nodules

is shown in Figure 3.25A–D and Table 3.9. A simple algorithm for evaluating nodules on HRCT is shown in Figure 3.26.

The following are a few important points to remember when attempting to identify the pattern of nodules:

(1) Subpleural nodules are present in both perilymphatic and random patterns, but should not be present in patients with centrilobular nodules. If the distribution is unclear, attention should be paid to the fissures and peripheral subpleural

Table 3.9	Characteristics of nodules based upon their distribution with respect to lung structures and the secondary pulmonary lobule		
Distribution	**Perilymphatic**	**Random**	**Centrilobular**
Pathophysiology	Primary lymphatic involvement or lymphatic drainage	Hematogenous spread	Bronchiolar, small vessel, or lymphatic disease
Nodule locations	Peribronchovascular, subpleural, interlobular septal, centrilobular	No specific distribution	Centrilobular only
Features	Patchy, clustered	Diffuse, uniform	Separated from pleura/fissures, evenly spaced, diffuse or patchy
Subpleural nodules present	Yes	Yes	No
Common diseases	Sarcoidosis, lymphangitic carcinomatosis	Miliary tuberculosis or fungal infection, metastases	Endobronchial infection or tumor, hypersensitivity pneumonitis, respiratory bronchiolitis, edema

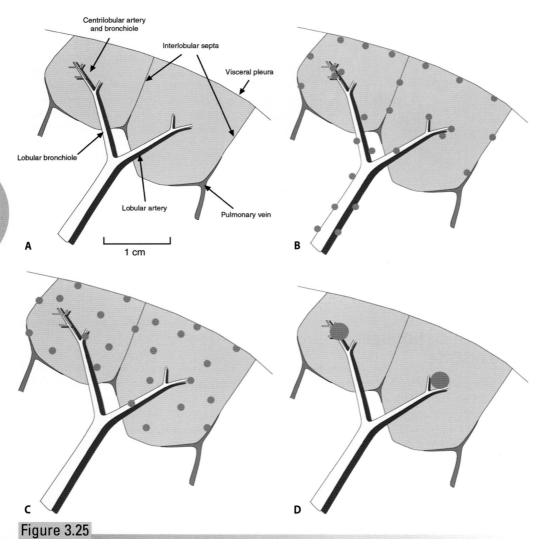

Figure 3.25

Comparison of distributions of nodules at the level of the secondary pulmonary lobule. A. Normal anatomy of the secondary pulmonary lobule. **B.** Perilymphatic nodules involve the subpleural lobule, interlobular septa, and the centrilobular peribronchovascular region. **C.** Random nodules involve the septa and pleural surfaces, but have no specific distribution with respect to the pulmonary lobule. **D.** Centrilobular nodules are found only at the center of the lobule.

interstitium to determine if nodules are present in these locations.

(2) A diffuse distribution is typical of a random pattern, whereas a patchy distribution is typical of perilymphatic nodules. Centrilobular nodules may be diffuse or patchy in distribution depending upon the cause. For instance, HP is often diffuse and endobronchial spread of infection is typically patchy.

(3) When centrilobular nodules are present, close inspection for the presence of TIB pattern should be made. When TIB is present, infection is very likely. When not present, the differential depends upon the attenuation and distribution of nodules.

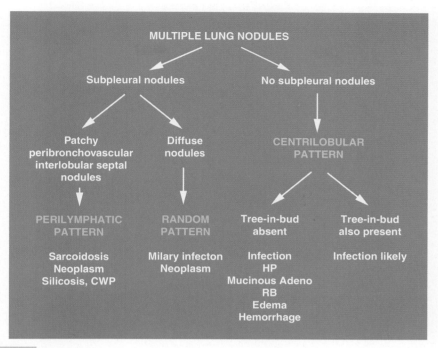

Figure 3.26

Algorithm for determining the distribution of small nodules on HRCT. CWP, coal worker's pneumoconiosis; HP, hypersensitivity pneumonitis; Adeno, adenocarcinoma; RB, respiratory bronchiolitis.

The symptoms present may also be helpful in diagnosis.

FURTHER READING

Aquino SL, Gamsu G, Webb WR, Kee SL. Tree-in-bud pattern: frequency and significance on thin section CT. *J Comput Assist Tomogr.* 1996;20:594-599.

Bendeck SE, Leung AN, Berry GJ, Daniel D, Ruoss SJ. Cellulose granulomatosis presenting as centrilobular nodules: CT and histologic findings. *AJR Am J Roentgenol.* 2001;177:1151-1153.

David M. Hansell, Alexander AB, et al. Fleischner Society: glossary of terms for thoracic imaging. *Radiology.* 2008;246:697-722.

Elicker B, Pereira CA, Webb R, Leslie KO. High-resolution computed tomography patterns of diffuse interstitial lung disease with clinical and pathological correlation. *J Bras Pneumol.* 2008;34:715-744.

Gruden JF, Webb WR, Naidich DP, McGuinness G. Multinodular disease: anatomic localization at thin-section CT-multireader evaluation of a simple algorithm. *Radiology.* 1999;210:711-720.

Gruden JF, Webb WR, Warnock M. Centrilobular opacities in the lung on high-resolution CT: diagnostic considerations and pathologic correlation. *AJR Am J Roentgenol.* 1994;162:569-574.

Lee KS, Kim TS, Han J, et al. Diffuse micronodular lung disease: HRCT and pathologic findings. *J Comput Assist Tomogr.* 1999;23:99-106.

Müller NL, Miller RR. Diseases of the bronchioles: CT and histopathologic findings. *Radiology.* 1995;196:3-12.

Murata K, Itoh H, Todo G, et al. Centrilobular lesions of the lung: demonstration by high-resolution CT and pathologic correlation. *Radiology.* 1986;161:641-645.

Okada F, Ando Y, Yoshitake S, et al. Clinical/pathologic correlations in 553 patients with primary centrilobular findings on high-resolution CT scan of the thorax. *Chest.* 2007;132:1939-1948.

Webb WR. High resolution lung computed tomography: normal anatomic and pathologic findings. *Radiol Clin North Am.* 1991;29:1051-1063.

Webb WR. Thin-section CT of the secondary pulmonary lobule: anatomy and the image—The 2004 Fleischner lecture. *Radiology.* 2006;239:322-338.

Increased Lung Attenuation: Ground Glass Opacity and Consolidation

Abnormalities characterized by increased lung opacity can be divided into two categories based upon their attenuation: ground glass opacity (GGO) and consolidation. Each of these findings tends to be nonspecific and has a long differential diagnosis. Clinical information, particularly the duration of symptoms, can limit the diagnosis when either of these findings is present.

GROUND GLASS OPACITY

On HRCT, GGO is characterized by hazy regions of increased lung opacity or attenuation in which vessels remain visible (Fig. 4.1). GGO represents the presence of abnormalities below the resolution of HRCT. It may reflect the presence of alveolar disease, interstitial disease, or a combination of both, and it may be a manifestation of lung infiltration, active inflammation, or fibrosis (Fig. 4.2). GGO may also result from atelectasis.

The differential diagnosis of GGO is broad and includes a variety of diseases in different disease categories. The duration of symptoms (i.e., acute or chronic) is important in limiting the initial differential diagnosis (Table 4.1). In general, the symptoms should be considered acute when they have been present for less than a few weeks and chronic if they have been present for 6 weeks or more.

GGO with Acute Symptoms

In a patient with acute symptoms, the most common causes of GGO include infection, most notably atypical infections such as viral pneumonia, *Pneumocystis jiroveci*, and atypical bacterial infections (e.g., Legionella, *Mycoplasma pneumoniae*, and *Chlamydia pneumoniae*); pulmonary edema, either hydrostatic or increased permeability edema; diffuse alveolar damage, the histologic abnormality present in patients with acute respiratory distress syndrome; pulmonary hemorrhage; and aspiration (Table 4.1). Additional causes include an acute presentation of hypersensitivity pneumonitis and acute eosinophilic pneumonia.

In the acute setting, the various causes of GGO are difficult to distinguish from one another based on their appearance. The specific distribution of GGO (diffuse, symmetric, patchy, nodular, or focal) is of limited use in narrowing the differential diagnosis (Fig. 4.3). Even processes

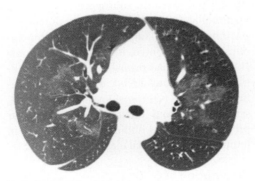

Figure 4.1

Ground glass opacity (GGO). Hazy regions of opacity are noted in the parahilar lung in this patient with acute pulmonary hemorrhage due to Wegener's granulomatosis. Vessels are well seen in the areas of opacity; this finding defines GGO.

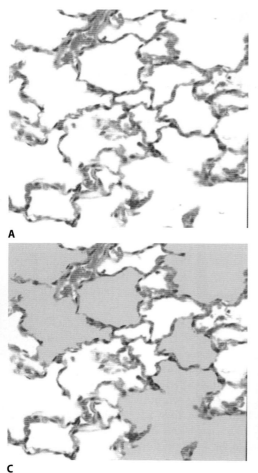

4

A

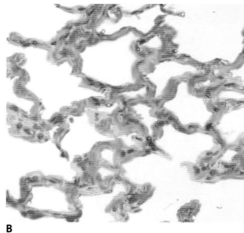

B

C

Figure 4.2

Causes of ground glass opacity (GGO). A. Normal alveoli. **B.** Simulated alveolar wall thickening in interstitial disease. Increased tissue within the volume scanned results in GGO. **C.** Simulated alveolar disease, with some alveoli filled with fluid. This results in increased attenuation, but because some alveoli remain aerated, consolidation does not result.

such as pulmonary edema, which are commonly symmetric or diffuse, can produce patchy, focal, or nodular opacities in some patients (Fig. 4.4), suggesting a specific diagnosis in a patient with acute symptoms and GGO aided by history (e.g., immunosuppression or AIDS, exposures, and known cardiac disease) and the specific presenting symptoms (e.g., fever, sputum production, and hemoptysis).

One HRCT finding that may be helpful in diagnosis is the presence of smooth interlobular septal thickening. When this finding is conspicuous and associated with GGO, pulmonary edema is the most likely diagnosis (Fig. 4.5). The presence of lung cysts associated with GGO suggests *Pneumocystis jiroveci* infection.

GGO with Chronic Symptoms

When GGO is associated with chronic symptoms, the differential diagnosis is different and very broad. Possible causes include hypersensitivity pneumonitis, nonspecific interstitial pneumonia (NSIP), desquamative interstitial pneumonia (DIP) and respiratory bronchiolitis (RB), lymphoid interstitial pneumonia (LIP) and follicular bronchiolitis, invasive pulmonary mucinous adenocarcinoma, organizing pneumonia (OP), eosinophilic pneumonia, sarcoidosis, lipoid pneumonia, and alveolar proteinosis. Several findings may be helpful in limiting the differential diagnosis (Table 4.2).

Distribution of GGO

When the distribution of GGO is strongly peripheral, an interstitial pneumonia is favored, most specifically NSIP or DIP, but eosinophilic pneumonia and OP may also show this appearance (Fig. 4.6). A peripheral distribution of findings with sparing of the immediate subpleural lung is highly suggestive of NSIP (Fig. 4.7).

Table 4.1	Differential diagnosis of GGO based upon symptom duration	
Acute	**Chronic**	
Infection (usually atypical)	Hypersensitivity pneumonitis	
Edema	Nonspecific interstitial pneumonia	
Diffuse alveolar damage	Desquamative interstitial pneumonia/respiratory bronchiolitis	
Hemorrhage	Lymphoid interstitial pneumonia/follicular bronchiolitis	
Aspiration	Invasive mucinous adenocarcinoma	
Hypersensitivity pneumonitis (acute)	Organizing pneumonia	
Acute eosinophilic pneumonia	Eosinophilic pneumonia	
	Sarcoidosis	
	Lipoid pneumonia	
	Alveolar proteinosis	

A patchy and geographic distribution of GGO, with significant involvement of the central lung, is not typical of an interstitial pneumonia (i.e., NSIP, DIP, LIP, and OP), but is occasionally seen with NSIP in patients with

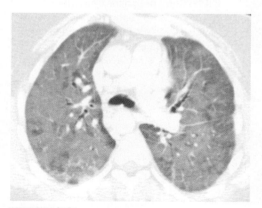

Figure 4.3

Acute drug reaction with pulmonary edema and diffuse ground glass opacity (GGO). The differential diagnosis of GGO is broad. In a patient with acute symptoms, the distribution of GGO is of limited value in helping distinguish among the various possible causes. The diagnosis is often determined by the clinical history, as in this patient with drug toxicity resulting from treatment of lymphoma.

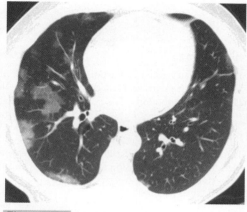

Figure 4.4

Acute pulmonary edema with patchy GGO. The distribution of GGO in the setting of acute symptoms is not particularly helpful in diagnosis. Even processes that are classically diffuse or symmetric, such as pulmonary edema, may occasionally present with focal or patchy abnormalities.

connective tissue disease or LIP. This distribution is more suggestive of other causes of GGO such as hypersensitivity pneumonitis (Fig. 4.8).

Associated Mosaic Perfusion and/or Air Trapping

If GGO is associated with significant mosaic perfusion and/or air trapping (involvement of multiple lobules in three or more lobes), the diagnosis of hypersensitivity pneumonitis is strongly favored (Fig. 4.9A, B). GGO associated

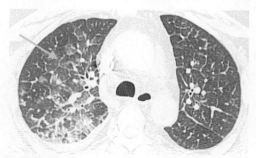

Figure 4.5

Pulmonary edema with a combination of ground glass opacity (GGO) and interlobular septal thickening. GGO in the acute setting is nonspecific, but when interlobular septal thickening (*arrow*) is a significant associated finding, pulmonary edema is the most likely etiology.

Table 4.2 Ground glass opacity with chronic symptoms. Utility of associated findings to suggest a particular diagnosis(es)

HRCT finding	Likely diagnosis(es)
Fibrosis (honeycombing, traction bronchiectasis, irregular reticulation)	Nonspecific interstitial pneumonia, hypersensitivity pneumonitis, usual interstitial pneumonia
Peripheral distribution	Nonspecific interstitial pneumonia, desquamative interstitial pneumonia
Peripheral distribution with sparing of the immediate subpleural interstitium	Nonspecific interstitial pneumonia
Patchy and geographic distribution	Hypersensitivity pneumonitis, nonspecific interstitial pneumonia
Significant mosaic perfusion and/or air trapping	Hypersensitivity pneumonitis
Centrilobular nodules	Hypersensitivity pneumonitis, respiratory bronchiolitis/desquamative interstitial pneumonia, follicular bronchiolitis/lymphoid interstitial pneumonia, invasive mucinous adenocarcinoma
Interlobular septal thickening	Alveolar proteinosis, invasive mucinous adenocarcinoma, lipoid pneumonia

4

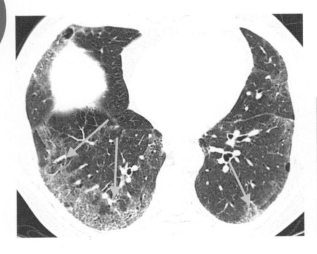

Figure 4.6

Desquamative interstitial pneumonia (DIP) with a peripheral distribution of ground glass opacity (GGO). In the chronic setting, GGO with a peripheral distribution (*arrows*) is suggestive of an interstitial pneumonia or more specifically nonspecific interstitial pneumonia, DIP, or usual interstitial pneumonia. This patient is a smoker with DIP.

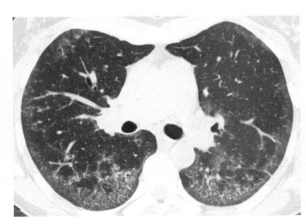

Figure 4.7

Nonspecific interstitial pneumonia (NSIP) with a peripheral distribution of ground glass opacity (GGO) and subpleural sparing. In this patient with NSIP, GGO shows a peripheral predominance, but the immediate subpleural lung is relatively spared. This distribution is typical of NSIP.

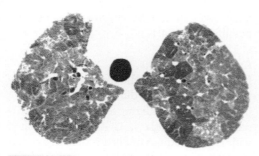

Figure 4.8

Hypersensitivity pneumonitis (HP) with a patchy and geographic distribution of ground glass opacity (GGO). In this patient with HP, the areas of GGO lack a peripheral predominance. This appearance is typical of HP.

with centrilobular nodules may be seen with hypersensitivity pneumonitis (Fig. 4.10), RB, follicular bronchiolitis, and invasive mucinous adenocarcinoma.

Crazy Paving

The combination of GGO and smooth interlobular septal thickening in the same lung regions is termed "crazy paving." This name refers to the appearance of irregularly shaped paving stones in an English garden.

While originally described as a typical HRCT finding in pulmonary alveolar proteinosis (Fig. 4.11), this finding is nonspecific

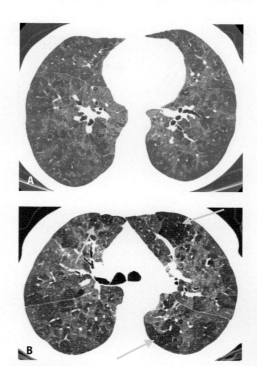

Figure 4.9

Hypersensitivity pneumonitis with patchy ground glass opacity (GGO) and air trapping. HRCT (**A**) shows nonspecific patchy GGO in a patient with chronic symptoms. Expiratory image (**B**) shows patchy air trapping (*arrows*). This combination of findings is strongly suggestive of hypersensitivity pneumonitis.

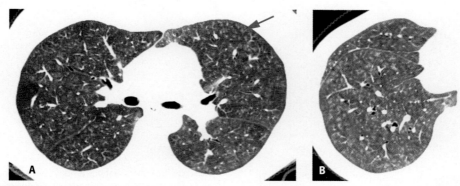

Figure 4.10

Hypersensitivity pneumonitis with ground glass opacity (GGO) and centrilobular nodules. A and **B.** When chronic GGO is associated with centrilobular nodules (**A**, *arrow*), the differential diagnosis includes hypersensitivity pneumonitis, respiratory bronchiolitis, follicular bronchiolitis, or invasive mucinous adenocarcinoma. Numerous centrilobular nodules of GGO are visible in (**B**).

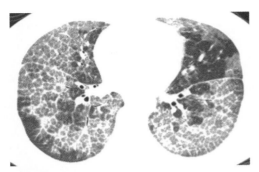

Figure 4.11

Pulmonary alveolar proteinosis with crazy paving. The combination of ground glass opacity (GGO) and smooth interlobular septal thickening in the same lung regions is termed "crazy paving." When associated with chronic symptoms, the differential diagnosis of crazy paving includes causes of chronic GGO, but alveolar proteinosis, which is otherwise rare, becomes an important consideration.

and may be seen in any disease resulting in GGO. In the acute setting, the differential diagnosis is identical to that of isolated GGO and includes edema, atypical infections (Fig. 4.12), diffuse alveolar damage, hemorrhage, acute hypersensitivity pneumonitis, and acute eosinophilic pneumonia. In a patient with chronic symptoms, the list of diagnostic possibilities is the same as for GGO, but alveolar proteinosis, which is otherwise

quite rare, should be considered a distinct possibility (Fig. 4.11).

Associated Fibrosis

In the presence of chronic symptoms, GGO may reflect one of two very different processes, active inflammatory or infiltrative disease, or microscopic lung fibrosis. If GGO is unassociated with HRCT findings of fibrosis such as traction bronchiectasis, irregular reticulation, or honeycombing, then it is likely that inflammatory or infiltrative disease is present (Fig. 4.13). On the other hand, if GGO is associated with signs of fibrosis in the same lung regions, then it is likely that the GGO represents (microscopic) lung fibrosis. In some patients, both inflammatory disease and fibrosis coexist.

Hypersensitivity pneumonitis and NSIP related to connective tissue disease or drug exposures are the most common diffuse fibrotic lung diseases to show GGO on HRCT (Fig. 4.14). Usual interstitial pneumonia and idiopathic pulmonary fibrosis may present with GGO as a significant finding, but in such patients, findings of fibrosis are generally visible in the same lung regions.

CONSOLIDATION

Consolidation is characterized on HRCT by homogeneous increased lung opacity, which

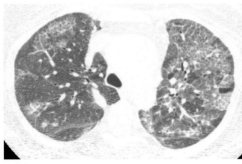

Figure 4.12

***Pneumocystis jiroveci* infection with crazy paving.** The differential diagnosis of crazy paving in the acute setting is identical to that of ground glass opacity and primarily includes edema, atypical infections, diffuse alveolar damage, and hemorrhage.

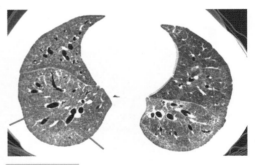

Figure 4.13

Nonspecific interstitial pneumonia with ground glass opacity (GGO) and traction bronchiectasis. When GGO is associated with signs of fibrosis, such as traction bronchiectasis (*arrows*) and reticulation, it is likely related to a chronic interstitial lung disease such as fibrotic nonspecific interstitial pneumonia secondary to scleroderma.

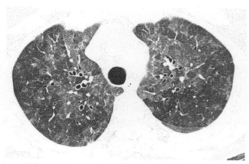

Figure 4.14

Hypersensitivity pneumonitis with ground glass opacity and chronic symptoms. Patchy central and peripheral areas of ground glass opacity are present in a patient with chronic symptoms. The most common causes of ground glass opacity in the chronic setting include hypersensitivity pneumonitis, nonspecific interstitial pneumonia, and desquamative interstitial pneumonia.

Table 4.3	Differential diagnosis of consolidation based upon symptom duration	
Acute	**Chronic**	
Infections	Organizing pneumonia	
Edema	Eosinophilic pneumonia	
Diffuse alveolar damage	Invasive mucinous adenocarcinoma	
Hemorrhage	Sarcoidosis	
Aspiration	Lymphoma (usually recurrent)	
Hypersensitivity pneumonitis	Lipoid pneumonia	
Acute eosinophilic pneumonia	Hypersensitivity pneumonitis	

results in obscuration of vessels (Fig. 4.15). Air bronchograms are often seen in affected regions. As with GGO, the abnormality may be alveolar or interstitial in origin, although filling of alveoli is most commonly responsible. As with GGO, the differential diagnosis is broad and depends primarily upon symptom duration (Table 4.3) and distribution.

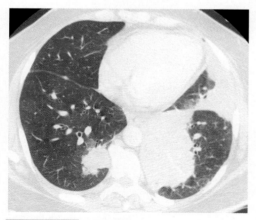

Figure 4.15

Consolidation. Patchy bilateral consolidation is present in a patient with invasive mucinous adenocarcinoma. Note that the vessels are obscured in the regions of abnormality.

Consolidation with Acute Symptoms

The differential diagnosis of consolidation in the acute setting is essentially the same as that of GGO with acute symptoms (Table 4.3), but acute consolidation is most commonly seen with pneumonia and aspiration. Other causes of acute consolidation include pulmonary edema, diffuse alveolar damage, and hemorrhage, but GGO is a more typical finding with these abnormalities.

Occasionally, interstitial lung diseases may present with acute symptoms and consolidation. This is most commonly seen with hypersensitivity pneumonitis and acute eosinophilic pneumonia. GGO is a more common manifestation of these diseases.

Distribution

A diffuse distribution of consolidation is common with edema, diffuse alveolar damage (the histological pattern associated with acute respiratory distress syndrome) (Fig. 4.16), certain infections, hemorrhage, and acute eosinophilic pneumonia. Of the infections, viral pneumonia, atypical bacterial (Legionella, *Mycoplasma pneumoniae*, and *Chlamydia pneumoniae*) pneumonia, and *Pneumocystis jiroveci* pneumonia are the most common to present with diffuse abnormalities, but these more commonly present with GGO. Other types of infections (bacterial, fungal, or mycobacterial) tend to be focal or patchy in distribution (Fig. 4.17). Aspiration may be focal or

4

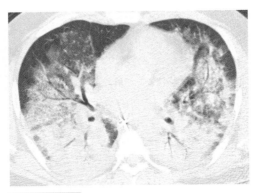

Figure 4.16

Acute respiratory distress syndrome with diffuse consolidation. In the acute setting, diffuse consolidation is nonspecific and may be seen with infection, diffuse alveolar damage (acute respiratory distress syndrome), edema, or hemorrhage. These entities are primarily distinguished clinically.

patchy and typically involves the lower lobes or posterior upper lobes.

Consolidation with Chronic Symptoms

In patients with chronic symptoms, the most frequent causes of consolidation are OP, chronic eosinophilic pneumonia, sarcoidosis, invasive mucinous adenocarcinoma, lymphoma, hypersensitivity pneumonitis, and lipoid pneu-

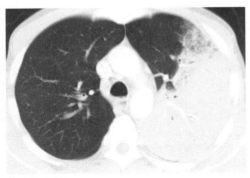

Figure 4.17

Bacterial pneumonia with focal consolidation. A focal distribution of consolidation in the acute setting is typically associated with pneumonia, aspiration, and hemorrhage. While nonspecific with regard to the type of infection, this is most typical of bacterial, mycobacterial, and fungal infections.

monia. The distribution of consolidation, and several other findings, may be helpful in narrowing the differential diagnosis.

Distribution

While distribution may be helpful in narrowing the list of possibilities (Table 4.4), it is unusual for distribution, by itself, to suggest a single diagnosis. All causes of chronic consolidation may present with a patchy, bilateral distribution of consolidation.

Extensive or diffuse chronic consolidation is most typical of invasive mucinous adenocarcinoma or, less likely, OP. A single, focal region of consolidation may be seen with invasive mucinous adenocarcinoma, lymphoma, lipoid pneumonia, or, rarely, OP. Lipoid pneumonia typically presents with patchy abnormalities in dependent regions of both lungs. A peribronchovascular distribution of consolidation may be seen with sarcoidosis, OP, or chronic eosinophilic pneumonia. Peripheral consolidation is typical of chronic eosinophilic pneumonia or OP, particularly in patients with polymyositis/dermatomyositis.

Table 4.4	Causes of chronic consolidation based upon distribution on HRCT
Distribution	**Causes of chronic consolidation**
Patchy	Any cause may show this pattern
Single, focal region	Invasive mucinous adenocarcinoma
	Lymphoma
	Lipoid pneumonia
	Organizing pneumonia
Diffuse consolidation	Invasive mucinous adenocarcinoma
	Organizing pneumonia
Peribronchovascular	Sarcoid
	Organizing pneumonia
	Chronic eosinophilic pneumonia
Peripheral	Chronic eosinophilic pneumonia
	Organizing pneumonia (polymyositis/ dermatomyositis)

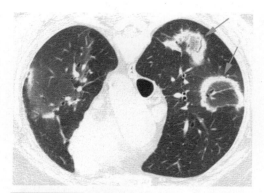

Figure 4.18

Organizing pneumonia with the atoll or reversed halo sign. The atoll or reversed halo sign is characterized by a peripheral rim of consolidation (*arrows*) surrounding a central area of ground glass opacity or clearing. This finding is highly specific for organizing pneumonia, in this case as a complication of chemotherapy.

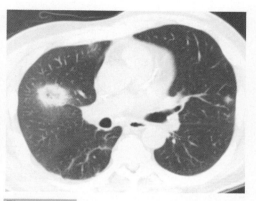

Figure 4.19

Fungal infection with the atoll sign. The atoll sign is specific for organizing pneumonia, but organizing pneumonia may be the result of multiple etiologies. Infection is one cause, most commonly fungal or viral infections.

The "Atoll or Reversed Halo Sign" and OP

The atoll sign is characterized by a ring of consolidation (sometimes incomplete) surrounding a central area of GGO or clearing (Fig. 4.18). It resembles a coral atoll, a circular coral reef with a sandy lagoon in its center. This sign has also been called the "reversed halo sign" because it is the opposite of the well-recognized "halo sign" (a dense nodule with a ring of GGO surrounding it). The atoll sign or reversed halo sign is highly suggestive of OP or its associated diseases (Table 4.5).

OP represents an organizing inflammatory reaction, typically associated with shortness of breath and fever of more than 6 weeks duration (see Chapter 9). It may be idiopathic, in which case it is called cryptogenic organizing pneumonia, or may be associated with one of its many possible causes including drug treatment, connective tissue disease, toxic inhalations, immunodeficiency, and graft versus host disease. Also, there are many diseases that may be associated, pathologically, with a significant component of OP and thus can have an identical appearance on HRCT. These include eosinophilic pneumonia, hypersensitivity pneumonitis, Wegener's granulomatosis, and some infections (most commonly fungal and viral) (Fig. 4.19).

OP classically shows patchy, bilateral focal regions of consolidation in a peripheral or peribronchovascular distribution. The atoll or reversed halo sign is seen in about 20% of patients with OP.

The "Galaxy Sign" and Sarcoidosis

Sarcoidosis may present with consolidation that represents confluent granulomatous lesions; air bronchograms may be visible. The consolidation tends to appear as a focal, patchy area or mass-like. Although this appearance is sometimes called "alveolar sarcoidosis," this term is a misnomer.

In most cases, the diagnosis of sarcoidosis is suggested when discrete, small nodules

Table 4.5	Differential diagnosis of organizing pneumonia
Causes of organizing pneumonia	**Diseases associated with organizing pneumonia**
Cryptogenic organizing pneumonia	Chronic eosinophilic pneumonia
Drugs	Hypersensitivity pneumonitis
Connective tissue disease	Infections (e.g., fungal infection)
Toxic inhalations	Wegener's granulomatosis
Immunodeficiencies	
Graft vs. host disease	

4

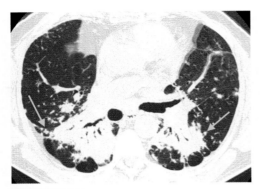

Figure 4.20

"Alveolar sarcoid." Mass-like areas of consolidation with air bronchograms, due to confluent interstitial granulomas, are seen in both upper lobes.
At the periphery of these areas, more discrete small pulmonary nodules are seen (*arrows*).
The consolidation represents confluent interstitial granulomas.

("*satellite nodules*") are seen at the periphery of the areas of consolidation (Fig. 4.20). The combination of focal consolidation or mass with satellite nodules has been termed the "*galaxy sign*." It may also be seen in patients with other granulomatous diseases, infections, silicosis, and coal worker's pneumoconiosis.

Lipoid Pneumonia with Low-Attenuation Consolidation

Lipoid pneumonia is a rare cause of consolidation. This disease results from repeated aspiration of fat-containing liquids. Areas of consolidation are usually located in the posterior lung, are irregular in shape, and often contain areas of low (fat) attenuation, measuring less than −30 Hounsfield units (Fig. 4.21). This appearance is nearly diagnostic of lipoid pneumonia.

DIFFERENTIAL DIAGNOSIS BASED UPON WHETHER GGO OR CONSOLIDATION IS PRESENT

Although many of the diseases discussed in this chapter may show either GGO or consolidation, some more commonly present with GGO while others more commonly present with consolidation (Table 4.6).

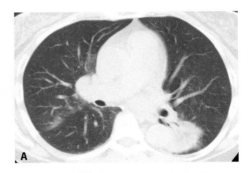

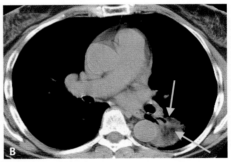

Figure 4.21

Lipoid pneumonia, fat attenuation consolidation. Lung windows **(A)** show nonspecific consolidation in a patient with focal, chronic consolidation. Soft tissue windows **(B)** show areas of fat attenuation (arrows) in consolidation compatible with lipoid pneumonia.

Table 4.6	Differential diagnosis based upon the predominant abnormality seen on HRCT: ground glass opacity or consolidation

Ground glass opacity	Consolidation
Viral, atypical, PCP infection	Bacterial, fungal, mycobacterial infection
Hemorrhage	Aspiration
Edema	Invasive mucinous adenocarcinoma
Hypersensitivity pneumonitis	Organizing pneumonia
Nonspecific interstitial pneumonia	Eosinophilic pneumonia
Desquamative interstitial pneumonia	Sarcoid
Alveolar proteinosis	Lymphoma
Acute eosinophilic pneumonia	

PCP, *Pneumocystis carinii* pneumonia.

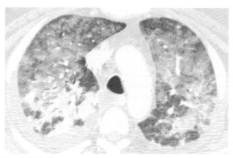

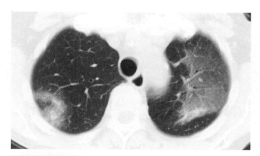

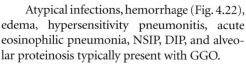

Figure 4.22

Pulmonary hemorrhage; diffuse ground glass opacity (GGO). While both GGO and consolidation are present, GGO is the predominant abnormality in this patient with diffuse pulmonary hemorrhage resulting from mitral stenosis.

Figure 4.24

Organizing pneumonia with patchy ground glass opacity (GGO). Organizing pneumonia usually presents with consolidation; however, it may occasionally present with GGO, particularly in the setting of immunosuppression.

Atypical infections, hemorrhage (Fig. 4.22), edema, hypersensitivity pneumonitis, acute eosinophilic pneumonia, NSIP, DIP, and alveolar proteinosis typically present with GGO.

Bacterial, fungal, or mycobacterial pneumonia, aspiration, OP, eosinophilic pneumonia, invasive mucinous adenocarcinoma, lymphoma (Fig. 4.23), and sarcoidosis most commonly present with consolidation.

Diffuse alveolar damage commonly presents with both GGO and consolidation, with the predominant HRCT abnormality depending upon the severity of the disease.

Nonetheless, it is important to recognize that overlap occurs. For instance, the majority of patients with OP present with consolidation, but occasionally GGO will be the major finding, particularly in patients with immunosuppression (Fig. 4.24). In contrast, hypersensitivity pneumonitis typically presents with GGO, but may be manifest with patchy consolidation, particularly when associated OP is present pathologically (Fig. 4.25).

4

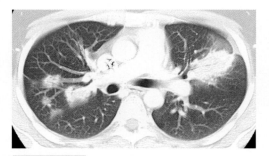

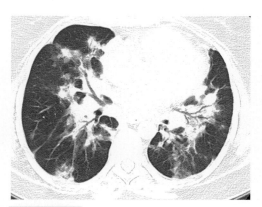

Figure 4.23

Recurrent non-Hodgkin's lymphoma with patchy consolidation. The two malignancies that may present with chronic consolidation include invasive mucinous adenocarcinoma and lymphoma. When lymphoma presents with consolidation, it is most commonly recurring after initial treatment.

Figure 4.25

Hypersensitivity pneumonitis with patchy consolidation. Hypersensitivity pneumonitis usually presents with ground glass opacity. It rarely may present with consolidation, particularly when pathologically there is significant associated organizing pneumonia.

FURTHER READING

Austin JH, Müller NL, Friedman PJ, et al. Glossary of terms for CT of the lungs: recommendations of the Nomenclature Committee of the Fleischner Society. *Radiology.* 1996;200:327-331.

Collins J. CT signs and patterns of lung disease. *Radiol Clin North Am.* 2001;39:1115-1135.

Elicker B, Pereira CA, Webb R, Leslie KO. High-resolution computed tomography patterns of diffuse interstitial lung disease with clinical and pathological correlation. *J Bras Pneumol.* 2008;34:715-744.

Engeler CE, Tashjian JH, Trenkner SW, Walsh JW. Ground-glass opacity of the lung parenchyma: a guide to analysis with high-resolution CT. *AJR Am J Roentgenol.* 1993;160:249-251.

Flaherty KR, Martinez FJ. Nonspecific interstitial pneumonia. *Semin Respir Crit Care Med.* 2006;27:652-658.

Hansell DM, Bankier AA, MacMahon H, et al. Fleischner Society: glossary of terms for thoracic imaging. *Radiology.* 2008;246:697-722.

Lee KS, Kim EA. High-resolution CT of alveolar filling disorders. *Radiol Clin North Am.* 2001;39:1211-1230.

Leung AN, Miller RR, Müller NL. Parenchymal opacification in chronic infiltrative lung diseases: CT-pathologic correlation. *Radiology.* 1993;188:209-214.

Lynch DA, Travis WD, Muller NL, et al. Idiopathic interstitial pneumonias: CT features. *Radiology.* 2005;236:10-21.

Miller WT Jr, Shah RM. Isolated diffuse ground-glass opacity in thoracic CT: causes and clinical presentations. *AJR Am J Roentgenol.* 2005;184:613-622.

Nowers K, Rasband JD, Berges G, Gosselin M. Approach to ground-glass opacification of the lung. *Semin Ultrasound CT MR.* 2002;23:302-323.

Polverosi R, Maffesanti M, Dalpiaz G. Organizing pneumonia: typical and atypical HRCT patterns. *Radiol Med.* 2006;111:202-212.

Remy-Jardin M, Giraud F, Remy J, Copin MC, Gosselin B, Duhamel A. Importance of ground-glass attenuation in chronic diffuse infiltrative lung disease: pathologic-CT correlation. *Radiology.* 1993;189:693-698.

Travis WD, Brambilla E, Noguchi M, et al. International Association for the Study of Lung Cancer/American Thoracic Society/European Respiratory Society International Multidisciplinary Classification of lung adenocarcinoma. *J Thorac Oncol.* 2011;6:244-285.

Travis WD, Hunninghake G, King TE Jr, et al. Idiopathic nonspecific interstitial pneumonia. *Am J Respir Crit Care Med.* 2008;15(177):1338-1347.

Webb WR. High resolution lung computed tomography: normal anatomic and pathologic findings. *Radiol Clin North Am.* 1991;29:1051-1063.

4

Decreased Lung Attenuation: Emphysema, Mosaic Perfusion, and Cystic Lung Disease

Focal or regional areas of decreased lung attenuation (i.e., increased lung lucency) can have a variety of causes and HRCT appearances. These include lung destruction due to emphysema, decreased lung perfusion, cyst formation, and airway dilatation. Airway dilatation, or bronchiectasis, is usually identifiable as such and will be discussed in the next chapter.

EMPHYSEMA

Emphysema reflects lung destruction that may be the end result of several different processes including cigarette smoking, enzyme deficiency, and drug abuse. Emphysema is categorized by the part of the secondary pulmonary lobule that is involved as centrilobular, panlobular, or paraseptal. Each of these has a different HRCT appearance and different possible causes (Table 5.1).

Centrilobular Emphysema

Centrilobular emphysema (CLE) is common and strongly associated with cigarette smoking.

In general, the severity of emphysema correlates with the length of time and amount a patient has smoked. Smoke induces lung destruction by causing chronic inflammation in and around small airways (respiratory bronchiolitis). Because these small airways are centrilobular in location, emphysema associated with smoking is predominantly centrilobular in distribution. As lung destruction becomes more extensive, emphysema may involve the entire pulmonary lobules.

On HRCT, CLE is visible as focal, air-attenuation cystic lucencies, a few millimeters to 1 cm in diameter, usually without a visible wall. These lucencies tend to predominate in the upper lobes and are most severe in the central lung regions. Small areas of CLE may be seen to surround the dot-like centrilobular artery (Fig. 5.1).

This appearance on HRCT is diagnostic of CLE and biopsy is not required for diagnosis if the patient has a smoking history. HRCT is able to detect very early stages of CLE and is often more sensitive than pulmonary function testing.

Table 5.1	Comparison of the different types of emphysema		
	Centrilobular	**Panlobular**	**Paraseptal**
Distribution	Upper lobes, central	Lower lobes, diffuse	Subpleural
HRCT appearance	Focal lucencies without visible walls	Generalized increase in lung lucency	Focal, round, well-defined lucencies with thin walls, in a single layer
Causes	Cigarette smoking	Alpha-1-antitrypsin deficiency, cigarette smoking, intravenous injection of oral Ritalin	Cigarette smoking or idiopathic

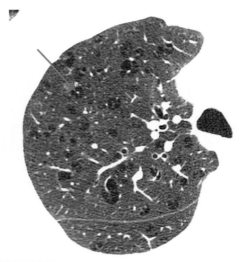

Figure 5.1

Centrilobular emphysema. HRCT in a smoker shows focal, upper lobe, central, air-attenuation lucencies without a recognizable wall. Note the centrilobular artery at the center of some of these lucencies (*arrow*).

Panlobular Emphysema

Panlobular emphysema (PLE) is commonly associated with alpha-1-antitrypsin deficiency, but may also be seen in association with cigarette smoking and intravenous injection of oral Ritalin. PLE involves all portions of the secondary pulmonary lobule equally. For this reason, it is generally unassociated with focal areas of lucency on HRCT, as is CLE. Instead, it shows generalized lung lucency with attenuated (small) vessels. Lung volume is increased. In other words, PLE results in a lung that is too big and too black and contains vessels that are too small. In cases of early PLE, the diagnosis may be difficult because focal abnormalities are not present.

PLE tends to be diffuse or lower lobe predominant or diffuse in distribution (Fig. 5.2A, B).

Paraseptal Emphysema

Paraseptal emphysema (PSE) may be associated with cigarette smoking or may be idiopathic. On HRCT, PSE is characterized by air-attenuation cysts, from a few millimeters to 2 cm or more in diameter, occurring in a single layer in the subpleural lung (Fig. 5.3). It is seen in the peripheral lung, adjacent to the mediastinum, and adjacent to fissures. The cysts of PSE are outlined by a discrete and thin wall. These walls may correspond to interlobular septa. Given its association with smoking, there is often coexistent CLE.

As discussed in Chapter 2, PSE should not be confused with honeycombing, which may have a similar appearance. There are several distinguishing features.

PSE occurs in a single layer, while honeycomb cysts are often in multiple layers. The walls of PSE are thinner than those of honeycombing, and the cystic spaces are usually larger. PSE is unassociated with signs of fibrosis such as traction bronchiectasis and irregular reticulation, which are typically seen with honeycombing. Honeycombing usually predominates at the lung bases, while PSE is most severe in the upper lobes. One caveat: both PSE and honeycombing may be seen in the same patient.

Bullous Emphysema

There is no specific pathologic type of emphysema termed "bullous emphysema," but this term is often used to refer to emphysema that is associated with large bullae. A bulla is defined as a sharply defined area of emphysema measuring more than 1 cm in diameter. Bulla walls are usually well seen on HRCT.

Bullae occur most commonly in patients with PSE or CLE. They are less frequent with PLE. Bullous emphysema is often asymmetrical.

MOSAIC PERFUSION

The term *mosaic perfusion* refers to the presence of geographic regions of varying lung attenuation due to regional differences in lung perfusion.

Approximately 50% of lung attenuation is derived from blood. Consequently, when blood flow is decreased to a specific region of lung, its attenuation appears decreased on HRCT. On HRCT, the attenuation of regions of mosaic (decreased) perfusion is intermediate between that of normal lung and room air.

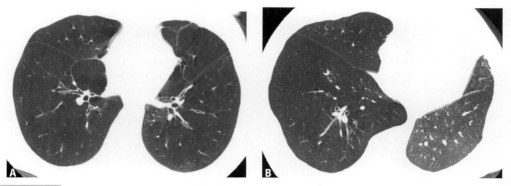

Figure 5.2

Panlobular emphysema. A. HRCT in a patient with alpha-1-antitrypsin deficiency shows basilar predominant, diffuse, increased lung lucency with small vessels. This appearance is typical of panlobular emphysema. **B.** In another patient with a left lung transplant for panlobular emphysema, the abnormal, markedly hyperinflated and lucent native right lung can be contrasted with a normal appearing transplanted left lung.

Mosaic perfusion may result from either airways disease or vascular disease; airways disease is most common as a cause. In cases of vascular disease, such as chronic pulmonary embolism, decreased perfusion is due to stenosis or occlusion of pulmonary arterial branches. In cases of airways disease, stenosis or obstruction of the abnormal airways results in decreased ventilation and hypoxia in the

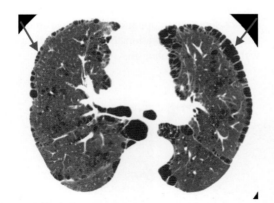

Figure 5.3

Paraseptal emphysema in a patient with a smoking history. Subpleural, air-density cysts (*arrows*) are present in a single layer. Note a thin wall at the periphery of the areas of emphysema. There is associated centrilobular emphysema in the central lung.

downstream lung. This leads to reflex vasoconstriction and decreased lung perfusion.

In patients with mosaic perfusion, the vessels in areas of lung lucency usually appear smaller on HRCT than those in normal lung regions. This finding is key in making the diagnosis of mosaic perfusion as a cause of patchy lung attenuation.

Mosaic Perfusion versus Ground Glass Opacity

When the lung shows patchy or geographic lung attenuation on HRCT (i.e., the lung has a "mosaic" appearance), one must first determine if the relatively opaque or the relatively lucent lung regions are abnormal. If the opaque lung is abnormal, the abnormality represents ground glass opacity. If the lucent lung is abnormal, the pattern represents mosaic perfusion. There are several features that help in making this distinction.

Geographic Areas of Decreased Lung Attenuation

With mosaic perfusion, regions of heterogeneous attenuation tend to be geographic and sharply demarcated (Fig. 5.4). Usually there is a sharp border between lung that is affected (relatively lucent) and unaffected (relatively opaque), reflecting normal geographic vascular supply. Ground glass opacity, on the other

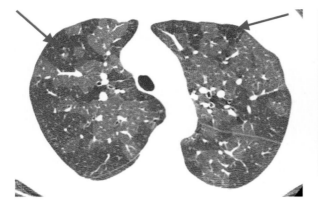

Figure 5.4

Mosaic perfusion. Heterogeneous lung density with geographic areas of decreased lung attenuation (*arrows*) is present in a patient with constrictive bronchiolitis due to neuroendocrine hyperplasia. This sharp demarcation between opaque and lucent lung suggests that the lucent lung is abnormal. Vessels in lucent regions appear small in comparison to vessels in the denser regions.

hand, usually has ill-defined borders because the responsible process results in variable involvement of the interstitium or alveoli (Fig. 5.5).

On occasion, however, ground glass opacity presents with geographic abnormalities. For instance, viral infections or alveolar proteinosis may present with geographic regions of ground glass opacity (Fig. 5.6). In these cases, there is usually a greater attenuation difference between opaque and lucent lung, whereas the difference is usually not as pronounced with mosaic perfusion.

Decreased Vessel Size in Lucent Lung Regions

As mosaic perfusion represents regional decreases in lung perfusion, the vessels in affected regions usually appear smaller than in areas of normal lung (Fig. 5.7). This finding is

more commonly seen with vascular causes of mosaic perfusion and is accentuated in severe cases. The absence of a difference in vessel size does not exclude mosaic perfusion as a cause of geographic attenuation.

Air Trapping on Expiratory Imaging

When mosaic perfusion is due to airways disease, lucent lung regions usually show air trapping on expiratory imaging (Fig. 5.8A, B). During expiration, normal lung shows an increase in attenuation of 100 to 200 HU. When airways disease is present, air trapping causes affected regions to show little or no increase in attenuation on expiratory images. Vascular causes of mosaic perfusion generally do not show air trapping on mosaic perfusion, although this may occasionally be seen in patients with pulmonary embolism.

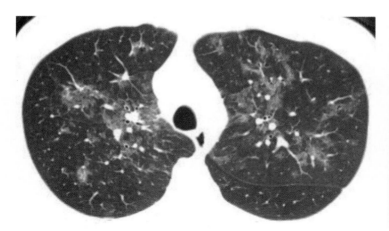

Figure 5.5

"Mosaic" ground glass opacity. Patchy perihilar areas of increased lung attenuation are present in a patient with pneumocystis pneumonia. The edges of the regions of ground glass opacity are ill-defined, rather than sharply demarcated. The vessels in regions of varying lung attenuation appear similar in size.

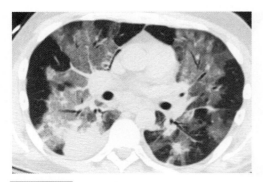

Figure 5.6

Geographic ground glass opacity in viral infection. While geographic areas of heterogeneous lung attenuation are usually due to mosaic perfusion, occasionally, ground glass opacity may have sharply demarcated borders. The marked difference in attenuation between affected and unaffected lung in this case would be unusual for mosaic perfusion, and frank consolidation is also visible.

Stability of Mosaic Attenuation Over Time

Ground glass opacity usually changes in distribution or severity over time, unless it is due to fibrosis. Mosaic perfusion, on the other hand, may be stable when followed on multiple HRCT examinations. When HRCT shows heterogeneous lung attenuation that has been stable on serial examinations, mosaic perfusion is the most likely etiology (Fig. 5.9A, B).

Differential Diagnosis

The differential diagnosis of mosaic perfusion is broad and includes many causes of airways or pulmonary vascular disease (Table 5.2). There may be other findings present such as nodules, tree-in-bud, bronchiectasis, airway wall thickening, air trapping, or pulmonary hypertension that suggest a specific diagnosis (Fig. 5.10A, B).

When mosaic perfusion is the predominant abnormality, and little else is visible on HRCT, the differential diagnosis includes asthma, hypersensitivity pneumonitis, constrictive bronchiolitis, chronic pulmonary embolism, and vasculitis.

Differentiating Airways versus Vascular Causes of Mosaic Perfusion

In most cases, a distinction can be made between mosaic perfusion resulting from airways disease and vascular disease. The presence of large airway abnormalities (bronchiectasis or bronchial wall thickening) suggests airways disease as the cause; the presence of pulmonary artery dilatation is more typical of vascular disease.

As discussed previously, vascular disease does not generally result in air trapping on expiratory imaging (Fig. 5.11A, B). The presence of at least one lucent region that is lobular (i.e., it can be recognized as corresponding to a secondary pulmonary lobule) suggests that airways disease is the cause.

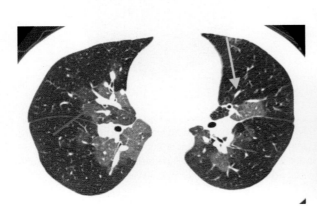

Figure 5.7

Mosaic perfusion due to chronic pulmonary embolism. Note the geographic appearance of the areas of increased lung lucency. The vessels are significantly smaller in the abnormally lucent lung (*yellow arrow*) as compared with the normal opaque lung (*red arrow*).

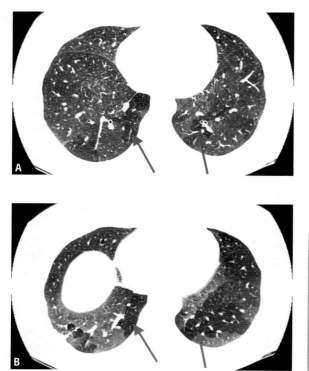

Figure 5.8

Mosaic perfusion in hypersensitivity pneumonitis. A. Geographic areas of decreased lung attenuation are present on the inspiratory images. **B.** On expiratory images, the normal (i.e., denser) lung shows the normal expected increase in attenuation, whereas the areas of mosaic perfusion (*arrows*) remain lucent.

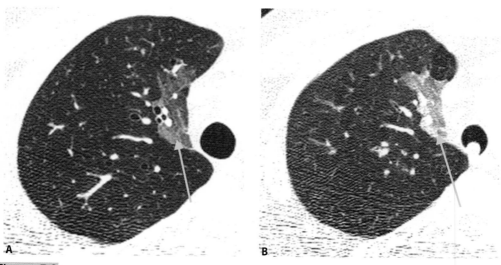

Figure 5.9

Mosaic perfusion, stability over time. HRCT in this patient showed heterogenous lung density, thought to represent ground glass opacity. On a 6-month follow-up CT (**A**), the heterogeneous regions of lung attenuation appeared identical. Expiratory images confirm air trapping in the lucent lung and a normal increase in density (*yellow arrow*) of the opaque lung (**B**) in this patient with constrictive bronchiolitis due to pulmonary graft versus host disease.

Table 5.2	Differential diagnosis of mosaic perfusion when it is an isolated or predominant abnormality

Asthma
Hypersensitivity pneumonitis
Constrictive bronchiolitis (bronchiolitis obliterans)
Chronic pulmonary embolism
Vasculitis

Occlusion of lobular bronchioles is common in patients with airways disease. Vascular disease, in contradistinction, typically demonstrates larger, often peripheral areas of decreased attenuation without a lobular appearance (Fig. 5.12A, B).

THE HEADCHEESE SIGN

The combination of ground glass opacity and mosaic perfusion in the same patient has been termed the *headcheese sign*, given its resemblance to a deli meat of the same name. Headcheese is a sausage made from the chopped and boiled parts of the head of an animal, usually a hog. It appears as a mosaic of different-appearing meats, of different colors and textures.

The combination of ground glass opacity and mosaic perfusion in the same patient, both in significant amounts, constitutes the headcheese sign. Three attenuations (or more) may also be present, representing a combination of normal lung, opaque lung (ground glass opacity), and lucent lung (mosaic perfusion) (Fig. 5.13). Geographic regions of differing lung attenuation, which resemble headcheese but in black and white, are typical on HRCT. The attenuation differences are accentuated on expiratory scans in which both the normal and opaque lung will become denser, but the areas of mosaic perfusion will stay lucent (Fig. 5.14A, B).

The headcheese sign is seen in patients with mixed obstructive and infiltrative disorders. The obstructive abnormality is manifested by mosaic perfusion associated with small airways disease. The infiltrative disorder results in ground glass opacity.

There are a limited number of disorders that have both a significant obstructive and infiltrative component (Table 5.3). These include hypersensitivity pneumonitis, respiratory bronchiolitis and desquamative interstitial pneumonia, follicular bronchiolitis and lymphoid interstitial pneumonia (LIP), sarcoidosis, and atypical infections. Also, it is possible for patients with the

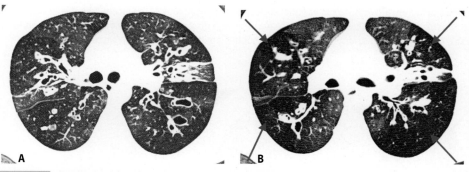

Figure 5.10

Mosaic perfusion in cystic fibrosis. A. HRCT shows heterogeneous lung attenuation on inspiration. Airway abnormalities are obvious. **B.** Expiratory HRCT shows patchy air trapping (*arrows*). There is extensive bronchiectasis and airway wall thickening present. In this case, mosaic perfusion should be ignored in terms of differential diagnosis and the emphasis should be placed on the large airway abnormalities.

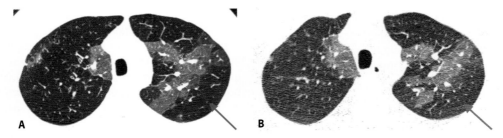

Figure 5.11

Mosaic perfusion without air trapping in chronic pulmonary embolism. Air trapping in a patient with mosaic perfusion indicates the presence of airways disease. In patients with mosaic perfusion resulting from vascular disease, air trapping is not usually present, as in this patient with chronic pulmonary embolism. There is an increase in attenuation of the more lucent lung when comparing inspiratory (**A**, *arrow*) and expiratory (**B**, *arrow*) images.

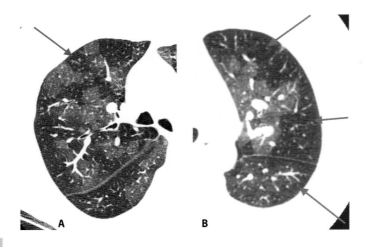

Figure 5.12

Mosaic perfusion: airways versus vascular disease. The morphology of the lucent lung in mosaic perfusion may differ between airways and vascular disease. In airways disease (**A**), the lucent lung often appears lobular (*arrow*) compared with the larger, peripheral, non-lobular appearance (*arrows*) in vascular disease (**B**).

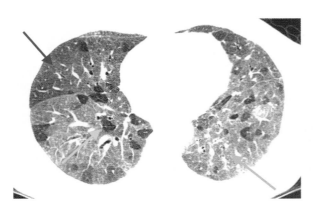

Figure 5.13

The "headcheese" sign in hypersensitivity pneumonitis. Three densities of lung are present: ground glass opacity (*blue arrow*), mosaic perfusion (*yellow arrow*), and normal lung (*red arrow*). This pattern is very suggestive of hypersensitivity pneumonitis.

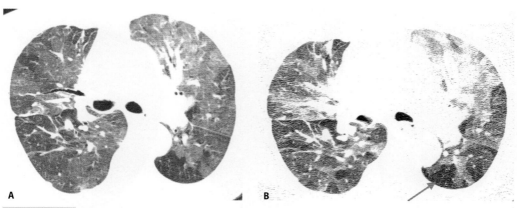

Figure 5.14

The "headcheese" sign. Inspiratory **(A)** and expiratory **(B)** HRCT in a patient with the "headcheese" sign resulting from hypersensitivity pneumonitis. During expiration **(B)**, the areas of decreased attenuation do not change in attenuation and remain lucent. Both the normal lung and ground glass opacity increase in density.

headcheese sign to have two entirely separate diseases such as pulmonary edema and asthma.

The importance of this sign is that the majority of patients who show it have hypersensitivity pneumonitis (Fig. 5.15). The other diseases in the differential diagnosis only rarely present with this pattern, and when they do, either the ground glass or mosaic perfusion is usually limited in its severity or distribution.

CYSTIC LUNG DISEASE

Lung cysts are defined, somewhat arbitrarily, as round, air-density structures, greater than 1 cm in size, and with a thin but recognizable wall.

Table 5.3	Differential diagnosis of the "headcheese" sign

Hypersensitivity (most common)
Respiratory bronchiolitis/desquamative interstitial
  pneumonia
Follicular bronchiolitis/lymphoid interstitial
  pneumonia
Atypical infections (e.g., viral)
Sarcoid
Two separate processes (e.g., edema and asthma)

On HRCT, a few lung cysts may be seen in occasional patients who are otherwise normal, but the presence of more than a few cysts suggests a primary cystic lung disease. Cystic lung diseases are rare and should not be confused with other causes of cysts such as emphysema (i.e., bullae are cysts), honeycombing (fibrosis with cystic regions of lung destruction), and bronchiectasis (Fig. 5.16A–D).

Cystic lung disease typically presents in one of several ways. Spontaneous

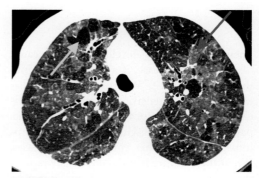

Figure 5.15

Headcheese sign in hypersensitivity pneumonitis. The combination of ground glass opacity (*red arrow*) and mosaic perfusion/air trapping (*yellow arrow*) is highly suggestive of hypersensitivity pneumonitis. There are other causes of the "headcheese" sign, but they are much less common.

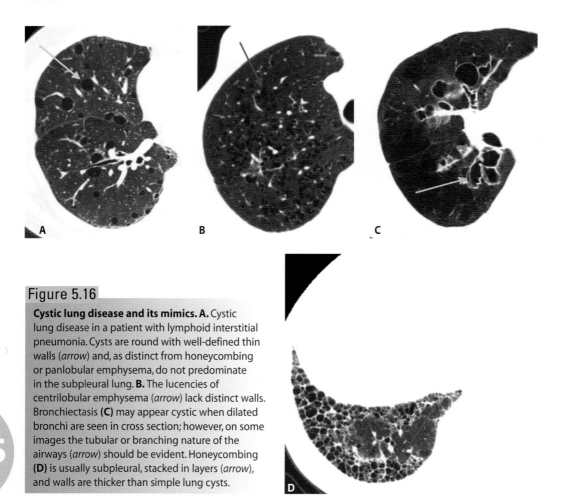

Figure 5.16

Cystic lung disease and its mimics. A. Cystic lung disease in a patient with lymphoid interstitial pneumonia. Cysts are round with well-defined thin walls (*arrow*) and, as distinct from honeycombing or panlobular emphysema, do not predominate in the subpleural lung. **B.** The lucencies of centrilobular emphysema (*arrow*) lack distinct walls. Bronchiectasis **(C)** may appear cystic when dilated bronchi are seen in cross section; however, on some images the tubular or branching nature of the airways (*arrow*) should be evident. Honeycombing **(D)** is usually subpleural, stacked in layers (*arrow*), and walls are thicker than simple lung cysts.

pneumothorax may develop with any cause of cystic lung disease, if a cyst ruptures into the pleural space. When cystic lung disease becomes extensive and replaces significant portions of normal lung parenchyma, patients may present with dyspnea and symptoms similar to other chronic lung diseases. When the cysts are diffuse and nearly replace the entire normal lung parenchyma, it may be difficult to distinguish them from extensive emphysema (Fig. 5.17A, B).

Cysts have visible walls, whereas CLE generally does not, although compressed lung or interlobular septa at the edges of areas of emphysema may resemble cyst walls. Pulmonary hypertension is not an uncommon sequela of extensive cystic lung disease.

Differential Diagnosis

The differential diagnosis of cystic lung disease includes Langerhans cell histiocytosis, lymphangioleiomyomatosis (LAM), LIP, pneumatoceles from prior infection such as pneumocystis pneumonia, treated cystic metastases, benign metastasizing leiomyoma, neurofibromatosis, barotrauma in scuba divers, pulmonary papillomatosis, and Birt-Hogg-Dubé disease (Table 5.4). These diseases are discussed in detail in other chapters. Langerhans cell histiocytosis and LAM produce the most extensive abnormalities and

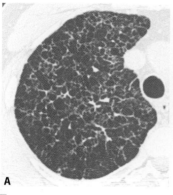
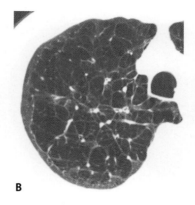

A   B

Figure 5.17

Cystic lung disease versus emphysema. When cystic lung disease is extensive, it may be difficult to distinguish from centrilobular emphysema. The presence of clearly defined walls suggests cystic lung disease. **A.** Cysts in a patient with Langerhans cell histiocytosis demonstrate discrete walls. Centrilobular emphysema (**B**) demonstrates lucencies without well-defined walls, although some areas of emphysema show thin walls, which likely represent interlobular septa.

Table 5.4	Differential diagnosis of primary cystic lung disease

Langerhans cell histiocytosis
Lymphangioleiomyomatosis
Lymphoid interstitial pneumonia
Pneumatoceles from prior infection
Treated cystic metastases
Benign metastasizing leiomyoma
Papillomatosis
Neurofibromatosis
Birt-Hogg-Dubé disease

5

in some cases the lungs may be nearly entirely replaced by cysts.

Langerhans cell histiocytosis is seen predominantly in cigarette smokers and HRCT may demonstrate nodules in association with

cysts. Cysts are irregular in shape, predominate in the upper lobes, and may be thick or thin walled. Associated nodules may be solid or cavitary (Figs. 5.17A and 5.18).

LAM is seen in women of childbearing age and is not commonly associated with nodules. Cysts are round in shape, thin walled, and as numerous in the lung bases as in the upper lobes. LAM is also seen in patients with tuberous sclerosis, usually women (Fig. 5.19A, B). Pleural effusions are common in LAM, but rare with LCH. Angiomyolipoma of the kidney may be associated.

Patients with LIP and the other causes of cystic lung disease usually have fewer cysts present. LIP is usually associated with a history of connective tissue disease or immunosuppression. Sjögren's disease, in particular, may present with cysts as the only

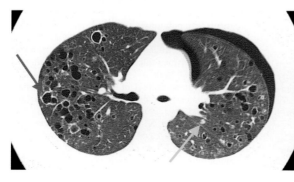

Figure 5.18

Langerhans cell histiocytosis. Irregularly shaped cysts are present, some of which have thin walls and others have thicker walls (*red arrow*). Nodules are also seen (*yellow arrow*). This patient presented with a pneumothorax.

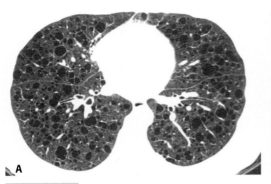
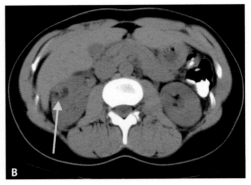

Figure 5.19

Lymphangioleiomyomatosis. A. In a patient with tuberous sclerosis, HRCT shows diffuse, round, well-defined cysts without associated nodules. **B.** An angiomyolipoma (*arrow*) is present in the right kidney.

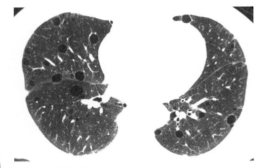

Figure 5.20

Lymphoid interstitial pneumonia. The cysts of lymphoid interstitial pneumonia are not nearly as numerous as those in Langerhans cell histiocytosis or lymphangioleiomyomatosis. Of the connective tissue diseases, lymphoid interstitial pneumonia is most commonly seen in association with Sjögren's disease.

manifestation of LIP (Fig. 5.20). Cysts are often associated with, or adjacent to, vessels.

FURTHER READING

Arakawa H, Webb WR. Air trapping on expiratory high-resolution CT scans in the absence of inspiratory scan abnormalities: correlation with pulmonary function tests and differential diagnosis. *AJR Am J Roentgenol.* 1998;170:1349-1353.

Arakawa H, Webb WR, McCowin M, Katsou G, Lee KN, Seitz RF. Inhomogeneous lung attenuation at thin-section CT: diagnostic value of expiratory scans. *Radiology.* 1998;206:89-94.

Austin JH, Müller NL, Friedman PJ, et al. Glossary of terms for CT of the lungs: recommendations of the Nomenclature Committee of the Fleischner Society. *Radiology.* 1996;200:327-331.

Foster WL Jr, Gimenez EI, Roubidoux MA, et al. The emphysemas: radiologic-pathologic correlations. *Radiographics.* 1993;13:311-328.

Hansell DM, Bankier AA, MacMahon H, et al. Fleischner Society: glossary of terms for thoracic imaging. *Radiology.* 2008;246:697-722.

Im JG, Kim SH, Chung MJ, Koo JM, Han MC. Lobular low attenuation of the lung parenchyma on CT: evaluation of forty-eight patients. *J Comput Assist Tomogr.* 1996;20:756-762.

Lynch DA. Imaging of small airways disease and chronic obstructive pulmonary disease. *Clin Chest Med.* 2008;29:165-179.

Müller NL, Miller RR. Diseases of the bronchioles: CT and histopathologic findings. *Radiology.* 1995;196:3-12.

Padley SPG, Adler BD, Hansell DM, Müller NL. Bronchiolitis obliterans: high-resolution CT findings and correlation with pulmonary function tests. *Clin Radiol.* 1993;47:236-240.

Park CS, Müller NL, Worthy SA, et al. Airway obstruction in asthmatic and healthy individuals: inspiratory and expiratory thin-section CT findings. *Radiology.* 1997;203:361-367.

Sherrick AD, Swensen SJ, Hartman TE. Mosaic pattern of lung attenuation on CT scans: frequency among patients with pulmonary artery hypertension of different causes. *AJR Am J Roentgenol.* 1997;169:79-82.

Thurlbeck WM, Müller NL. Emphysema: definition, imaging, and quantification. *AJR Am J Roentgenol.* 1994;163:1017-1025.

Webb WR. Thin-section CT of the secondary pulmonary lobule: anatomy and the image—The 2004 Fleischner lecture. *Radiology.* 2006;239:322-338.

Worthy SA, Müller NL, Hartman TE, Swensen SJ, Padley SP, Hansell DM. Mosaic attenuation pattern on thin-section CT scans of the lung: differentiation among infiltrative lung, airway, and vascular diseases as a cause. *Radiology.* 1997;205:465-470.

SPECIFIC DISEASES

6

Airways Diseases

Airways disease may have a variety of causes, including inhalation of organic or inorganic materials, systemic diseases, infections, tumors, and congenital defects. Airways diseases are broadly categorized by the size of airways involved as large airways disease or small airways disease.

Bronchi are large airways and contain cartilage in their walls. Small airways, or bronchioles, are less than about 3 mm in diameter and lack cartilage in their walls. While large and small airways abnormalities often occur in combination, most diseases show predominant involvement of either one or the other. This chapter focuses on the HRCT findings of airways diseases, typical patterns of airways disease, and a discussion of common airways diseases.

LARGE AIRWAYS DISEASES

HRCT Findings

HRCT findings indicative of large airways disease include airway dilatation, airway inflammation or infiltration with wall thickening, and mucoid impaction of the airway lumen.

Airway Dilatation

Irreversible dilatation of the bronchi is termed *bronchiectasis*. Bronchiectasis is usually defined by an increased *bronchoarterial ratio* (BA, described below) or specific contour abnormalities that indicate the presence of bronchial dilatation. Bronchiectasis has a variety of causes (Table 6.1), including infections, chronic

inflammatory disease, bronchial obstruction, and morphologic bronchial abnormalities.

A transient increase in bronchial diameter may be seen in patients who have atelectasis or inflammatory lung disease; this is sometimes referred to using the oxymoronic term "reversible bronchiectasis."

BA Ratio and the "Signet Ring Sign"

The ratio of the diameter of the internal bronchial lumen to the diameter of the adjacent pulmonary artery branch is termed the BA ratio. A normal BA ratio is approximately 0.7.

A BA ratio greater than 1.0 is usually considered abnormal (Fig. 6.1), but this may sometimes be seen as a normal finding in elderly

Table 6.1	Differential diagnosis of bronchiectasis
Infection (viral, bacterial, mycobacterial, fungal)	
Asthma	
Aspiration	
Constrictive bronchiolitis	
Collagen vascular disease	
Allergic bronchopulmonary aspergillosis	
Cystic fibrosis	
Immunodeficiency	
Primary ciliary dyskinesia	
Marfan syndrome	
Inflammatory bowel disease	
Alpha-1-antitrypsin	
Yellow nail lymphedema syndrome	
Young syndrome	
Tracheobronchomegaly	
Williams-Campbell syndrome	

6

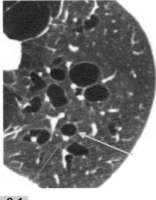

Figure 6.1

Bronchiectasis with a bronchoarterial ratio >1.5. The diameter of the lumen of the bronchus (*yellow arrow*) is significantly greater than the adjacent artery (*red arrow*) in a patient with a disorder of bronchial cartilage. While a bronchoarterial ratio of 1–1.5 is occasionally seen in normal patients, a ratio >1.5 is almost always abnormal.

patients and patients living at high altitudes (e.g., Denver, the mile-high city).

A BA ratio greater than 1.5 is usually specific for airway dilatation. In patients with a BA ratio between 1.0 and 1.5, the presence of airway wall thickening or impaction, or mosaic perfusion and air trapping, makes it likely that airways disease is present. The term *signet ring sign* refers to the presence of airway

dilatation with an increased BA ratio. The ring represents a dilated airway, whereas the signet or stone represents the smaller adjacent artery.

One caveat: the BA ratio may be elevated in patients with normal bronchi and abnormally small arteries. This may be seen in processes such as alpha-1-antitrypsin deficiency or chronic pulmonary embolism.

Contour Abnormalities in the Diagnosis of Bronchiectasis

Bronchiectasis is classified into three categories depending upon the severity and morphology of airway dilatation. These specific contour abnormalities may be used to diagnose the presence of bronchiectasis.

1. *Cylindrical bronchiectasis* (Fig. 6.2A, B) is the least severe form of bronchiectasis. It is characterized by relatively mild dilatation of the bronchi. The contour of the dilated bronchi is smooth and cylindrical. Bronchi have parallel wall and do not taper as they extend into the lung periphery. This type of bronchiectasis is nonspecific and may be seen with most causes of airways disease. In some patients, cylindrical bronchiectasis may resolve; in other words, this is often the appearance of "reversible bronchiectasis."
2. *Varicose bronchiectasis* (Fig. 6.3) is due to more severe, long-standing, or recurrent

6

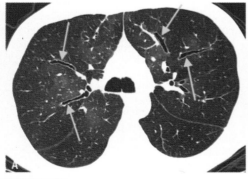 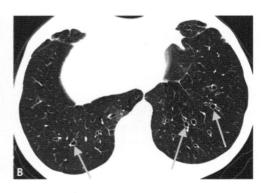

Figure 6.2

Cylindrical bronchiectasis. Mild bronchial dilatation is present without evidence of strictures or saccular dilatations. When the bronchi lie within the axial plane **(A)** they appear tubular, with parallel walls (*arrows*). When they are oriented perpendicular to the axial plane **(B)** they appear circular (*arrows*), and the signet ring sign is characteristically present.

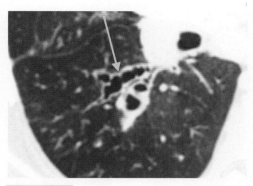

Figure 6.3
Varicose bronchiectasis. Bronchial dilatation with an irregular contour and wall thickening (*arrow*) are present. This appearance, while nonspecific, reflects a more severe and long-standing process.

airway injury. The contour of the bronchial walls appears irregular with focal areas of dilatation intermixed with regions of narrowing. This form of bronchiectasis may be seen with most causes of bronchiectasis, including chronic infection, inflammation, and lung fibrosis. It may be referred to as having a "string of pearls" appearance.

3. *Cystic bronchiectasis* (Fig. 6.4) is the most severe form of airway dilatation and is seen

only with long-standing, severe causes of airways inflammation. Morphologically, it is characterized by relatively large saccular dilatations of the airways that often contain air/fluid levels. It may be focal or diffuse. The differential diagnosis of cystic bronchiectasis is more focused, given that only a limited number of diseases cause severe, chronic inflammation in the large airways. It is sometimes described as having a "cluster of grapes" appearance.

Airway Inflammation with Wall Thickening
Airway wall thickening is commonly seen in patients with bronchiectasis. Wall thickening without bronchial dilatation can be seen in patients with acute or chronic bronchitis due to infection and in inflammatory airways diseases (Fig. 6.5).

In a normal subject, the bronchial wall appears thin, with a ratio of the thickness of the bronchial wall to the diameter of the bronchus of around 0.1 to 0.2. When this ratio is increased, bronchial wall thickening is usually present. However, keep in mind that this measurement may be normal in patients with bronchial wall thickening associated with bronchial dilatation (i.e., bronchiectasis).

Often the diagnosis of bronchial wall thickening is subjective and based on experience or on a comparison of bronchi in one

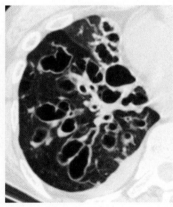

Figure 6.4
Cystic bronchiectasis. The bronchi are markedly enlarged with multiple saccular dilatations and air/fluid levels. This appearance reflects severe, chronic airways inflammation and is seen with a limited number of diseases.

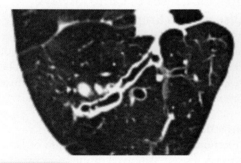

Figure 6.5
Bronchial wall thickening in varicose bronchiectasis. The bronchial wall in this patient with atypical mycobacterial infection is >5 mm in maximum thickness. In some regions, the ratio of the thickened wall to the air-filled lumen is greater than 1:1.

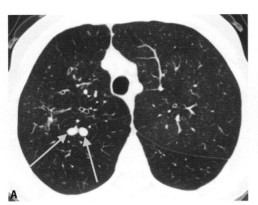
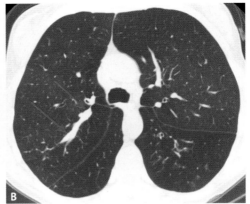

Figure 6.6

Airway impaction. When an airway is completely impacted with mucus, its appearance varies depending upon its orientation. **A.** Airways perpendicular to the axial plane will appear circular (*arrows*). **B.** Airways parallel to the axial plane will appear tubular (*arrows*).

lung region to those in another. Airways disease is often patchy in distribution, which allows this comparison to be made.

Airway Lumen Impaction

Airway impaction is characterized by filling of the airway lumen by secretions, infectious debris, or other substances. Depending upon the orientation of the airways with respect to the image, airway impaction will appear as circular or tubular structures (Fig. 6.6A, B) that connect to more central bronchi.

Specific Causes of Large Airways Disease and Bronchiectasis

There is a broad differential diagnosis for large airways diseases (Table 6.1). The discussion of causes of specific large airways diseases will be restricted to those that tend to produce diffuse or extensive bilateral abnormalities.

Infectious Diseases

Infection is the most common cause of large airways disease. Any type of infection may be associated with airway dilatation and inflammation, although bacterial and mycobacterial infections are most common. Childhood infections are a common cause of bronchiectasis.

Airway abnormalities seen in bacterial, mycobacterial, and fungal infections are usually associated with patchy lung consolidation,

centrilobular nodules, or tree-in-bud (TIB) opacities. Viral infections may present with findings of large airways abnormalities as an isolated abnormality (Fig. 6.7) or in association with lung parenchymal findings. Bronchiectasis associated with ongoing or remote infection is often lobar, multilobar, or patchy.

In most cases, the findings of large airways disease associated with acute infection are mild and reversible. The presence of more

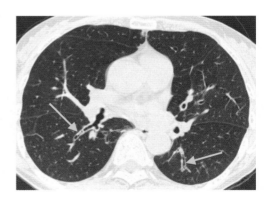

Figure 6.7

Viral infection with bronchial dilatation and wall thickening (arrows). Among acute infections, viral organisms are most likely to produce isolated abnormalities of the large airways such as in this patient with dilated and thickened airways (*arrows*).

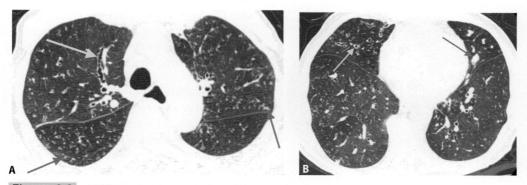

Figure 6.8

Atypical mycobacterial infection. A. Varicose bronchiectasis (*yellow arrow*) is associated with small clusters of centrilobular nodules or tree-in-bud (*red arrows*). **B.** Bronchiectasis (*yellow arrow*) and bronchial impaction (*red arrow*) are typically most severe in the right middle lobe and lingua.

extensive or severe abnormalities, such as varicose bronchiectasis, should suggest a remote (i.e., childhood) infection or a different etiology.

Severe or chronic airway infection may be seen with tuberculosis or nontuberculous mycobacterial infection (Fig. 6.8A, B), chronic aspiration, or acquired or congenital abnormalities that impair immunity or ciliary clearance (discussed below). Constrictive bronchiolitis (CB) may also predispose patients to chronic airway infection and mucostasis.

Allergic Bronchopulmonary Aspergillosis

Allergic bronchopulmonary aspergillosis (ABPA) is a disorder seen predominantly in asthmatics or patients with cystic fibrosis (CF). It is a hypersensitivity reaction to Aspergillus that colonizes the lumen of the airways, without invasion into the lung parenchyma. The diagnosis of ABPA is predominantly clinical, but typical HRCT findings may also be diagnostic.

The most characteristic HRCT finding in patients with ABPA is unilateral or asymmetric, central (parahilar), cylindrical or varicose bronchiectasis, associated with mucoid impaction (Fig. 6.9). The mid- or upper lungs are typically involved. High-attenuation (100 HU) mucous plugs are particularly suggestive of this diagnosis. The finding, seen in about 25% of patients with ABPA, reflects concentration of calcium salts and metallic ions by the fungus.

While large airways abnormalities usually predominate, small airways may also be affected in ABPA. Small airway abnormalities appear as bronchiolectasis, centrilobular nodules, and TIB opacities.

Cystic Fibrosis

CF is a congenital disorder that results in impaired clearance of bronchial secretions. This predisposes patients to chronic mucostasis and airway infection. While classically presenting in

Figure 6.9

Allergic bronchopulmonary aspergillosis.
Asymmetric central bronchiectasis and mucoid impaction is seen in the upper lobes (*arrows*). No significant abnormalities were visible in the lower lobes. This distribution of varicose or cystic bronchiectasis is most typical of allergic bronchopulmonary aspergillosis and tuberculosis.

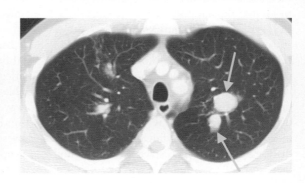

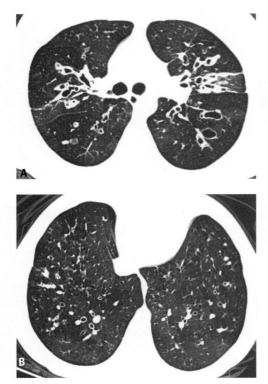

Figure 6.10

Cystic fibrosis. Extensive varicose and cystic bronchiectasis, bronchial wall thickening, and mucous impaction are noted in the upper lobes **(A)**. The process is symmetric and relatively spares the lower lobes **(B)**. This pattern is most typical of cystic fibrosis.

6

a young patient population (less than 20 years of age), a greater understanding of the genetic heterogeneity and variable penetrance of this disease has led to the diagnosis of patients presenting later in life. Also, improvement in treatment has allowed many young patients with CF to survive into adulthood.

Typical HRCT findings include symmetric, upper lobe predominant, central bronchiectasis, bronchial wall thickening, and luminal impaction (Fig. 6.10A, B). The right upper lobe is often involved first, and most severely. The bronchiectasis varies in severity, but varicose or cystic bronchiectasis is most characteristic in advanced cases. Findings of small airways disease (bronchiolectasis, centrilobular nodules, and TIB) are often present in association

with the large airways findings. Mosaic perfusion and air trapping are usually present. Hilar enlargement may be due to reactive lymphadenopathy or pulmonary arterial enlargement.

Immunodeficiency

Congenital or acquired immunodeficiency predisposes patients to chronic airways infection. Congenital immunodeficiencies that commonly lead to large airways disease include agammaglobulinemia, hypogammaglobulinemia, and common variable immunodeficiency. The findings are similar to other causes of chronic large airways disease and include bronchiectasis (often cystic), bronchial wall thickening, and mucoid impaction. The distribution tends to be symmetric and lower lobe predominant.

The most common acquired disorder to result in large airways disease is the acquired immunodeficiency syndrome (AIDS). *AIDS-related airways disease* is most likely due to chronic airway infection by pyogenic organisms. It manifests as symmetric bilateral bronchiectasis, usually lower lobe predominant, bronchial wall thickening, and impaction. While cystic bronchiectasis is rare, varicose bronchiectasis is common and its presence reflects the chronicity of findings.

Primary Ciliary Dyskinesia

Primary ciliary dyskinesia or *immotile cilia syndrome* is a congenital disorder causing reduced or absent ciliary motion. This leads to abnormal mucociliary clearance affecting the lungs, sinuses, inner ear, and reproductive systems. Situs inversus is seen in 50% of patients, in which case the disease is termed *Kartagener syndrome*. Impaired airway mucociliary clearance results in chronic mucostasis, recurrent infections, and bronchiectasis.

The HRCT findings are very similar to those seen with congenital immunodeficiency. Abnormalities usually are symmetric and affect the lower lobes. Cystic or varicose bronchiectasis is typical and associated with airway wall thickening and mucous impaction. Findings of small airways disease may also be present, but do not predominate. Kartagener syndrome is associated with situs inversus (Fig. 6.11A, B).

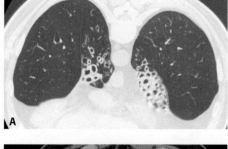

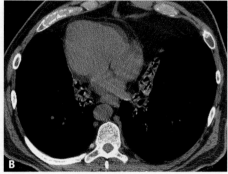

Figure 6.11

Kartagener syndrome. Prone HRCT **(A)** shows extensive bilateral lower lobe cystic bronchiectasis and collapse. Supine HRCT image **(B)** shows situs inversus and dextrocardia.

Williams-Campbell Syndrome

Williams-Campbell syndrome is a rare congenital disorder characterized by the absence of cartilage in the fourth through sixth order bronchi. It typically presents in children, but a rare initial presentation in adults has been described. Lack of supporting cartilage causes weakness and dilatation of affected bronchi. Over time, this eventually leads to chronic mucostasis and infection.

Cystic bronchiectasis with a mid- to lower lung predominance is characteristic. Focal mid-lung bronchiectasis may be present or there may be more extensive dilatation beginning in the central lung and extending peripherally. As is typical of other disorders of cartilage, there may be severe cystic bronchiectasis with relatively little airway inflammation. The airways typically show significant increase in size during inspiration and collapse on expiration. This is in contrast

to immunodeficiency syndromes and primarily ciliary disorders.

Tracheobronchomegaly

Tracheobronchomegaly or *Mounier-Kuhn syndrome* is another rare condition in which there is atrophy of portions of the tracheal and bronchial walls.

Typical HRCT findings include thinning of the walls of the trachea and bronchi. The airways are dilated and show dynamic collapse during expiration. Scalloping of the walls of the affected airways may be seen because of restriction of the lumen by cartilage rings (Fig. 6.12A, B). As with Williams-Campbell

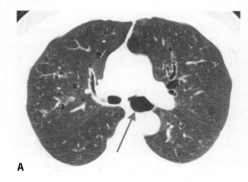

A

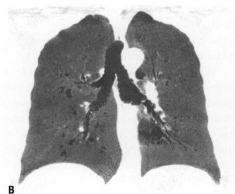

B

Figure 6.12

Tracheobronchomegaly. Marked dilatation of the left main bronchus (*red arrow*) is noted in association with bronchiectasis predominantly within the central lung regions **(A)**. There is a relative paucity of airways inflammation and wall thickening. Coronal reformatted minimum intensity projection image **(B)** shows scalloping of the tracheal wall and thin-walled bronchiectasis in the central lung regions.

6

syndrome, there may be a relative lack of inflammatory abnormalities, even in cases of severe dilatation.

Other Causes of Large Airways Disease

There are many other causes of diffuse or extensive bilateral large airways disease including connective tissue disease, recurrent and chronic aspiration, CB, Marfan syndrome, alpha-1-antitrypsin deficiency, yellow nail lymphedema syndrome, and Young syndrome. Most of these disorders present with nonspecific findings and the diagnosis is often based on the clinical presentation. Recurrent or chronic aspiration often shows consolidation and/or fibrosis involving the dependent lung regions. Marfan syndrome may show bullous emphysema out of proportion to the patient's age. Alpha-1-antitrypsin deficiency shows diffuse lung lucency with a lower lobe predominance.

HRCT Diagnosis of Large Airways Diseases and Bronchiectasis

Some HRCT findings may be used to suggest a specific diagnosis or to limit the diagnostic possibilities.

Cylindrical bronchiectasis is a nonspecific finding, and in patients who show this finding, the diagnosis is usually based on a combination of the clinical presentation, sputum analysis, and/or pathologic findings.

Varicose bronchiectasis suggests a chronic process and is not typically seen in acute processes such as viral infection. Some examples of diseases that may produce varicose bronchiectasis include mycobacterial infections, chronic aspiration, and lung fibrosis (traction bronchiectasis). Varicose bronchiectasis is common in ABPA and CF.

The differential diagnosis of cystic bronchiectasis is more limited and depends upon the overall distribution of bronchiectasis. Diseases that lead to mid- or upper lung cystic bronchiectasis include CF, ABPA, and tuberculosis (Fig. 6.13). Lower lobe predominant cystic bronchiectasis may be due to long-standing or remote infection, CB, primary ciliary dyskinesia (Fig. 6.14), immunodeficiency, and abnormalities of the cartilage including tracheobronchomegaly and Williams-Campbell syndrome.

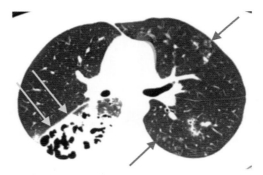

Figure 6.13

Tuberculosis. Focal cystic bronchiectasis is seen in the superior segment of the right lower lobe (*yellow arrows*). Small clusters of centrilobular nodules (*red arrows*) are seen elsewhere, reflecting endobronchial spread of tuberculosis.

HRCT is otherwise limited in its ability to distinguish the various causes of bronchiectasis, although a few additional features may be helpful. High-density mucous within areas of bronchiectasis is suggestive of ABPA

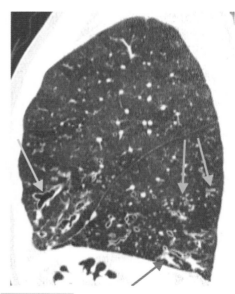

Figure 6.14

Primary ciliary dyskinesia. Sagittal reformatted volumetric HRCT shows lower lobe predominant bronchiectasis (*yellow arrow*), airway impaction (*red arrow*), and centrilobular nodules (*blue arrows*). This distribution is typical of constrictive bronchiolitis, immunodeficiency, primary ciliary dyskinesia, and congenital cartilage disorders.

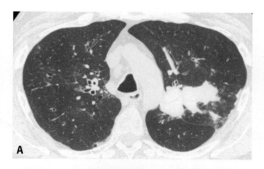

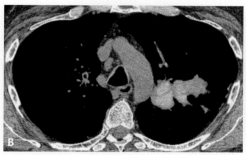

Figure 6.15

Allergic bronchopulmonary aspergillosis.
A. Lung window shows a tubular branching structure in the left upper lobe representing focal bronchiectasis and mucoid impaction. **B.** Soft tissue window shows that the mucus in the lumen of this dilated bronchus is high in attenuation. This strongly suggests allergic bronchopulmonary aspergillosis.

(Fig. 6.15A, B). Situs inversus suggests primary ciliary dyskinesia. A paucity of airway inflammation in the presence of severe bronchiectasis suggests either CB or a cartilage abnormality (Fig. 6.16).

SMALL AIRWAYS DISEASES

HRCT Findings
Analogous to large airways disease, HRCT findings indicative of small airways disease include bronchiolectasis, bronchiolar inflammation with wall thickening, and bronchiolar impaction (TIB). Other findings of small airways disease include centrilobular nodules and mosaic perfusion with air trapping. Also, keep in mind that patients with small airways disease commonly show large airway abnormalities as well.

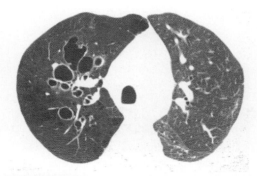

Figure 6.16

Williams-Campbell syndrome. HRCT in a patient with Williams-Campbell syndrome, status-post left lung transplant. The native right lung shows extensive cystic bronchiectasis and diffuse lung lucency. Note the lack of inflammation and airway wall thickening.

Bronchiolectasis and TIB
Bronchiolectasis is defined as dilatation of small airways (Fig. 6.17). There are no specific criteria for bronchiolectasis on HRCT, but normal airways should not be visualized in the peripheral 1 to 2 cm of the lung. When they are seen in this location, bronchiolectasis is likely present.

Dilated bronchioles may be air filled or filled with secretions. Bronchiolectasis with luminal impaction results in the appearance of "TIB." TIB is an important finding in making the diagnosis of small airways disease.

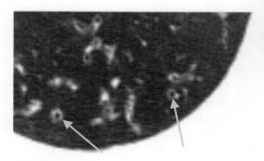

Figure 6.17

Bronchiolectasis. Dilatation of small peripheral airways (*arrows*) is seen in a patient with cystic fibrosis. Airways are seen in the peripheral 1–2 cm of the lung, which is not normal, and their lumens are significantly larger than the adjacent arteries.

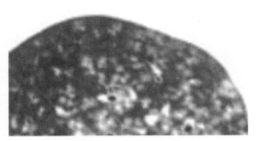

Figure 6.18

Centrilobular nodules of soft tissue attenuation. Centrilobular nodules of soft tissue attenuation are most typical of endobronchial spread of infection or tumor, or aspiration. The nodules spare the subpleural lung. This patient has a bacterial bronchopneumonia.

Centrilobular Nodules

Impaction of small airways may appear as soft tissue attenuation centrilobular nodules (Fig. 6.18). Infectious or inflammatory diseases involving the bronchiole may result in infiltration of the surrounding lung. This may also result in the appearance of centrilobular nodules. Centrilobular nodules may be of soft tissue attenuation or of ground glass opacity.

Mosaic Perfusion and Air Trapping

Mosaic perfusion is caused by decreased blood flow to localized lung regions. In the case of airways disease, hypoxia from airway narrowing or occlusion results in reflex vasoconstriction and reduced perfusion. HRCT shows focal regions of decreased attenuation; vessels within these regions appear relatively small. When due to small airways disease, mosaic perfusion is often associated with air trapping. The HRCT features of mosaic perfusion are discussed in greater detail in Chapter 5.

Mosaic perfusion may be seen with both small and large airways disease, but is more commonly seen with the former. Mosaic perfusion and air trapping in the setting of large airways disease are segmental or lobar in distribution (Fig. 6.19) or may involve an entire lung. Small airways disease typically demonstrates lobular regions of increased lung lucency (Fig. 6.20), although when extensive it can involve larger regions of the lung (Fig. 6.21A, B).

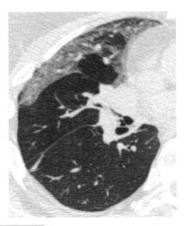

Figure 6.19

Air trapping due to central airways stenosis. Expiratory HRCT in a lung transplant recipient with a stricture of the bronchus intermedius shows focal air trapping involving the right middle and lower lobes. A portion of the anterior right upper lobe shows a normal increase in attenuation on expiration. Air trapping that involves a segment, lobe, or lung suggests large airways disease.

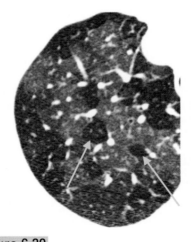

Figure 6.20

Mosaic perfusion due to small airways disease. Inspiratory HRCT shows very well-defined lobular regions of decreased lung attenuation (*arrows*) in a patient with constrictive bronchiolitis. A lobular distribution of mosaic perfusion or air trapping suggests small airways disease.

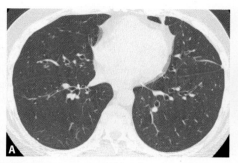 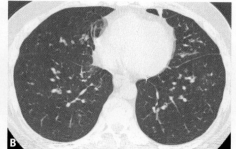

Figure 6.21

Constrictive bronchiolitis with a diffuse distribution. Rarely small airways disease may have a diffuse and uniform distribution. This is most typical of constrictive bronchiolitis. In such cases, inspiratory HRCT **(A)** shows diffusely increased lung lucency and attenuated vessels. Expiratory images **(B)** show diffuse air trapping that may be difficult to distinguish from a poor expiratory effort.

HRCT Classification of Small Airways Disease

The HRCT classification of small airways disease is based on the recognition of specific findings. Four major patterns of small airways disease are shown in Table 6.2. Recognition of one of these patterns allows for formulation of a focused differential diagnosis that may be further refined using clinical information.

Bronchiolitis with Centrilobular Nodules of Ground Glass Opacity

Pathologically, centrilobular nodules of ground glass opacity represent either inflammation or fibrosis surrounding the centrilobular bronchiole. Impaction of bronchioles is typically absent. The nodules tend to be fairly homogeneous in size and may be diffuse or patchy in distribution (Fig. 6.22).

The differential diagnosis of bronchiolitis with centrilobular ground glass opacity nodules (Table 6.3) includes hypersensitivity pneumonitis (HP), respiratory bronchiolitis (RB), follicular bronchiolitis (FB), pneumoconioses, and atypical infections. Langerhans cell histiocytosis, other infections, and endobronchial spread of tumor rarely present with centrilobular ground glass nodules as the predominant abnormality; soft-attenuation nodules are more common.

Some patients with this pattern have a clinical history that suggests a specific diagnosis. HP, the most common cause of this pattern, has an identifiable exposure in 50% of patients. When an exposure is present, this HRCT pattern is considered diagnostic of HP. In smokers, RB or Langerhans cell histiocytosis is most likely. FB is seen in patients with connective tissue disease or immunocompromise. Patients with a pneumoconiosis have a long-term exposure history. Patients with acute symptoms are most likely to have either an atypical infection or HP.

Table 6.2   HRCT patterns of small airways disease

HRCT finding	Pathophysiology	Common diseases
Centrilobular nodules of ground glass opacity	Peribronchiolar inflammation or fibrosis	Hypersensitivity pneumonitis, respiratory bronchiolitis, follicular bronchiolitis, atypical infections, pneumoconioses
Centrilobular nodules of soft tissue attenuation	Bronchiolar impaction with spread into adjacent alveoli	Endobronchial infection, tumor, aspiration
Tree-in-bud opacities	Infectious mucoid impaction of bronchioles	Endobronchial infection, aspiration
Mosaic perfusion or air trapping	Bronchiolar narrowing or occlusion	Asthma, hypersensitivity pneumonitis, constrictive bronchiolitis

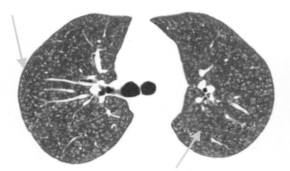

Figure 6.22

Centrilobular nodules of ground glass attenuation. Symmetric, similar-sized nodules of ground glass opacity are present in a patient with subacute hypersensitivity pneumonitis. Note sparing of the subpleural regions (*arrows*) and even spacing of the nodules; this is typical of a centrilobular distribution of nodules.

Bronchiolitis with Centrilobular Nodules of Soft Tissue Attenuation

Soft tissue attenuation centrilobular nodules are a reflection of endobronchial impaction with adjacent consolidation (Fig. 6.23). The process begins in the centrilobular region, eventually spreading outward, and may involve the entire pulmonary lobule. Consolidation in adjacent lobules may coalesce to form larger, confluent regions of consolidation. The distribution of this consolidation is typically segmental or subsegmental.

Soft tissue attenuation centrilobular nodules tend to be patchy and heterogeneous in size. The differential diagnosis (Table 6.4) includes diseases that spread via the small airways (Fig. 6.24), including infections (bacterial, mycobacterial, fungal, and viral) and tumor (invasive mucinous adenocarcinoma). Aspiration without pneumonia is also included in this category. Infection and aspiration typically present with acute symptoms, whereas tumor typically presents with chronic symptoms.

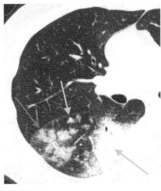

Figure 6.23

Centrilobular nodules of soft tissue attenuation in invasive mucinous adenocarcinoma. The centrilobular distribution of nodules on this HRCT is indicated by relative sparing of the subpleural lung (*yellow arrow*). As the process extends outward from the centrilobular region, it may reach the pleural surface (*red arrow*). When adjacent lobules coalesce, confluent areas of consolidation may be present (*blue arrow*).

Table 6.3	Differential diagnosis of centrilobular nodules of ground glass opacity

Hypersensitivity pneumonitis
Respiratory bronchiolitis
Follicular bronchiolitis
Pneumoconioses
Atypical infections
Langerhans cell histiocytosis (usually soft tissue nodules)
Bacterial, mycobacterial infections (usually soft tissue nodules)
Endobronchial spread of tumor (usually soft tissue nodules)

Table 6.4	Differential diagnosis of centrilobular nodules of soft tissue attenuation

Endobronchial spread of infection (bacterial, mycobacterial, fungal)
Endobronchial spread of tumor (invasive mucinous adenocarcinoma)
Aspiration

6

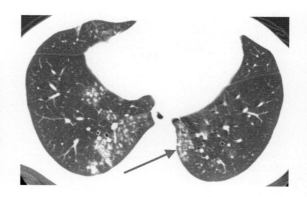

Figure 6.24

Bronchopneumonia with soft tissue attenuation centrilobular nodules. Nodules are patchy, asymmetric, and heterogeneous in size. Note that the nodules are separated from the pleural surface (*red arrow*). This appearance is typical of endobronchial spread with bronchiolar impaction such as in this patient with bacterial bronchopneumonia.

Bronchiolitis with TIB Opacities

On HRCT, TIB manifests as tubular, branching opacities with associated nodules (Fig. 6.25). Pathologically, this represents impaction of lobular bronchioles with infectious material. The importance of TIB is that it almost always represents infection (Table 6.5), although it is not specific with regard to the type of infection. TIB is most commonly seen with bacterial and mycobacterial infections; however, it may also be seen with fungal and viral infections.

Chronic causes of airways infection may demonstrate TIB; these include CF, ciliary disorders, and immunodeficiency. In such cases, large airways findings are also usually present (Fig. 6.26). Two additional causes of TIB include diffuse panbronchiolitis (Fig. 6.27) and ABPA (Fig. 6.28A, B). The etiology of diffuse panbronchiolitis is unclear, but it is likely that chronic infection plays a significant role. Noninfectious causes of airways disease rarely produce TIB; causes include FB and invasive mucinous adenocarcinoma.

Bronchiolitis with Mosaic Perfusion or Air Trapping

Mosaic perfusion associated with airways disease reflects bronchiolar narrowing or occlusion and reflex vasoconstriction. It is a nonspecific finding and may be seen with any cause of small or large airways disease. In most cases, other findings predominate. For instance, mosaic perfusion may be seen in patients with atypical mycobacterial infections, but in this disease bronchiectasis, nodules, and TIB are usually the most significant findings (Fig. 6.29).

When mosaic perfusion or air trapping is the only or predominant finding (Fig. 6.30), the differential diagnosis (Table 6.6) is quite limited and includes asthma, hypersensitivity pneumonia, and CB as common causes.

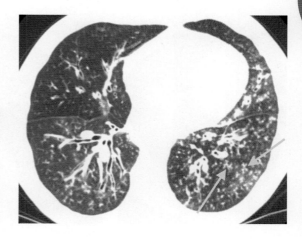

Figure 6.25

Tree-in-bud sign. Several good examples of the tree-in-bud are visible, with branching, tubular opacities (*yellow arrows*) representing dilated and impacted bronchioles. This finding is highly specific for infection as in this case of bacterial bronchopneumonia. Patchy, bilateral centrilobular nodules of soft tissue attenuation are also present.

Table 6.5	Differential diagnosis of the tree-in-bud sign

Bacterial infection
Mycobacterial infection
Fungal infection
Viral infection
Cystic fibrosis
Allergic bronchopulmonary aspergillosis
Primary ciliary dyskinesia
Immunodeficiency
Diffuse panbronchiolitis
Follicular bronchiolitis
Invasive mucinous adenocarcinoma
Aspiration

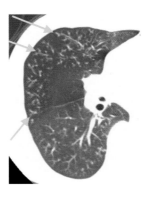

Figure 6.27

Diffuse panbronchiolitis with the tree-in-bud. Centrilobular nodules and tree-in-bud opacities (*arrows*) are classic findings of diffuse panbronchiolitis. This disease is most common in Asian patients.

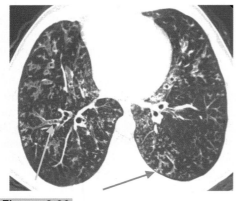

Figure 6.26

Primary ciliary dyskinesia. Tree-in-bud opacities are visible (*red arrow*). Bronchiectasis and large airways inflammation are also present (*yellow* arrow).

Specific Small Airways Diseases

Infections

Infections commonly involve the small airways and are discussed in greater detail in Chapter 14. The HRCT manifestations depend upon the mechanism of spread of the infection. Endobronchial spread is the most common mechanism by which infections disseminate and is characteristic of bacterial bronchopneumonia and mycobacterial and fungal infections.

In these cases, bronchiolar impaction is the initial abnormality, appearing on HRCT as soft tissue attenuation centrilobular nodules (Fig. 6.31) or TIB. The infection subsequently

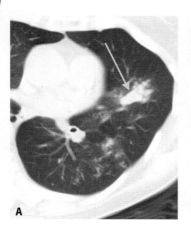
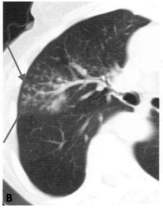

A

B

Figure 6.28

Allergic bronchopulmonary aspergillosis (ABPA). A. ABPA is most commonly seen in asthmatics and in most cases large airways findings of bronchiectasis and bronchial impaction (*arrow*) predominate. **B.** Small airways abnormalities such as tree-in-bud opacities (*arrows*) may also be present.

6

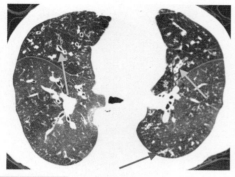

Figure 6.29

Mosaic perfusion associated with other findings of airways disease. HRCT shows focal areas of decreased lung attenuation representing mosaic perfusion in a patient with atypical mycobacterial infection. However, other findings of airways disease are the predominant abnormality, including bronchiectasis (*yellow arrows*), bronchial wall thickening, and tree-in-bud opacities (*red arrow*). In this case, the mosaic perfusion should be ignored and diagnosis is driven by the other findings.

spreads into the alveoli adjacent to the center of the pulmonary lobule. As this occurs, the nodules become larger until eventually they involve the entire pulmonary lobule or multiple lobules. When consolidation in adjacent lobules coalesces, confluent areas of consolidation will

develop. These findings are often associated with bronchiolar wall thickening and dilatation.

Peribronchiolar inflammation without bronchiolar impaction is another pattern of small airway infection and is characteristic of atypical infections. It is manifested by centrilobular nodules of ground glass opacity (Fig. 6.32). As the abnormality progresses, patchy areas of ground glass opacity and eventually consolidation will develop, representing more generalized areas of infection and diffuse alveolar damage. Bronchial/bronchiolar wall thickening and dilatation with mosaic perfusion/air trapping may be associated findings.

Hypersensitivity Pneumonitis
HP is discussed in greater detail in Chapter 13. It represents a reaction to inhaled organic antigens. Airway abnormalities are most evident in the subacute stage of HP. Centrilobular nodules of ground glass opacity are characteristically visible on HRCT and represent peribronchiolar inflammation and cellular infiltration. The centrilobular nodules are often diffuse or symmetric in distribution (Fig. 6.33), similar to the distribution of nodules in RB, FB, and atypical infections.

HP commonly presents with mosaic perfusion and/or air trapping due to bronchiolitis and bronchiolar narrowing. This finding may

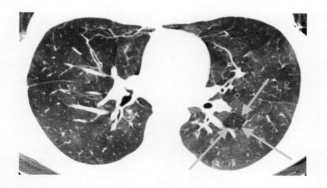

Figure 6.30

Mosaic perfusion as the predominant finding. Patchy bilateral mosaic perfusion is present, associated with only minimal airway wall thickening. Note the lobular distribution (*arrows*) of some areas of mosaic perfusion. When mosaic perfusion is the predominant abnormality in small airways disease, the differential diagnosis includes constrictive bronchiolitis, asthma, and hypersensitivity pneumonitis. This patient has constrictive bronchiolitis from smoke inhalation during a fire.

Table 6.6	Differential diagnosis of isolated mosaic perfusion

Asthma
Hypersensitivity pneumonitis
Constrictive bronchiolitis
Vascular diseases (chronic pulmonary
  thromboembolism, vasculitis)

be seen in isolation or may be associated with nodules. When seen in isolation, the differential diagnosis includes CB and asthma. Air trapping and mosaic perfusion are also commonly present in association with fibrosis in patients with chronic HP. In fact, this combination is highly suggestive of HP.

Respiratory Bronchiolitis and Desquamative Interstitial Pneumonia

RB is a disease of cigarette smokers in which cellular infiltration and/or inflammation occurs around bronchioles as a reaction to smoke inhalation. This is discussed in greater detail in Chapter 11. The classic HRCT finding of RB is centrilobular nodules of ground glass opacity (Fig. 6.34), a finding it shares with HP. RB may also show mosaic perfusion and/or air trapping; however, the severity of these findings is less than with HP.

Desquamative interstitial pneumonia (DIP), also a smoking-related disease, is closely related to RB. RB and DIP, in fact, are thought to represent different points on a spectrum of the same pathological process. Thus, HRCT features of both may coexist. When there is overlap, HRCT may

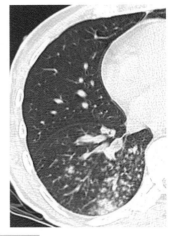

Figure 6.31

Bronchopneumonia with centrilobular nodules of soft tissue attenuation. Focal centrilobular nodules of soft tissue attenuation are seen in the right lower lobe. Note the sparing of the subpleural regions and the heterogeneous size of the nodules. In the acute setting, these findings are suggestive of either infection or aspiration.

demonstrate peripheral or generalized ground glass opacity with or without associated cysts or emphysema.

Follicular Bronchiolitis

FB is seen in patients with connective tissue disease or immunocompromise and is characterized by cellular bronchiolitis with lymphoid follicle formation in relation to the bronchioles. This is discussed in greater detail in Chapter 17. Similar to RB, the characteristic finding of FB is centrilobular nodules of ground glass opacity (Fig. 6.35).

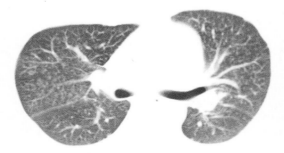

Figure 6.32

Viral infection with centrilobular nodules of ground glass opacity. While some overlap exists, atypical infections are more likely to produce centrilobular nodules of ground glass attenuation in comparison to bacterial, mycobacterial, and fungal infections. The density of these nodules reflects peribronchiolar inflammation without bronchiolar impaction.

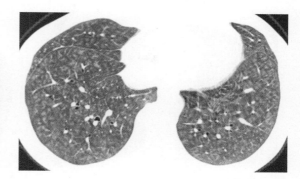

Figure 6.33

Hypersensitivity pneumonitis (HP) with ground glass opacity (GGO) centrilobular nodules. When centrilobular nodules of GGO are present, HP is the most likely diagnosis. When there is a clear exposure, such as in this patient with an exposure to birds, the HRCT is considered diagnostic of HP.

Also similar to RB, FB may have associated mosaic perfusion and/or air trapping; however, it is rarely as severe as in patients with HP. Lymphoid interstitial pneumonia is a more generalized lymphoproliferative disorder seen in the same groups of patients as FB. FB and lymphoid interstitial pneumonia are thought to represent different distributions or severity of the same disease.

Invasive Pulmonary Mucinous Adenocarcinoma

The multifocal or diffuse type of invasive mucinous adenocarcinoma commonly involves the small airways via endobronchial spread. This will be discussed in greater detail in Chapter 17. This mechanism of spread shares many similarities with endobronchial spread of infection.

The initial manifestation is that of bronchiolar impaction with tumor or mucin and fluid produced by the tumor, manifesting as centrilobular nodules, often of soft tissue attenuation. The tumor, which primarily spreads along alveolar walls, eventually can involve the entire pulmonary lobules, producing confluent areas of consolidation (Fig. 6.36). The consolidation is often due to mucin and fluid-filling alveoli, rather than tumor.

Asthma

Asthma is characterized by recurrent or chronic airway hyperreactivity. The primary features of this disease are small airways obstruction and chronic inflammation. The initial diagnosis is usually made in young patients (less than 40 years) with typical symptoms, physical

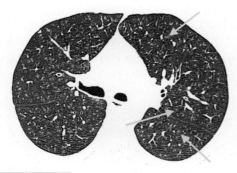

Figure 6.34

Respiratory bronchiolitis with ground glass opacity (GGO) centrilobular nodules. Centrilobular nodules of GGO (*arrows*) seen in smokers suggest respiratory bronchiolitis. Note the sparing of the subpleural regions.

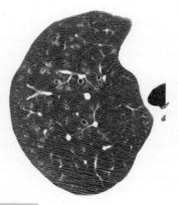

Figure 6.35

Follicular bronchiolitis with ground glass opacity (GGO) centrilobular nodules. HRCT through the right upper lobe shows centrilobular nodules of GGO in a patient with follicular bronchiolitis associated with connective tissue disease.

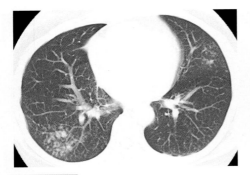

Figure 6.36

Invasive mucinous adenocarcinoma with centrilobular nodules. Patchy bilateral centrilobular nodules are present. Note sparing of the subpleural lung and even spacing of the nodules. Many of the nodules are of soft tissue attenuation.

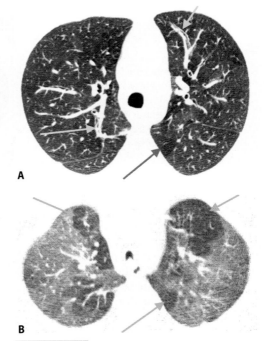

A

B

Figure 6.37

Asthma. Inspiratory HRCT **(A)** shows mosaic perfusion (*red arrow*) and mild bronchial wall thickening (*yellow arrows*) as the predominant findings in this patient with asthma. Note air trapping (*blue arrows*) on the dynamic expiratory image **(B)** in the same distribution as the mosaic perfusion on inspiration.

examination findings, and an obstructive defect on pulmonary function tests that is at least partially reversible. Patients with asthma are not commonly imaged, because the diagnosis in most cases is straightforward, and symptoms in the majority of patients are well controlled on currently available therapies.

The HRCT findings of asthma are typically mild and include bronchial wall thickening, mild bronchiectasis, and mosaic perfusion or air trapping (Fig. 6.37A, B). As mosaic perfusion and air trapping are often the predominant findings, the differential includes HP and CB.

Constrictive Bronchiolitis

CB is also known as obliterative bronchiolitis or bronchiolitis obliterans. Pathologically, constrictive bronchiolitis is characterized by fibrosis of the bronchiolar wall and peribronchiolar tissues with bronchiolar obstruction.

There are multiple causes of constrictive bronchiolitis, the most common of which is prior severe viral infection. Other etiologies include connective tissue disease, drug toxicity, toxic inhalations such as chlorine gas and smoke, graft versus host disease, chronic rejection in lung transplant

recipients, and neuroendocrine hyperplasia (Table 6.7). The end result of these insults is irreversible obstruction of the small airways by fibrosis.

Fibrosis of the small airways cannot be directly visualized on HRCT. The secondary

Table 6.7	Cause of constrictive bronchiolitis
Post-viral infection	
Connective tissue disease	
Drug toxicity	
Toxic inhalations	
Graft vs. host disease	
Chronic rejection in lung transplant recipients	
Neuroendocrine hyperplasia	

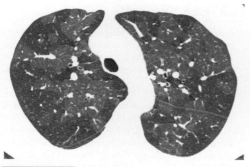

Figure 6.38

Constrictive bronchiolitis due to neuroendocrine hyperplasia. Inspiratory HRCT shows heterogeneous lung density with sharply demarcated regions of decreased lung attenuation compatible with mosaic perfusion. Note the lobular nature of these regions, highly suggestive of small airways disease.

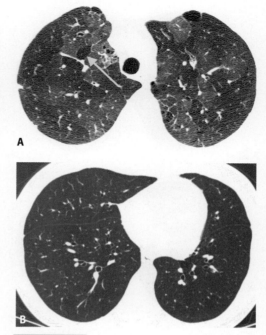

A

B

Figure 6.40

Constrictive bronchiolitis, spectrum of lung involvement. A. Patchy lobular mosaic perfusion (*arrow*). Only minimal bronchiectasis is present in this relatively mild case of constrictive bronchiolitis from connective tissue disease. **B.** Diffuse lung involvement is seen in a lung transplant recipient with constrictive bronchiolitis from chronic rejection. Diffuse lung lucency is present reflecting diffuse lung involvement. This may be difficult to distinguish from normal.

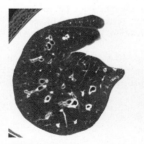
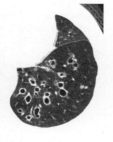

Figure 6.39

Bronchiolitis obliterans associated with rheumatoid arthritis. Diffuse lung lucency is noted with associated bronchiectasis and bronchial wall thickening. This is an example of severe, long-standing constrictive bronchiolitis with near-complete lung involvement.

effects of airway obstruction are the primary HRCT findings of CB. These findings include mosaic perfusion and/or air trapping (Fig. 6.38). Bronchial wall thickening, bronchiectasis, and bronchiolar impaction may be seen in severe, long-standing disease (Fig. 6.39).

The extent of lung involvement in CB varies significantly, ranging from scattered lobules to diffuse lung involvement (Fig. 6.40A, B). Unilateral CB with decreased lung volume and reduction in the size of pulmonary artery branches may be referred to as *Swyer-James syndrome*.

HP and asthma usually show a limited distribution of mosaic perfusion and air trapping; thus, when findings of mosaic perfusion or air trapping are extensive, CB is the favored diagnosis. On the other hand, diffuse lung involvement by CB may be difficult to appreciate or distinguish from panlobular emphysema. Furthermore, diffuse air trapping on expiratory images may be difficult

6

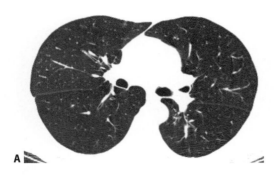

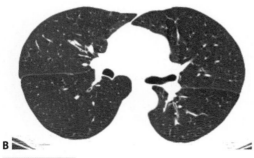

Figure 6.41

Constrictive bronchiolitis with a diffuse distribution. A diffuse distribution of constrictive bronchiolitis appears as extensive lung lucency on inspiratory HRCT **(A)**. Diagnosis of diffuse involvement may be challenging as there is no normal lung with which to compare the affected regions. Correlation with expiratory images **(B)**, showing no change, and pulmonary function tests is helpful to confirm diffuse constrictive bronchiolitis.

to differentiate from a poor expiratory effort (Fig. 6.41A, B). Correlation with pulmonary function tests may be helpful to confirm the presence of extensive small airways disease in questionable cases.

FURTHER READING

Arakawa H, Webb WR. Air trapping on expiratory high-resolution CT scans in the absence of inspiratory scan abnormalities: correlation with pulmonary function tests and differential diagnosis. *AJR Am J Roentgenol.* 1998;170:1349-1353.

Cartier Y, Kavanagh PV, Johkoh T, et al. Bronchiectasis: accuracy of high-resolution CT in the differentiation of specific diseases. *AJR Am J Roentgenol.* 1999;173:47-52.

Im JG, Kim SH, Chung MJ, Koo JM, Han MC. Lobular low attenuation of the lung parenchyma on CT: evaluation of forty-eight patients. *J Comput Assist Tomogr.* 1996;20:756-762.

Kang EY, Miller RR, Müller NL. Bronchiectasis: comparison of preoperative thin-section CT and pathologic findings in resected specimens. *Radiology.* 1995;195:649-654.

Kang EY, Woo OH, Shin BK, et al. Bronchiolitis: classification, computed tomographic and histopathologic features, and radiologic approach. *J Comput Assist Tomogr.* 2009;33:32-41.

Lynch DA. Imaging of small airways disease. *Clin Chest Med.* 1993;14:623-634.

Lynch DA. Imaging of small airways disease and chronic obstructive pulmonary disease. *Clin Chest Med.* 2008;29:165-179.

McGuinness G, Naidich DP, Leitman BS, McCauley DI. Bronchiectasis: CT evaluation. *AJR Am J Roentgenol.* 1993;160:253-259.

Müller NL, Miller RR. Diseases of the bronchioles: CT and histopathologic findings. *Radiology.* 1995;196:3-12.

O'Donnell AE. Bronchiectasis. *Chest.* 2008;134:815-823.

Padley SPG, Adler BD, Hansell DM, Müller NL. Bronchiolitis obliterans: high-resolution CT findings and correlation with pulmonary function tests. *Clin Radiol.* 1993;47:236-240.

Park CS, Müller NL, Worthy SA, et al. Airway obstruction in asthmatic and healthy individuals: inspiratory and expiratory thin-section CT findings. *Radiology.* 1997;203:361-367.

Shah RM, Sexauer W, Ostrum BJ, et al. High-resolution CT in the acute exacerbation of cystic fibrosis: evaluation of acute findings, reversibility of those findings, and clinical correlation. *AJR Am J Roentgenol.* 1997;169:375-380.

Ward S, Heyneman L, Lee MJ, et al. Accuracy of CT in the diagnosis of allergic bronchopulmonary aspergillosis in asthmatic patients. *AJR Am J Roentgenol.* 1999;173:937-942.

Pulmonary Vascular Diseases

Vascular diseases of the lung may affect arteries, veins, and/or capillaries. They are primarily evaluated using modalities such as echocardiography, contrast-enhanced CT, or conventional angiography, but in selected cases, HRCT may give an insight not provided by other imaging studies.

HRCT provides an accurate assessment of lung parenchymal abnormalities, but may also allow for a limited assessment of abnormalities directly involving the pulmonary arteries, pulmonary veins, and heart. This chapter focuses upon the pulmonary manifestations of pulmonary vascular disease.

PULMONARY HYPERTENSION

HRCT Findings

Pulmonary hypertension (PH) may be seen with a variety of diseases that affect the lung parenchyma, pulmonary arteries, pulmonary veins, and heart. While pulmonary artery (PA) pressures cannot be directly estimated using HRCT, it may show signs that suggest the presence and relative severity of PH (Table 7.1).

Enlargement of the Main PA

Main PA diameter correlates with the presence or absence of pulmonary arterial hypertension. This correlation is significantly more accurate in patients without parenchymal lung disease than in those with lung disease.

PA diameter should be measured perpendicular to the long axis of the vessel. This may be challenging using HRCT with spaced sections. The threshold above which PH can be said to be present varies in the literature. A threshold diameter of 3.3 cm is relatively specific for this diagnosis. The PA should also be smaller than the adjacent aorta (Fig. 7.1).

Increased Right Ventricular Size

Right ventricular (RV) size may be difficult to assess on HRCT images obtained without contrast injection; however, in many cases the location of the interventricular septum may be estimated even on non-contrast images (Fig. 7.2). The transverse diameter of the RV should be less than the left ventricle. PH is a common cause of RV enlargement.

Increased Size of the Right Atrium, Superior Vena Cava, and Inferior Vena Cava

In the setting of PH, the right atrium (Fig. 7.3), superior vena cava, and inferior vena cava are often enlarged due to tricuspid regurgitation.

Table 7.1	HRCT findings that may be associated with pulmonary hypertension
Enlargement of the main pulmonary artery	
Increased right ventricular size	
Increased right atrial size	
Increased size of superior/inferior vena cava	
Mosaic perfusion	
Centrilobular nodules	

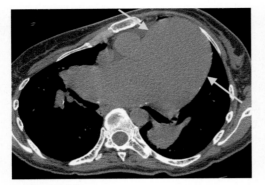

Figure 7.1

Main pulmonary artery enlargement. There is marked dilatation of the main pulmonary artery (*arrows*) in a patient with idiopathic pulmonary arterial hypertension.

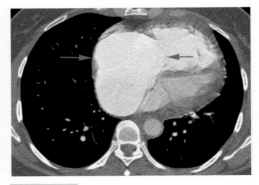

Figure 7.3

Right atrial enlargement. The right atrium (*arrows*) is markedly dilated in a patient with idiopathic pulmonary arterial hypertension. This finding is often due to tricuspid regurgitation resulting from dilatation of the right ventricle.

The size of these structures can usually be determined on non-contrast images. There are no specific size thresholds to use, and enlargement is mainly determined by reader experience. These signs are the least specific for PH as enlargement may be caused by multiple other etiologies.

Mosaic Perfusion

Heterogeneous lung attenuation due to regional alterations in blood flow is termed

mosaic perfusion (see Chapter 5). Mosaic perfusion may be seen with either airways disease or vascular disease, the former being significantly more likely. Mosaic perfusion may be seen with any cause of PH, but is most common with chronic pulmonary thromboembolic disease.

The appearance of mosaic perfusion may help to distinguish airways and vascular causes. Vascular disease usually presents with larger, peripheral, non-lobular regions of decreased lung attenuation (Fig. 7.4). Small airways disease

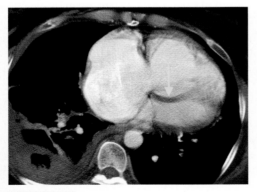

Figure 7.2

Right ventricular enlargement. The diameter of the right ventricle is significantly greater than that of the left ventricle in a patient with pulmonary hypertension due to chronic pulmonary thromboembolism. Bowing of the interventricular septum toward the left ventricle (*arrow*) is also seen.

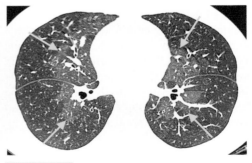

Figure 7.4

Mosaic perfusion. Heterogeneous lung attenuation is present with peripheral lung appearing decreased in attenuation and central lung regions (*arrows*) appearing to be of increased attenuation. In this case, the lower attenuation lung is abnormal, resulting from decreased perfusion due to vasculitis.

typically shows smaller patchy regions of mosaic perfusion, some of which appear lobular.

Centrilobular Nodules

The distal pulmonary arteries are centrilobular in location, and diseases that affect the pulmonary arterial system may manifest as centrilobular nodules. Centrilobular nodules from a vascular etiology are often of ground glass opacity (Fig. 7.5). These may be seen in association with pulmonary arterial hypertension of any cause, but they are most common with idiopathic pulmonary arterial hypertension (IPAH), capillary hemangiomatosis, pulmonary veno-occlusive disease, and vasculitis. They often reflect the presence of pulmonary edema or hemorrhage, or cholesterol granulomas, which are an indication of previous hemorrhage.

Centrilobular nodules are not specific for a vascular etiology as they may also be seen with pulmonary edema or hemorrhage (Fig. 7.6) of any cause and airways diseases such as hypersensitivity pneumonitis. In a patient with known PH, however, they are likely due to the vascular disease.

Diseases Associated with PH

The differential diagnosis of PH is very broad (Table 7.2). HRCT may be obtained in the

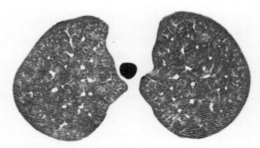

Figure 7.6

Centrilobular nodules of ground glass opacity. The nodules in this patient represented pulmonary hemorrhage due to systemic lupus erythematosus. Nodules of this type commonly have causes other than pulmonary hypertension. These include edema and hemorrhage unrelated to pulmonary vascular disease, hypersensitivity pneumonitis, and respiratory bronchiolitis.

diagnostic evaluation of a patient with PH of unknown cause. One major role of HRCT in this setting is the detection of diffuse lung disease, primarily emphysema and lung fibrosis. Contrast-enhanced CT may also be obtained to evaluate for chronic pulmonary thromboembolism (CPTE).

There are many causes of PH that are not well evaluated using HRCT. These are unified

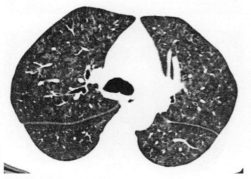

Figure 7.5

Centrilobular nodules of ground glass opacity in pulmonary hypertension. Ill-defined centrilobular ground glass opacity nodules are often seen in primary and secondary causes of pulmonary hypertension. They may represent focal areas of edema, hemorrhage, or cholesterol granuloma formation.

Table 7.2	Differential diagnosis of pulmonary hypertension

Parenchymal lung disease (emphysema, fibrosis, cystic lung disease)
Hypoxemia without parenchymal lung disease
Chronic pulmonary thromboembolism
Fibrosing mediastinitis
Left-sided heart disease
Congenital systemic to pulmonary shunts
Vasculitis
Liver disease
Human immunodeficiency virus infection
Drugs
Sickle cell anemia
Idiopathic pulmonary arterial hypertension
Familial pulmonary arterial hypertension
Pulmonary veno-occlusive disease
Capillary hemangiomatosis
Intravenous injection of oral medications

7

Table 7.3	Causes of pulmonary hypertension that may be associated with findings suggestive of a specific diagnosis
Disease	**HRCT finding**
Parenchymal lung disease	Fibrosis, emphysema, or cystic lung disease
Chronic pulmonary thromboembolism	Pulmonary artery filling defects or occlusion; mosaic perfusion
Idiopathic pulmonary arterial hypertension	Dilated main pulmonary artery; centrilobular nodules of ground glass opacity
Pulmonary veno-occlusive disease	Smooth interlobular septal thickening; dilated main pulmonary artery; normal sized pulmonary veins
Pulmonary capillary hemangiomatosis	Centrilobular nodules of ground glass opacity; progression of findings after treatment with vasodilators
Intravenous injection of oral medications	Diffuse, small, homogeneous, branching centrilobular nodules
Sickle cell disease	Dense bones, rugger jersey spine
Liver disease	Small, nodular liver
Left heart disease	Left atrial or ventricular dilatation; smooth interlobular septal thickening (pulmonary edema)

by a relative lack of lung abnormalities or the presence of nonspecific lung findings. Examples include systolic or diastolic left ventricular dysfunction, valvular heart disease, cardiovascular shunts, hypoventilation disorders, and sleep disorders. The discussion of specific diseases associated with PH will be restricted to those that commonly show lung abnormalities on HRCT (Table 7.3).

Parenchymal Lung Disease

PH may result from parenchymal lung disease because of hypoxia (with vasoconstriction) or obliteration of the pulmonary capillary bed. The most common lung parenchymal processes to result in PH are emphysema (Fig. 7.7A, B) and diffuse lung fibrosis (Fig. 7.8A, B). Cystic lung disease is a rare cause of PH.

Lung fibrosis causing PH is most commonly due to idiopathic pulmonary fibrosis, connective tissue disease, or sarcoidosis. Chronic airways disease, such as cystic fibrosis, and cystic lung disease, such as lymphangioleiomyomatosis or Langerhans histiocytosis, may also be associated with PH. As lung disease associated with PH is typically extensive, it should be evident on HRCT. The lack of significant abnormality on HRCT makes a lung etiology of PH unlikely. In general, the severity of lung disease correlates with the degree of PH.

Sarcoidosis and connective tissue disease–related interstitial lung disease (Fig. 7.9A–C)

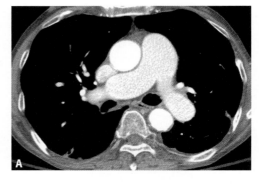

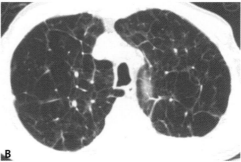

Figure 7.7

Pulmonary hypertension due to emphysema.
A. The main pulmonary artery is enlarged in this patient with pulmonary hypertension. **B.** On lung windows, extensive centrilobular emphysema is visible.

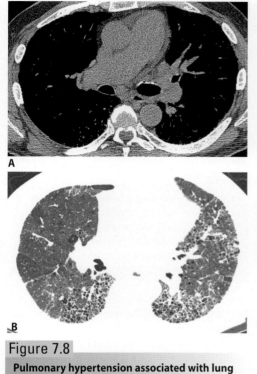

Figure 7.8

Pulmonary hypertension associated with lung fibrosis. Mild main pulmonary artery enlargement **(A)** is associated with fibrosis **(B)** in this patient with idiopathic pulmonary fibrosis.

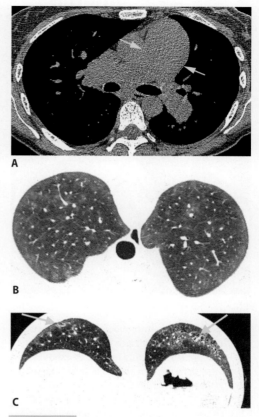

Figure 7.9

Pulmonary hypertension in connective tissue disease. This patient with scleroderma and pulmonary hypertension shows enlargement of the main pulmonary artery (arrow) **(A)**. A prone scan through the upper lobes **(B)** shows lobular areas of ground glass opacity, perhaps pulmonary edema or hemorrhage related to pulmonary hypertension. In the lower lobes **(C)** mild fibrosis is present (*arrows*); it is too mild to explain the pulmonary hypertension. This patient likely has vasculitis contributing to pulmonary hypertension.

may show PH disproportionate to the extent of lung disease. In these cases, vasculitis, thrombosis, stenosis, or occlusion of small pulmonary arteries likely contribute. Of note, in the presence of lung disease, there is a poor correlation between main PA diameter and the severity of PH. This is in contrast to IPAH and other diseases without significant lung manifestations in which pulmonary arterial diameter shows better correlation with the presence and severity of PH.

Chronic Pulmonary Thromboembolism

The diagnosis of CPTE may be challenging. Patients present with nonspecific symptoms and initial objective examinations, such as pulmonary function tests, are nonspecific. Contrast-enhanced CT pulmonary angiography, while effective in the setting of acute pulmonary thromboembolism, has limited sensitivity in the diagnosis of CPTE.

Despite this fact, contrast-enhanced CT is often obtained as the first imaging test in the evaluation of suspected CPTE. Findings that may be seen include eccentric filling defects in pulmonary arteries with or without calcification, artery wall thickening, and PA webs. Enlargement of the main PA, right ventricle, and right atrium are common findings. Narrowing of the distal pulmonary arterial branches and bronchial artery enlargement may also be seen.

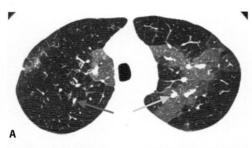

A

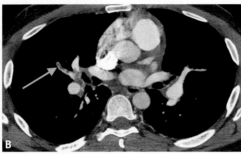

B

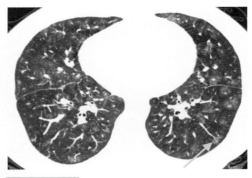

Figure 7.11

Idiopathic pulmonary arterial hypertension. Centrilobular nodules of ground glass opacity (*arrow*) are seen in a patient with pulmonary arterial hypertension. These nodules may be seen with both primary and secondary causes of pulmonary hypertension and often reflect edema or hemorrhage.

Figure 7.10

Chronic pulmonary thromboembolism. A. Mosaic perfusion is present with lucent regions of lung reflecting decreased perfusion. Note that the vessels are significantly larger in areas of normal lung (*yellow arrow*) than in lucent lung regions (*red arrow*). **B.** CT with contrast shows irregular filling defects in pulmonary artery branches (*blue arrow*).

The principal lung parenchymal finding of CPTE is mosaic perfusion due to vascular stenoses and/or occlusions. Mosaic perfusion tends to be more severe in CPTE than in other causes of pulmonary arterial hypertension. The distribution of mosaic perfusion is peripheral and usually affects larger geographic areas of lung as compared with airways disease (Fig. 7.10A, B). Lobular areas of decreased lung attenuation are not typical.

Idiopathic Pulmonary Arterial Hypertension

IPAH is a disease that typically affects young females with a peak onset of 30 to 40 years of age. It is a diagnosis of exclusion, but occurs in an age group in which other causes of pulmonary arterial hypertension are uncommon. Plexogenic arteriopathy, a disordered proliferation of capillary-like vessels, is the typical histologic abnormality in these patients,

although it may also be seen with other causes of PH.

Enlargement of the main PA is a common finding in IPAH and is seen in greater than 90% of patients with this disease. Centrilobular nodules of ground glass opacity may be present (Fig. 7.11). These may represent focal hemorrhage or edema, cholesterol granulomas, or perhaps plexogenic lesions. When present in this clinical setting, centrilobular nodules should be assumed to be related to the PAH and not due to an alternative disease such as hypersensitivity pneumonitis.

Other findings that may be seen in IPAH include mosaic perfusion, interlobular septal thickening, and air trapping. These are typically mild in severity and not useful in diagnosis. Significant mosaic perfusion, in particular, is atypical for IPAH and suggests an alternative disease, particularly pulmonary thromboembolic disease.

Pulmonary Veno-occlusive Disease

Pulmonary veno-occlusive disease (PVOD) is a rare cause of PH characterized by idiopathic obliteration of the pulmonary venules, which leads to pulmonary edema, hemorrhage, and/or venous infarcts proximal to the level of obstruction. This disease is seen in patients of various ages, but most commonly presents in

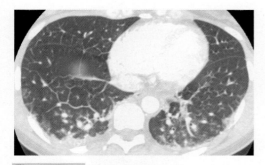

Figure 7.12

Pulmonary veno-occlusive disease. Smooth interlobular septal thickening is present in a patient with pulmonary veno-occlusive disease (PVOD). This finding represents pulmonary edema and in a patient with pulmonary hypertension without left-sided heart disease suggests PVOD.

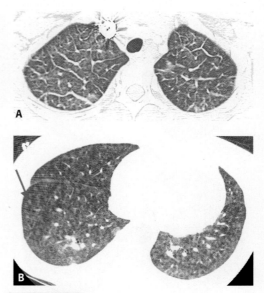

Figure 7.13

Pulmonary veno-occlusive disease. A. Smooth interlobular septal thickening is present in a patient with pulmonary veno-occlusive disease (PVOD). **B.** After treatment, the septal thickening resolved and centrilobular nodules of ground glass opacity were evident (*arrow*). This represents an overlap of PVOD and capillary hemangiomatosis.

children and young adults. It portends a poor prognosis with an average survival of 2 years after presentation. Clinically PVOD closely mimics IPAH, and in some cases HRCT may be the only examination to suggest the correct diagnosis. This distinction is clinically important as some patients with PVOD worsen clinically with vasodilatory therapy.

The most characteristic finding of PVOD is smooth interlobular septal thickening (Fig. 7.12), resembling pulmonary edema from heart failure. This finding is suggestive of PVOD in patients with known PH and no evidence of left-sided heart disease. Ground glass opacity may also be present in a diffuse, patchy, or lobular distribution. Centrilobular nodules of ground glass opacity can also be seen and may reflect the overlap between this disease and capillary hemangiomatosis (Fig. 7.13A, B). Supportive findings include enlargement of the main PA and normal sized or small pulmonary veins.

Pulmonary Capillary Hemangiomatosis

Pulmonary capillary hemangiomatosis (PCH) is a rare cause of PH characterized by an idiopathic proliferation of capillaries within the alveolar walls. It has a similar demographic to PVOD. In fact, PCH and PVOD may be part of a spectrum of the same disease, as there is significant overlap of these entities both clinically

and pathologically. As with PVOD, PCH is often confused clinically with IPAH. As with PVOD, symptoms may worsen after the initiation of vasodilatory therapy.

The most characteristic HRCT finding of PCH is centrilobular nodules of ground glass opacity (Fig. 7.14A, B). These resemble the nodules seen in IPAH, and it is unclear if HRCT is able to make a distinction between these two entities. Other findings include ground glass opacity, pleural effusions, and lymphadenopathy. The presence of smooth interlobular septal thickening may also be seen and likely represents an overlap with PVOD.

Intravenous Injection of Oral Medications

Oral medications contain binders, such as talc or cellulose, that are not absorbed through the gastrointestinal tract. When these medications are injected intravenously, the binders may embolize to the lungs and deposit in small pulmonary arterial branches. Over time, these

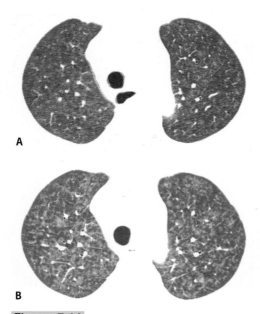

A

B

Figure 7.14

Capillary hemangiomatosis. A. Centrilobular nodules of ground glass opacity are seen in a patient with pulmonary arterial hypertension. **B.** After the initiation of vasodilator therapy, the patient clinically worsened and the nodules became larger and denser.

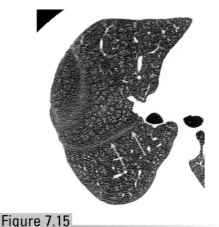

Figure 7.15

Talcosis. Diffuse, small centrilobular nodules are noted. Note sparing of the subpleural lung (*yellow arrows*) reflecting their centrilobular distribution. Some of the centrilobular opacities have a branching appearance (*red arrow*). These are due to injected material embolized in small pulmonary arterial branches and an associated inflammatory reaction and fibrosis.

may induce an inflammatory lung response that causes vascular and lung fibrosis. While this entity is commonly called *talcosis*, talc is but one of many materials contained in oral medications that may cause this disease.

Centrilobular nodules or branching structures are the earliest HRCT manifestations of the intravenous injection of oral medications. These may resemble tree-in-bud opacities (Fig. 7.15). In contrast to infectious causes of tree-in-bud, the nodules or branching opacities are diffuse in distribution, small, and not associated with significant consolidation. Diffuse or symmetric ground glass opacity may also be present, but this finding is nonspecific. Over time, fibrosis may develop in areas affected by nodules. This fibrosis may progress even after the cessation of injection. When fibrosis occurs, irregular reticulation, traction bronchiectasis, and progressive massive fibrosis are seen.

Panlobular emphysema is another manifestation of the intravenous injection of oral

medications. This is most closely associated with the intravenous injection of oral methylphenidate (Ritalin). HRCT shows a diffuse increase in lung lucency and attenuated vessels with a basilar predominance.

Miscellaneous Diseases

There are many other causes of PH including familial pulmonary arterial hypertension, left-sided heart disease, hypoxemia without parenchymal lung disease, vasculitis, liver disease, human immunodeficiency virus, congenital systemic to pulmonary shunts, drugs, sickle cell anemia, and other rare congenital disorders. In most cases, lung findings are either absent or nonspecific and making a correct diagnosis depends on the clinical history. There may be extrapulmonary findings that suggest a specific diagnosis, such as dense bones in patients with sickle cell disease. Findings suggestive of the appropriate diagnosis may be outside the chest, such as a cirrhotic liver. Left-sided heart disease may be accompanied by chamber dilatation or evidence of pulmonary edema such as smooth interlobular septal thickening.

7

VASCULITIS

The term vasculitis refers to a group of systemic disorders that cause inflammation of vessel walls and may eventually lead to vessel dilatation, stenosis, or hemorrhage. Some vasculitis syndromes may have pulmonary manifestations.

Vasculitis is classified by the size of vessels involved: large, medium, or small (Table 7.4). Large vessel vasculitis includes giant cell and Takayasu's arteritis. Medium vessel vasculitis includes polyarteritis nodosa and Kawasaki's disease. Small vessel vasculitis includes Wegener's granulomatosis (also known as granulomatosis with polyangiitis) and microscopic polyangiitis. Other vasculitides that may show pulmonary involvement include Goodpasture syndrome, Churg-Strauss granulomatosis, Behçet's disease, and connective tissue disease.

HRCT Findings

In patients with pulmonary vasculitis, HRCT may show abnormalities of pulmonary arteries or lung parenchyma. In general, large vessel vasculitis shows predominant involvement of the pulmonary arteries and their branches, while small vessel vasculitis shows predominant pulmonary parenchymal involvement. Medium vessel vasculitis only rarely affects the pulmonary arteries or lungs.

Pulmonary arterial involvement may be manifested by stenosis, dilatation, thrombosis, or aneurysm. PA dilatation and aneurysm may eventually lead to rupture and hemorrhage. When stenosis predominates, mosaic perfusion may be present, reflecting regional decreases in blood flow.

Parenchymal manifestations of vasculitis include pulmonary hemorrhage, infarcts, and/or inflammation. Pulmonary hemorrhage results in ground glass opacity or consolidation that is often diffuse, but may, in selected cases, be focal, patchy, or centrilobular. Infarcts and inflammation may appear on HRCT as nodules with or without cavitation. These nodules vary in size from less than 1 to 10 cm or more. Consolidation may also be present.

The vasculitis syndromes that most commonly present with pulmonary manifestations are discussed below.

Table 7.4	Classification of pulmonary vasculitides and their most common HRCT findings	
Size of vessels involved	**Associated diseases**	**HRCT findings**
Large	Takayasu's arteritis	Pulmonary artery wall thickening, thrombosis, stenosis, or obstruction
		Infarcts
		Mosaic perfusion
	Giant cell arteritis	Same as Takayasu's
Medium	Polyarteritis nodosa	Pulmonary involvement rare
	Kawasaki's disease	Pulmonary involvement rare
Small	Wegener's granulomatosis (granulomatosis with polyangiitis)	Nodules often with cavitation
		Hemorrhage
		Patchy consolidation
	Microscopic polyangiitis	Hemorrhage
Miscellaneous	Goodpasture syndrome	Hemorrhage
	Churg-Strauss granulomatosis	Peripheral/lobular consolidation or ground glass opacity
		Centrilobular nodules
		Interlobular septal thickening
	Behçet's disease	Pulmonary artery aneurysms
		Hemorrhage
	Connective tissue disease	Mosaic perfusion

7

Specific Vasculitis Syndromes

Giant Cell and Takayasu's Arteritis

These are both large vessel vasculitides that predominantly affect the large systemic thoracic arteries, including branches of the aorta and carotid arteries. Takayasu's arteritis typically affects women under the age of 40, whereas giant cell arteritis affects patients over the age of 40. Involvement of pulmonary arteries may result in wall thickening, thrombosis, stenosis, or obstruction (Fig. 7.16A, B). Associated mosaic perfusion or infarcts may also be present. Pulmonary arterial aneurysms are less common and likely due to post-stenotic dilatation.

Behçet's Disease

Behçet's disease is a rare disorder characterized by deposition of immune complexes in vessel walls. It presents clinically with oral aphthous ulcers, genital ulcers, uveitis, and skin lesions. It typically occurs in young adults of Turkish or Japanese descent.

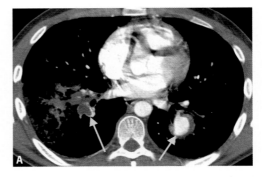

A

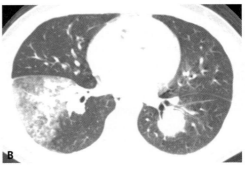

B

Figure 7.17

Behçet's disease. A. Post-contrast CT shows pulmonary artery aneurysms (*arrows*) with both peripheral and central thrombus. **B.** Lung window ground glass opacity around the aneurysm in the right lower lobe from acute hemorrhage.

Behçet's disease shows a predilection for pulmonary arterial involvement and is characterized by PA aneurysms that may rupture and produce hemorrhage (Fig. 7.17A, B). PA thrombosis and thrombosis of thoracic veins (i.e., superior vena cava and brachiocephalic veins) also occur.

Hughes-Stovin syndrome is likely a forme fruste of Behçet's disease in which PA aneurysms and systemic venous thrombosis predominate, but the other clinical manifestations of Behçet's disease are absent. Pulmonary hemorrhage may also occur because of small vessel abnormalities.

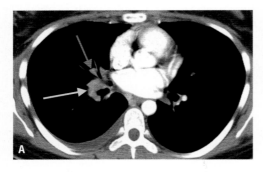

A

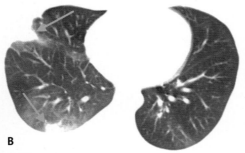

B

Figure 7.16

Takayasu's arteritis. A. Post-contrast CT shows occlusion of the right lower lobe (*yellow arrow*) and right middle lobe (*red arrow*) pulmonary arteries. **B.** Lung windows show infarcts (*blue arrows*) in the affected lobes.

Wegener's Granulomatosis (Granulomatosis with Polyangiitis)

Wegener's granulomatosis (also now referred to as granulomatosis with polyangiitis) is the most common vasculitis to have pulmonary parenchymal manifestations. The most frequently

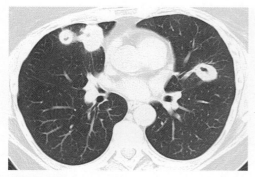

Figure 7.18

Wegener's granulomatosis (granulomatosis with polyangiitis). Several nodules are seen, ranging from 1 to 3 cm in size. Early cavitation is present in two of the nodules. This is the most common manifestation of Wegener's granulomatosis.

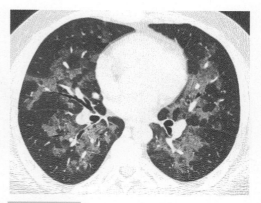

Figure 7.19

Wegener's granulomatosis (granulomatosis with polyangiitis). Symmetric bilateral ground glass opacity is seen as a manifestation of pulmonary hemorrhage in a patient presenting with hemoptysis.

affected organs include the upper respiratory tract, lungs, and kidneys. Serum antineutrophilic cytoplasmic antibody is positive in up to 90% of patients.

The most common HRCT manifestation is pulmonary nodules. These are variable in size from less than 1 cm to large masses and are limited in number when compared with diseases such as miliary tuberculosis, metastases, or sarcoidosis. They have a variable distribution but are usually bilateral. Cavitation is common, particularly with larger nodules (Fig. 7.18).

Ground glass opacity may also be seen in patients with Wegener's granulomatosis, representing pulmonary hemorrhage (Fig. 7.19). The ground glass opacity may be focal, patchy, or diffuse. Consolidation is a less frequent finding and may be a manifestation of hemorrhage or organizing pneumonia (OP). OP is not uncommonly seen pathologically in association with Wegener's. When consolidation is due to OP, it is often peribronchovascular and subpleural (Fig. 7.20).

Microscopic Polyangiitis

Microscopic polyangiitis is a systemic small vessel vasculitis that occurs in middle-aged men. It commonly affects the kidneys, but lung involvement may be seen in up to 30% of patients. Its most common lung manifestation is that of pulmonary hemorrhage. Ground glass opacity and/or consolidation may be

present in a variable distribution, similar to Wegener's granulomatosis.

MISCELLANEOUS VASCULAR DISEASES

Hepatopulmonary Syndrome

Liver dysfunction may result in pulmonary vascular dilatation, causing hypoxemia. This is termed hepatopulmonary syndrome (HPS).

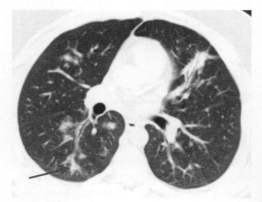

Figure 7.20

Wegener's granulomatosis (granulomatosis with polyangiitis). Patchy, bilateral, peribronchovascular consolidation is present. Pathologically these abnormalities corresponded to areas of organizing pneumonia. This is a rare manifestation of Wegener's granulomatosis.

7

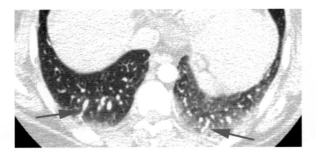

Figure 7.21

Hepatopulmonary syndrome. Enhanced HRCT at the lung bases in a 33-year-old woman with liver disease, platypnea, and orthodeoxia. Dilated vessels (*arrows*) in the posterior lung are typical of hepatopulmonary syndrome.

It is hypothesized that nitric oxide or other vasoactive substances, not metabolized by the liver, have a vasodilatory effect upon the lungs that causes these abnormalities. Patients with liver disease may present with a clinical syndrome that includes hypoxemia, platypnea (dyspnea with sitting up) and orthodeoxia (desaturation with sitting up). Dilated vessels at the lung bases are better perfused with sitting, and shunting increases in this position.

In patients with HPS, HRCT typically shows dilated vessels, 1 to 2 mm in diameter, in the lung periphery, particularly in the lower lobes (Fig. 7.21). The dilated vessels in patients with HPS may extend to the pleural surface. The severity of vascular dilatation correlates with the severity of hypoxemia, but not all patients with HPS will show this finding. In 15% of cases of HPS, frank arteriovenous fistulas are present. Angiography is likely more sensitive than HRCT in the detection of these abnormalities.

Metastatic Calcification

Metastatic calcification occurs in disorders that lead to abnormal calcium or phosphorus metabolism. It is most frequently seen in patients with renal failure. Other disorders with which it is associated include hyperparathyroidism, osseous malignancies, and hypervitaminosis D. In these conditions, calcium is deposited within the lung interstitium adjacent to pulmonary vessels. Most patients are asymptomatic, even with extensive disease; however, this disorder may occasionally lead to symptoms and even death.

Typical HRCT findings include centrilobular nodules of ground glass opacity. The nodules are symmetric bilaterally and variable in size but may eventually involve the entire pulmonary lobule (Fig. 7.22A, B). The process is usually upper lobe predominant. Frank calcification may or may not be seen.

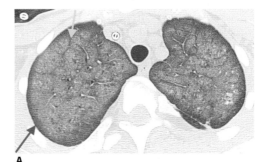

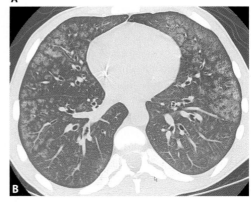

Figure 7.22

Metastatic calcification. A. Symmetric bilateral ground glass opacity is present. Note sparing of the subpleural region (*red arrow*) reflecting a centrilobular distribution. Linear areas of sparing represent the interlobular septa at the periphery of the lobules (*yellow arrow*). **B.** Findings in the mid-lung are much less severe but show the lobular nature of the ground glass opacity.

FURTHER READING

Bergin CJ, Rios G, King MA, Belezzuoli E, Luna J, Auger WR. Accuracy of high-resolution CT in identifying chronic pulmonary thromboembolic disease. *AJR Am J Roentgenol.* 1996;166:1371-1377.

Connolly B, Manson D, Eberhard A, et al. CT appearance of pulmonary vasculitis in children. *AJR Am J Roentgenol.* 1996;167:901-904.

Cordier JF, Valeyre D, Guillevin L, et al. Pulmonary Wegener's granulomatosis. A clinical and imaging study of 77 cases. *Chest.* 1990;97:906-912.

Engelke C, Schaefer-Prokop C, Schirg E, Freihorst J, Grubnic S, Prokop M. High-resolution CT and CT angiography of peripheral pulmonary vascular disorders. *Radiographics.* 2002;22:739-764.

Hansell DM. Small-vessel diseases of the lung: CT-pathologic correlates. *Radiology.* 2002; 225:639-653.

Hiller N, Lieberman S, Chajek-Shaul T, Bar-Ziv J, Shaham D. Thoracic manifestations of Behcet disease at CT. *Radiographics.* 2004;24:801-808.

Hoffman GS, Kerr GS, Leavitt RY, et al. Wegener granulomatosis: an analysis of 158 patients. *Ann Intern Med.* 1992;116:488-498.

Lee KN, Lee HJ, Shin WW, Webb WR. Hypoxemia and liver cirrhosis (hepatopulmonary syndrome) in eight patients: comparison of the central and peripheral pulmonary vasculature. *Radiology.* 1999;211:549-553.

Lee KS, Kim TS, Fujimoto K, et al. Thoracic manifestation of Wegener's granulomatosis: CT findings in 30 patients. *Eur Radiol.* 2003;13:43-51.

Marten K, Schnyder P, Schirg E, Prokop M, Rummeny EJ, Engelke C. Pattern-based differential diagnosis in pulmonary vasculitis using volumetric CT. *AJR Am J Roentgenol.* 2005;184:720-733.

Ng CS, Wells AU, Padley SP. A CT sign of chronic pulmonary arterial hypertension: the ratio of main pulmonary artery to aortic diameter. *J Thorac Imaging.* 1999;14:270-278.

Primack SL, Müller NL, Mayo JR, Remy-Jardin M, Remy J. Pulmonary parenchymal abnormalities of vascular origin: high-resolution CT findings. *Radiographics.* 1994;14:739-746.

Reuter M, Schnabel A, Wesner F, et al. Pulmonary Wegener's granulomatosis: correlation between high-resolution CT findings and clinical scoring of disease activity. *Chest.* 1998;114:500-506.

Schwickert HC, Schweden F, Schild HH, et al. Pulmonary arteries and lung parenchyma in chronic pulmonary embolism: preoperative and postoperative CT findings. *Radiology.* 1994;191:351-357.

Seo JB, Im JG, Chung JW, et al. Pulmonary vasculitis: the spectrum of radiological findings. *Br J Radiol.* 2000;73:1224-1231.

Tunaci A, Berkmen YM, Gokmen E. Thoracic involvement in Behcet's disease: pathologic, clinical, and imaging features. *AJR Am J Roentgenol.* 1995;164:51-56.

Weir IH, Müller NL, Chiles C, et al. Wegener's granulomatosis: findings from computed tomography of the chest in 10 patients. *Can Assoc Radiol J.* 1992;43:31-34.

Pulmonary Edema, Diffuse Alveolar Damage, the Acute Respiratory Distress Syndrome, and Pulmonary Hemorrhage

PULMONARY EDEMA

Fluid accumulation in the lungs may be the result of changes in pulmonary venous hydrostatic pressure, increased permeability of capillary endothelium, or a combination of these two. The HRCT features of these two processes show significant overlap and are often difficult to distinguish. The most important role of HRCT is in making a distinction between edema and other causes of pulmonary symptoms, such as pneumonia.

Hydrostatic Pulmonary Edema

An alteration of the hydrostatic or oncotic pressure within pulmonary capillaries may result in pulmonary edema. Increased hydrostatic pressure is significantly more common and usually results from pulmonary venous hypertension due to left heart disease. Left heart failure and valvular heart disease are the most frequent causes. Decreased oncotic pressure due to low albumin may also result in edema accumulation, but this is less common.

The HRCT findings of hydrostatic pulmonary edema associated with pulmonary venous hypertension are shown in Table 8.1. Hydrostatic pulmonary edema may be interstitial or alveolar. These may both be associated with vascular congestion in which the pulmonary veins are enlarged, particularly in the upper lobes, and both are typically diffuse or symmetrical.

Interstitial Pulmonary Edema

Edema fluid may accumulate within the interlobular septa, subpleural interstitium, and peribronchovascular interstitium.

On HRCT, edema fluid within the interlobular septa appears as smooth interlobular septal thickening (Fig. 8.1). Keep in mind that a few interlobular septa may be seen in normal patients. However, when multiple, easily seen, interlobular septa are visible, the septa are abnormally thickened. Interlobular septal thickening can be diagnosed if visible reticular

Table 8.1	HRCT findings of pulmonary venous hypertension
Stage of pulmonary venous hypertension	**HRCT finding**
Vascular congestion	Enlarged pulmonary veins Upper lobe vessels particularly involved
Interstitial edema	Smooth interlobular septal thickening Subpleural edema (thickening of fissures) Peribronchovascular interstitial thickening Typically diffuse or symmetric
Alveolar edema	Ground glass opacity and consolidation Typically diffuse or symmetric

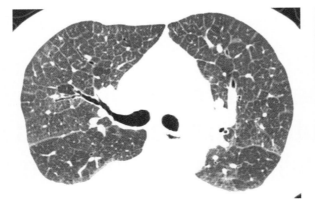

Figure 8.1

Pulmonary edema with smooth interlobular septal and fissural thickening. Multiple, smooth, thin, interconnecting linear opacities are noted, outlining polygonal structures, which can be identified as pulmonary lobules because of their characteristic size and shape and the presence of a centrilobular artery. These are the interlobular septa that marginate the pulmonary lobule. Pulmonary edema is the most common cause of this finding. Thickening of the major fissures is also seen.

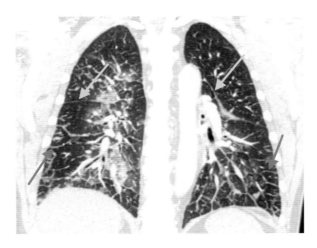

Figure 8.2

Pulmonary edema with interlobular septal and fissural thickening. Coronal reformatted CT shows thickening of the fissures (*yellow arrows*). This represents fluid in the subpleural interstitium. Smooth interlobular septal thickening is also noted (*red arrows*) in this patient with interstitial pulmonary edema.

opacities outline what can be recognized as pulmonary lobules because of their typical size and polygonal shape. Centrilobular arteries may be seen as small dots at the center of these polygonal structures. Interlobular septal thickening as a result of edema is often best seen in the upper lobes, because septa are best developed in this location. Subpleural edema (Fig. 8.2), equivalent to interlobular septal thickening, may be seen as thickening of fissures.

Edema fluid may also accumulate in the peribronchovascular interstitium. This may be the result of lymphatic drainage of edema fluid to the hila. On HRCT, thickening of the interstitium surrounding the central bronchi gives the appearance of bronchial wall thickening and a corresponding increase in the diameter of pulmonary arteries (Fig. 8.3).

Smooth interlobular septal and peribronchovascular interstitial thickening are often

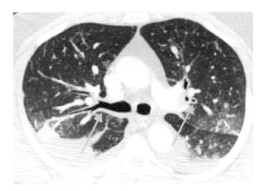

Figure 8.3

Pulmonary edema with peribronchovascular interstitial thickening. Fluid is seen in the interstitium adjacent to or surrounding the bronchi and arteries (*arrows*). This is easily confused with bronchial wall thickening. Note the lack of narrowing of the lumen of the bronchi. Ground glass opacity and pleural effusion are also present.

8

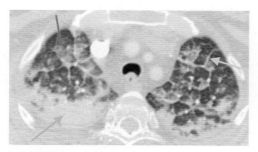

Figure 8.4

Interstitial and alveolar pulmonary edema.
Smooth interlobular septal thickening (*yellow arrow*)
is seen as a manifestation of interstitial pulmonary
edema. Additionally, there is patchy bilateral ground
glass opacity (*red arrow*) and consolidation (*blue
arrow*) compatible with alveolar edema. Abnormalities
of both interstitial and alveolar edema often coexist.

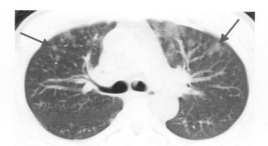

Figure 8.6

Pulmonary edema with centrilobular nodules.
Ill-defined centrilobular nodules of ground glass
opacity (*arrows*) are seen in the anterior lungs
bilaterally. This is not an uncommon manifestation
of edema and is often seen in association with
other findings of alveolar edema.

seen in association with findings of alveolar
edema (Fig. 8.4). Their distribution is quite
variable, but findings tend to be bilateral and
relatively symmetric. While edema is often
most severe in the dependent lung regions,
this is not a constant feature.

Alveolar Edema

Severe pulmonary edema results in alveolar
flooding. Ground glass opacity and consolidation are the most common findings (Fig. 8.5).
Ground glass opacity nodules may also be seen
in a centrilobular distribution (Fig. 8.6). Findings
of both interstitial and alveolar edema frequently
coexist. Ground glass opacity may be associated

with smooth interlobular septal or peribronchovascular interstitial thickening. A combination
of ground glass opacity and interlobular septal
thickening in the same lung regions, the crazy
paving sign, is not uncommon (Fig. 8.7).

Distribution of Hydrostatic Edema

The distribution of these abnormalities is
typically diffuse or symmetric. More severe
abnormalities may be seen in the dependent

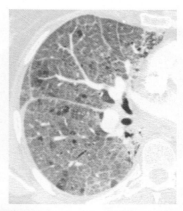

Figure 8.7

Pulmonary edema with crazy paving.
A combination of ground glass opacity and smooth
interlobular septal thickening is seen in the right
lung. This finding is nonspecific, but pulmonary
edema is one of the most common causes of this
pattern in the acute setting.

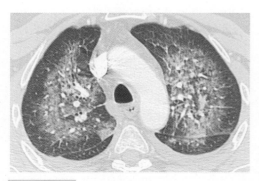

Figure 8.5

**Pulmonary edema with symmetric ground glass
opacity.** Symmetric parahilar ground glass opacity
is seen as a manifestation of pulmonary edema.
Edema is classically symmetric in distribution.

8

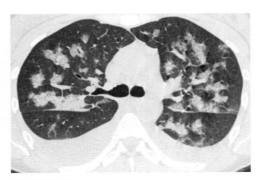

Figure 8.8

Pulmonary edema with lobular opacities.
Lobular areas of ground glass opacity are present.
The process is symmetric and associated with
pleural effusions. Occasionally, causes of alveolar
disease such as pulmonary edema may be very
geographic such as in this case.

lung because of the normal hydrostatic gradient, but this is not always present.

A patchy or lobular distribution of abnormalities may sometimes be present (Fig. 8.8), and in some patients, edema may be asymmetric (Fig. 8.9). Causes of asymmetric or focal pulmonary edema include the following:

1. *Patient position.* Pulmonary edema may occur in dependent lung regions because

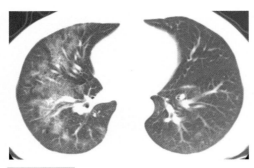

Figure 8.9

Asymmetric pulmonary edema. While edema
is typically a symmetric process, unilateral or
asymmetric edema is not uncommon. This patient
was placed in a right side down decubitus position
for a surgical procedure, explaining the unilateral
right-sided edema. Patchy ground glass opacity
and crazy paving are visible.

of gravitational effects. Patient positioning may have an influence on the location of pulmonary edema. For example, right-sided pulmonary edema may be seen in patients who lay on their right side while sleeping.

2. *Asymmetric emphysema/bullous disease.* Emphysema, particularly when associated with bulla, may be asymmetric. Edema will show relative sparing of areas of emphysema and will appear more severe on the contralateral side.

3. *Mitral regurgitation.* Focal right upper lobe pulmonary edema may occur in the setting of mitral regurgitation, particularly when associated with acute papillary muscle rupture after a myocardial infarction. The regurgitant jet is directed into the right superior pulmonary vein.

4. *Pulmonary embolism or vascular obstruction.* In patients with pulmonary embolism or other causes of pulmonary artery obstruction, edema predominates in well-perfused lung regions and may appear patchy.

5. *Neurogenic pulmonary edema.* An unusual distribution of pulmonary edema may be seen in patients with intracranial abnormalities associated with trauma, hemorrhage, or seizure. The exact mechanism by which this occurs is poorly understood, but it often occurs in patients without heart disease. Approximately 50% of patients show focal bilateral upper lobe abnormalities, while the remainder of the cases are indistinguishable from other causes of pulmonary edema. Opacities may show rapid shifting from one location to another, a feature uncommon in pulmonary edema from other causes.

Differential Diagnosis

In the acute setting, pulmonary edema is the most common cause of isolated smooth interlobular septal thickening. Lymphangitic spread of tumor is another cause of this abnormality, but such patients often have a history of malignancy or have chronic and progressive symptoms.

Interlobular septal thickening that is not an isolated or predominant feature is

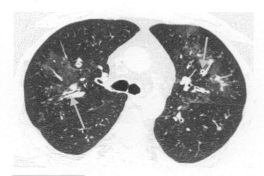

Figure 8.10

Bronchial wall thickening in a patient with airways disease. Thickening of the bronchial wall may resemble fluid in the peribronchovascular interstitium. When narrowing of the airway lumen is present (*arrows*), bronchial wall thickening is the likely etiology.

nonspecific and should be ignored in formulating a differential diagnosis. Some septal thickening is present in a variety of lung diseases.

Peribronchovascular interstitial thickening is easily confused with bronchial wall thickening from bronchial inflammation. When mucous impaction or luminal narrowing is present, bronchial inflammation is the most likely cause (Fig. 8.10).

Ground glass opacity and consolidation are nonspecific findings in the acute setting and may be seen with infection, aspiration, diffuse alveolar damage (DAD), and hemorrhage. The diagnosis is driven by the clinical presentation, rather than the HRCT findings. When ground glass opacity is associated with significant smooth interlobular septal thickening, however, pulmonary edema is the most likely etiology.

Increased Permeability Edema Without DAD

Increased permeability edema results from injury to the capillary endothelium with increased capillary permeability. It is usually associated with DAD. Increased permeability edema unassociated with DAD is uncommon and usually is seen in association with drugs, transfusion reactions, toxic shock syndrome, air embolism, and Hantavirus pulmonary syndrome. The HRCT findings closely mimic those of hydrostatic pulmonary edema with smooth interlobular septal thickening and ground glass opacity.

Increased Permeability Edema with DAD

Increased permeability edema is often, but not always, associated with DAD. The histologic findings in DAD vary with the time interval between injury and biopsy. The acute, exudative stage shows pulmonary edema, hyaline membranes, and acute interstitial inflammation. In the subacute, proliferative, or organizing stage, there is fibroblast proliferation within the interstitium and airspaces. In the chronic, fibrotic stage, typically 2 weeks or more after the injury, there is progressive fibrosis with collagen deposition. When edema and DAD coexist, the HRCT appearance is usually that of DAD.

DAD is the primary pathologic finding seen in patients with acute respiratory distress syndrome (ARDS). However, not all patients with DAD will meet criteria for ARDS; thus, DAD is a more accurate term to use when describing HRCT abnormalities. ARDS is a clinical syndrome characterized by the following:

1. Known inciting cause
2. Acute onset of symptoms
3. Bilateral opacities on chest x-ray
4. Pulmonary artery wedge pressure ≤18 mm Hg or absence of clinical evidence of left atrial hypertension
5. Ratio of partial pressure of oxygen in arterial blood to fraction of inspired oxygen (Pao_2/Fio_2) ≤200

The causes of DAD and ARDS are the same. They can be divided into systemic processes and processes that directly involve the lungs. Systemic processes resulting in DAD and ARDS include sepsis, shock, disseminated intravascular coagulation, drugs, pancreatitis, and severe burns. Processes that involve the lungs and result in DAD and ARDS include pneumonia, aspiration, trauma, and toxic inhalations. DAD without a known inciting cause is termed *acute interstitial pneumonia* or

Table 8.2	HRCT findings of diffuse alveolar damage
Early	Diffuse or symmetric ground glass opacity and consolidation May show peripheral distribution Lack of interlobular septal thickening
Late	Fibrosis (irregular reticulation, traction bronchiectasis, honeycombing) Anterior/subpleural distribution

Hamman-Rich syndrome. This is discussed in more detail in Chapter 9.

The HRCT findings of DAD/ARDS (Table 8.2) resemble hydrostatic pulmonary edema, although some differences exist. Diffuse or symmetric consolidation and ground glass opacity are most characteristic (Fig. 8.11). In early stages of DAD, these abnormalities may have a peripheral distribution, but abnormalities eventually become diffuse and confluent. Abnormalities are usually more severe in the dependent lung (Fig. 8.11). Asymmetric or focal abnormalities may be seen in patients with a pulmonary cause of DAD/ARDS, such as pneumonia. Interlobular septal thickening is characteristically absent.

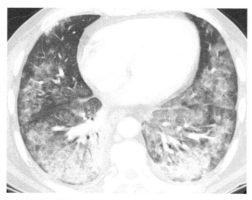

Figure 8.11

Acute respiratory distress syndrome. Diffuse consolidation and ground glass opacity are present in a patient with diffuse alveolar damage and acute respiratory distress syndrome (ARDS) resulting from sepsis. While a nonspecific pattern, this appearance is typical of ARDS. Note more severe involvement of the periphery of the lung and in dependent lung regions.

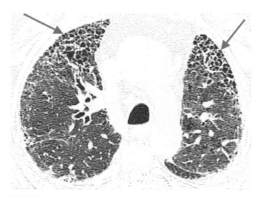

Figure 8.12

Post-ARDS fibrosis. Patients who survive an episode of acute respiratory distress syndrome may develop fibrosis as a sequela. This fibrosis typically has an anterior distribution. Typical findings include irregular reticulation, traction bronchiectasis, and/or honeycombing (*arrows*).

In patients who survive, consolidation may eventually be replaced by ground glass opacity, reticulation, traction bronchiectasis, honeycombing, and architectural distortion. Fibrosis in patients with DAD/ARDS classically has an anterior and peripheral distribution (Fig. 8.12). It is hypothesized that dependent atelectasis protects the posterior lung from developing fibrosis that is due to barotrauma and high inspired oxygen levels.

On HRCT, the differential diagnosis of DAD includes other causes of extensive consolidation such as hydrostatic pulmonary edema, infection, and hemorrhage. There is significant overlap of the findings in these diseases and, not infrequently, more than one process is present. Early DAD may have a peripheral distribution as opposed to pulmonary edema, which is typically diffuse or central. Significant smooth interlobular septal thickening suggests pulmonary edema rather than DAD. Centrilobular nodules of soft tissue attenuation, airways inflammation, and tree-in-bud opacities suggest infection.

PULMONARY HEMORRHAGE

Pulmonary hemorrhage may be diffuse or focal. Focal pulmonary hemorrhage is usually due to localized lung abnormalities, and an identifiable

8

cause may be visualized. Diffuse pulmonary hemorrhage is often due to systemic processes, and making a specific diagnosis based upon HRCT findings is challenging. As the HRCT findings overlap significantly with those of other diseases, correlation with the patient's clinical symptoms is important. Patients with pulmonary hemorrhage may present with hemoptysis, but this is not always the case.

Focal Pulmonary Hemorrhage

Findings of focal hemorrhage include consolidation, ground glass opacity, and centrilobular nodules. The cause of the focal pulmonary hemorrhage may be associated with specific HRCT abnormalities that lead to diagnosis (Fig. 8.13). Examples of diagnosable causes of focal hemorrhage include bronchiectasis, malignancy, trauma, pneumonia, cavitary lung disease, mycetoma, and thromboembolic disease. The pulmonary abnormality determines the likely diagnosis.

HRCT may also be useful in localizing the approximate site of hemorrhage prior to angiography or bronchoscopy. Volumetric HRCT is optimal in this setting.

Diffuse Pulmonary Hemorrhage

Diffuse pulmonary hemorrhage is rare and most commonly secondary to systemic disorders

Table 8.3	Causes of diffuse pulmonary hemorrhage

Vasculitis (Wegener's granulomatosis, microscopic polyangiitis, immune complex vasculitis, Henoch-Schönlein purpura)
Connective tissue disease
Drugs
Goodpasture syndrome
Antiphospholipid syndrome
Anticoagulation and coagulation disorders
Idiopathic pulmonary hemosiderosis

(Table 8.3). Examples include Goodpasture syndrome, idiopathic pulmonary hemosiderosis (IPH), pulmonary vasculitis (Chapter 7), connective tissue disease (Chapter 10), drugs (Chapter 15), and disorders of coagulation or their treatment. In many of these cases, diffuse hemorrhage may be the only lung manifestation of disease, and findings that suggest a specific diagnosis are absent.

HRCT findings include diffuse or symmetric ground glass opacity progressing to consolidation (Fig. 8.14). Ground glass may be lobular in distribution. Additionally, centrilobular nodules of ground glass opacity may be present in isolation or may be associated with more diffuse hemorrhage (Fig. 8.15). Smooth interlobular septal thickening may be seen in

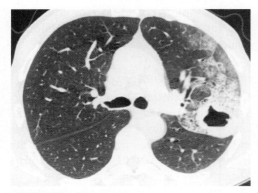

Figure 8.13

Focal pulmonary hemorrhage. HRCT may be used to identify a source of bleeding in patients with hemoptysis. Focal ground glass opacity and consolidation are present in the left upper lobe surrounding a cavitary bronchogenic carcinoma.

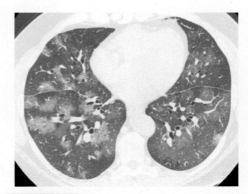

Figure 8.14

Diffuse pulmonary hemorrhage. Patchy bilateral ground glass opacity is seen as a manifestation of diffuse pulmonary hemorrhage in a patient with systemic lupus erythematosus.

8

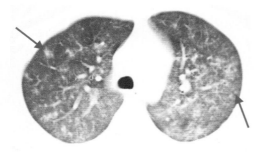

Figure 8.15

Pulmonary hemorrhage with centrilobular nodules. Nodules of ground glass opacity (*arrows*) may be a manifestation of pulmonary hemorrhage and are often associated with more generalized ground glass opacity. The centrilobular distribution may reflect bleeding around the centrilobular artery or blood spreading via the airways.

association with ground glass opacity (i.e., the crazy paving pattern) (Fig. 8.16). Isolated septal thickening is uncommon.

HRCT findings show significant overlap with other causes of diffuse ground glass opacity such as pulmonary edema, DAD, and atypical infections.

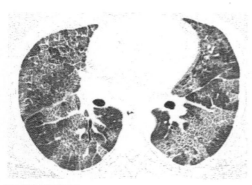

Figure 8.16

Pulmonary hemorrhage with crazy paving. A combination of ground glass opacity and smooth interlobular septal thickening is seen in a patient with pulmonary hemorrhage from vasculitis. Other causes of the crazy paving pattern in the acute setting include edema, atypical infection, and diffuse alveolar damage.

Goodpasture Syndrome

This is an autoimmune disorder characterized by antibodies against the glomerular basement membrane. It primarily affects the kidneys and lungs. A pulmonary capillaritis results, with pulmonary hemorrhage.

The combination of renal and pulmonary disease in Goodpasture syndrome is most common in young males, 20 to 30 years of age. Isolated renal disease may be seen in elderly females, 60 to 70 years of age.

The HRCT findings are identical to other causes of pulmonary hemorrhage. Ground glass opacity and consolidation are most often diffuse, but may be asymmetric or focal.

Idiopathic Pulmonary Hemosiderosis

IPH is a rare disease of unknown origin characterized by recurrent episodes of diffuse pulmonary hemorrhage without associated glomerulonephritis or a serologic abnormality. IPH most commonly occurs in children or young adults. IPH may sometimes be associated with conditions such as milk allergy, immunoglobulin A gammopathy, and exposure to toxic mold.

IPH is a diagnosis of exclusion in which there is no evidence of other causes of pulmonary hemorrhage, such as Wegener's granulomatosis (also termed granulomatosis with polyangiitis). HRCT findings are the same as Goodpasture syndrome and other causes of diffuse pulmonary hemorrhage.

Immune Complex Small Vessel Vasculitis

Systemic diseases may be associated with circulating immune complexes. When these deposit in the walls of pulmonary vessels, capillaritis results that may lead to diffuse pulmonary hemorrhage. Circulating immune complexes are characteristic of collagen vascular disease, Henoch-Schönlein purpura, mixed cryoglobulinemia, antiphospholipid syndrome, IgA nephropathy, and Behçet's syndrome. The HRCT findings are identical to other causes of diffuse pulmonary hemorrhage.

FURTHER READING

Akyar S, Ozbek SS. Computed tomography findings in idiopathic pulmonary hemosiderosis. *Respiration.* 1993;60:63-64.

Cheah FK, Sheppard MN, Hansell DM. Computed tomography of diffuse pulmonary haemorrhage with pathological correlation. *Clin Radiol.* 1993;48:89-93.

Collard HR, Schwarz MI. Diffuse alveolar hemorrhage. *Clin Chest Med.* 2004;25:583-592.

Desai SR, Wells AU, Rubens MB, Evans TW, Hansell DM. Acute respiratory distress syndrome: CT abnormalities at long-term follow-up. *Radiology.* 1999;210:29-35.

Gluecker T, Capasso P, Schnyder P, et al. Clinical and radiologic features of pulmonary edema. *Radiographics.* 1999;19:1507-1531.

Goodman LR. Congestive heart failure and adult respiratory distress syndrome. New insights using computed tomography. *Radiol Clin North Am.* 1996;34:33-46.

Goodman LR, Fumagalli R, Tagliabue P, et al. Adult respiratory distress syndrome due to pulmonary and extrapulmonary causes: CT, clinical, and functional correlations. *Radiology.* 1999;213:545-552.

Hartman TE, Müller NL, Primack SL, et al. Metastatic pulmonary calcification in patients with hypercalcemia: findings on chest radiographs and CT scans. *AJR Am J Roentgenol.* 1994;162:799-802.

Ioachimescu OC, Sieber S, Kotch A. Idiopathic pulmonary haemosiderosis revisited. *Eur Respir J.* 2004;24:162-170.

Johkoh T, Ikezoe J, Nagareda T, et al. Metastatic pulmonary calcification: early detection by high-resolution CT. *J Comput Assist Tomogr.* 1993;17:471-473.

Ketai LH, Godwin JD. A new view of pulmonary edema and acute respiratory distress syndrome. *J Thorac Imaging.* 1998;13:147-171.

Mayberry JP, Primack SL, Müller NL. Thoracic manifestations of systemic autoimmune diseases: radiographic and high-resolution CT findings. *Radiographics.* 2000;20:1623-1635.

Primack SL, Miller RR, Müller NL. Diffuse pulmonary hemorrhage: clinical, pathologic, and imaging features. *AJR Am J Roentgenol.* 1995;164:295-300.

Storto ML, Kee ST, Golden JA, Webb WR. Hydrostatic pulmonary edema: high-resolution CT findings. *AJR Am J Roentgenol.* 1995;165:817-820.

8

The Interstitial Pneumonias

The interstitial pneumonias (IPs), or idiopathic interstitial pneumonias (IIPs), are a heterogeneous group of diffuse lung diseases characterized by varying degrees of lung inflammation and fibrosis. They are best thought of as reactions to lung injury, presenting with specific histologic patterns. They are loosely unified by several characteristics including clinical presentation, radiographic manifestations, and pathologic appearance and may be idiopathic or associated with specific diseases. In this chapter, we intend to provide a general understanding of the IPs and the idiopathic clinical disorders with which they may be associated.

CLASSIFICATION

The IPs were originally classified by Liebow in the 1960s. They have been redefined and reclassified several times as an understanding of their patterns has been refined. While some of the terms in the original classification have remained the same, others have been changed or deleted. For instance, giant cell IP was part of the original classification of IPs, but has since been recognized to be a specific entity, namely hard metal pneumoconiosis; it is no longer considered an IP.

It is important to recognize that the IPs are defined as histologic patterns and not diseases. Each pattern may be the result of an idiopathic clinical syndrome (thus representing an IIP) or may be associated with a specific disease, and not be idiopathic. The current classification is shown in Table 9.1.

The IPs include usual interstitial pneumonia (UIP), nonspecific interstitial pneumonia (NSIP), organizing pneumonia (OP), desquamative interstitial pneumonia (DIP), lymphoid interstitial pneumonia (LIP), and diffuse alveolar damage (DAD) with acute interstitial pneumonia (AIP). DIP, along with respiratory bronchiolitis interstitial lung disease (RB-ILD), is usually related to smoking and is also discussed in Chapter 11. LIP is best thought of as a lymphoproliferative disorder that will be discussed in detail in Chapter 17.

HRCT IN THE IPs

In the interpretation of HRCT in a patient with a suspected IP, it is important to understand the relationship between the imaging pattern and the pathology and clinical syndrome present. In classic cases, the HRCT pattern may be used to predict the pathologic pattern.

Take, for example, UIP. When classic findings of UIP are present on HRCT (i.e., we say a "UIP pattern" is present), there is a high degree of certainty that a surgical lung biopsy will also show UIP. However, several different diseases may be associated with a UIP pattern. If idiopathic, UIP is considered to represent idiopathic pulmonary fibrosis (IPF). On the other hand, UIP may be associated with connective tissue diseases, drug toxicity, and asbestosis. These may be indistinguishable radiographically and pathologically. Clinical correlation is important in distinguishing the various causes of a UIP pattern.

Table 9.1 Classification of interstitial pneumonia

Histologic pattern	Idiopathic clinical syndrome	Associated diseases or conditions
Usual interstitial pneumonia	Idiopathic pulmonary fibrosis	Connective tissue disease, drug toxicity, asbestosis
Nonspecific interstitial pneumonia (NSIP)	Idiopathic NSIP	Connective tissue disease, drug toxicity, hypersensitivity pneumonitis
Organizing pneumonia	Cryptogenic organizing pneumonia	Drugs, infections, toxic inhalations
Desquamative interstitial pneumonia (DIP)/respiratory bronchiolitis interstitial lung disease	Idiopathic DIP	Cigarette smoking, toxic fumes
Diffuse alveolar damage	Acute interstitial pneumonia	Known causes of acute respiratory distress syndrome
Lymphoid interstitial pneumonia (LIP)	Idiopathic LIP	Connective tissue disease, immunodeficiency

The IPs are a common cause of diffuse lung disease and should be considered as a possible etiology whenever a patient has chronic symptoms or findings of fibrosis or lung infiltration on HRCT. The HRCT findings vary depending upon the degree of inflammation or fibrosis that is present. Cases that are predominantly inflammatory result in ground glass opacity and consolidation. Cases that are predominantly fibrotic are associated with irregular reticulation, traction bronchiectasis, and/or honeycombing.

Most of the IPs present at the extremes of this spectrum (Fig. 9.1A, B), although there may be significant components of both inflammation and fibrosis present in selected cases. UIP is a pattern characterized predominantly by fibrosis. NSIP may be fibrotic, cellular, or a combination of both. The remaining IPs are predominantly inflammatory, although they may show progression to fibrosis in some cases.

Distribution can be helpful in distinguishing the IPs from alternative causes of diffuse lung disease (Fig. 9.2A, B). UIP, NSIP, and DIP often demonstrate a subpleural predominance of abnormalities, with involvement of the lung bases, including the costophrenic angles. Other causes of diffuse lung disease, such as hypersensitivity pneumonitis (HP), are often diffuse or

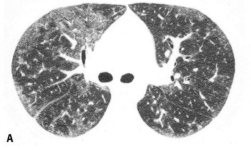
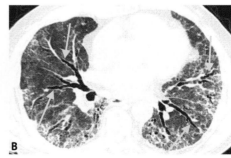

A   B

Figure 9.1

Inflammation versus fibrosis on HRCT. The interstitial pneumonias present with varying degrees of inflammation and fibrosis. Two patients with nonspecific interstitial pneumonia from connective tissue disease are depicted. **A.** HRCT shows ground glass opacity without definite signs of fibrosis, representing potentially reversible inflammatory abnormalities. **B.** HRCT shows fibrosis as manifested by traction bronchiectasis (*arrows*) and irregular reticulation. These findings reflect irreversible lung scarring that would be unresponsive to treatment.

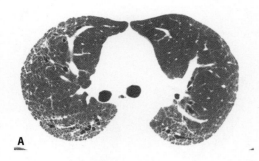

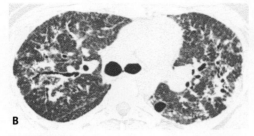

Figure 9.2

Distribution of HRCT abnormalities in diagnosis.
A. In this patient with fibrotic nonspecific interstitial pneumonia (NSIP) related to scleroderma, HRCT shows a peripheral and subpleural predominance of abnormalities. **B.** HRCT in a patient with sarcoidosis shows central and peribronchial abnormalities, with relative sparing of the subpleural lung. In the setting of chronic symptoms, a subpleural and basilar predominance of abnormalities suggests usual interstitial pneumonia, NSIP, or desquamative interstitial pneumonia. A diffuse or central axial distribution is atypical for an interstitial pneumonia and suggests alternative diseases such as hypersensitivity pneumonitis or sarcoidosis.

central in axial distribution and show sparing of the inferior costophrenic angles.

USUAL INTERSTITIAL PNEUMONIA

UIP (Table 9.2) is common and accounts for approximately 50% of cases of IP. Pathologically, patients with UIP have irreversible fibrosis with heterogeneous involvement of the lung. Areas of normal lung are intermixed with areas of end-stage fibrosis. As UIP represents irreversible fibrosis, affected lung regions do not show improvement with immunosuppressive medications.

The most common disease associated with UIP is IPF, but there are several specific diseases that may also result in this pattern.

HRCT Findings

In patients with UIP, HRCT typically shows reticulation with a subpleural and basilar predominance. The reticular opacities are often irregular in appearance. Traction bronchiectasis is often associated with the reticular opacities. Honeycombing is present in about 70% of cases and is critical in making a definite diagnosis of UIP (Fig. 9.3A–D). Honeycombing results in the presence of clustered, cystic airspaces, with well-defined walls, usually 3 to 10 mm in diameter, and predominating in the subpleural lung. As with the overall extent of abnormalities, honeycombing, when present, is most severe and extensive at the lung bases (Fig. 9.4A–E).

Table 9.2	Features of usual interstitial pneumonia
Frequency	Most common interstitial pneumonia; 50% of cases
HRCT findings	Subpleural, basilar predominant
	Honeycombing
	Other signs of fibrosis (traction bronchiectasis, irregular reticulation)
	Absence of mosaic perfusion, air trapping, diffuse nodules, ground glass opacity outside of areas of fibrosis
Idiopathic syndrome	Idiopathic pulmonary fibrosis
Associated diseases	Connective tissue disease
	Drug toxicity (rare)
	Asbestosis (rare)
	Hypersensitivity pneumonitis (usually has HRCT findings atypical for usual interstitial pneumonia [UIP])
	Sarcoidosis (usually has HRCT findings atypical for UIP)

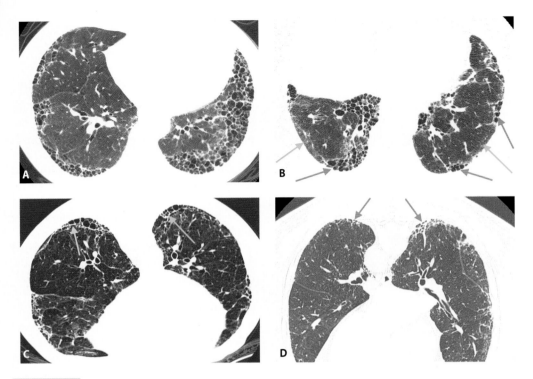

Figure 9.3

Usual interstitial pneumonia (UIP). A. Extensive subpleural and basilar predominant honeycombing is noted in a patient with a UIP pattern associated with idiopathic pulmonary fibrosis. **B.** Subpleural honeycombing (*red arrows*) is present in a patchy distribution. This is interspersed with areas of relatively normal lung (*blue arrows*). **C.** Prone HRCT shows honeycombing (*arrows*) in a patient with UIP. Honeycombing may be in a single (*yellow arrow*) or multiple (*blue arrow*) layers. **D.** Early UIP shows mild subpleural reticulation and honeycombing. A confident diagnosis of honeycombing (*arrows*) can be made in this case despite the mild abnormalities.

In patients with early or mild UIP, only reticulation or reticulation with traction bronchiectasis is visible on HRCT. With progressive or severe lung involvement, honeycombing is also present.

Ground glass opacities are common in UIP, but are less extensive than areas of fibrosis. Ground glass opacity is usually seen in lung regions that also show findings of fibrosis (i.e., reticulation, traction bronchiectasis, or honeycombing) and, in UIP, typically reflects the presence of microscopic fibrosis.

Although the upper lobes are usually abnormal in patients with UIP, findings of fibrosis predominate in the lung bases, and the posterior costophrenic angles are almost always involved. The findings of fibrosis are often patchy in distribution, but involve the posterior and subpleural lung to the greatest degree.

When typical HRCT findings of UIP are present on HRCT, the appearance is termed a *UIP pattern*. According to criteria recently agreed upon by American, European, Japanese, and Latin American societies (Table 9.3), the HRCT diagnosis of a ***UIP pattern*** can be based on (1) the presence of a basal and subpleural predominance of abnormalities, (2) reticular opacities, (3) honeycombing with or without traction bronchiectasis, and (4) an absence of findings inconsistent with this diagnosis. This combination of findings predicts a pathologic diagnosis of UIP in 95% to 100% of cases. However, keep in mind that not all cases of UIP will meet these criteria. These criteria are specific, but likely not very sensitive.

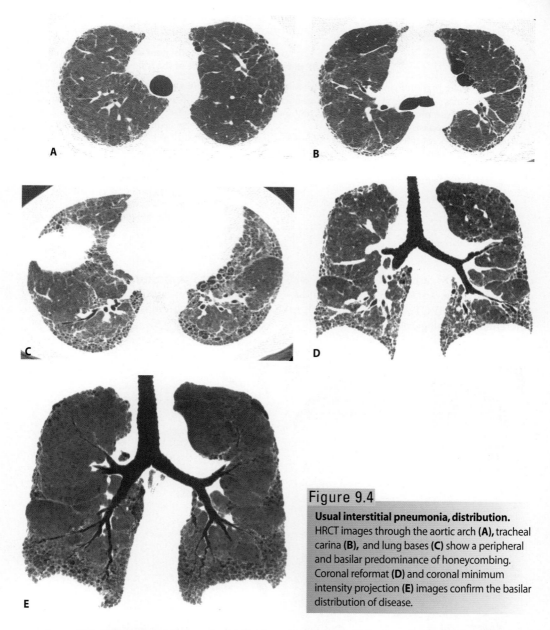

A

B

C

D

E

Figure 9.4

Usual interstitial pneumonia, distribution. HRCT images through the aortic arch **(A)**, tracheal carina **(B)**, and lung bases **(C)** show a peripheral and basilar predominance of honeycombing. Coronal reformat **(D)** and coronal minimum intensity projection **(E)** images confirm the basilar distribution of disease.

A *possible UIP pattern* is based on all of these, but without honeycombing being present.

HRCT findings that are considered *inconsistent with a UIP pattern* include (1) an upper or mid-lung predominance of abnormalities, (2) a peribronchovascular predominance of abnormalities, (3) extensive ground glass opacity, exceeding reticulation in extent, (4) profuse micronodules, bilateral, and upper lobe, (5) discrete cysts, not representing honeycombing, (6) mosaic perfusion or air trapping, bilateral, and in three or more lobes, and (7) segmental or lobar consolidation. Each of these findings is typical of an IP other than UIP or a different lung disease. Any one of these is sufficient for determining if the HRCT is inconsistent with a UIP pattern (see Figs. 9.12–9.15).

When HRCT findings are considered diagnostic of a UIP pattern, the differential diagnosis includes IPF (Fig. 9.5A), connective tissue

Table 9.3 ATS/ERS/JRS/ALAT criteria for HRCT diagnosis of usual interstitial pneumonia

UIP pattern	Possible UIP pattern	Inconsistent with UIP pattern (any one of the following may be present)
Subpleural, basilar predominance Reticular opacities Honeycombing with or without traction bronchiectasis Absence of features considered "inconsistent" with UIP	Subpleural, basilar predominance Reticular opacities No honeycombing Absence of features considered "inconsistent" with UIP	Upper or mid-lung predominance Peribronchovascular predominance Extensive ground glass opacity (exceeding reticulation in extent) Profuse micronodules (bilateral predominantly upper lobe) Discrete cysts (not representing honeycombing) Mosaic perfusion or air trapping (bilateral, ≥3 lobes) Segmental or lobar consolidation

UIP, usual interstitial pneumonia.

disease (Fig. 9.5B), asbestosis (Fig. 9.5C), and drug toxicity (Fig. 9.5D). These are often indistinguishable on HRCT and may be difficult to differentiate pathologically.

Idiopathic Pulmonary Fibrosis

IPF is a common cause of diffuse fibrotic lung disease and is the most common cause of a UIP pattern (Fig. 9.6).

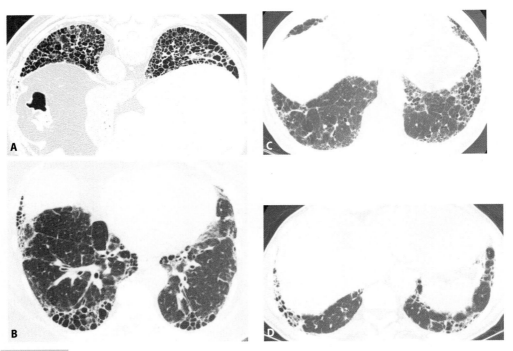

Figure 9.5

Usual interstitial pneumonia (UIP), differential diagnosis. Four examples of UIP on HRCT are shown. Subpleural, basilar predominant fibrosis with honeycombing is seen in patients with UIP secondary to idiopathic pulmonary fibrosis **(A)**, connective tissue disease **(B)**, asbestosis **(C)**, and drug toxicity **(D)**. When presenting with a UIP pattern, these diseases are often indistinguishable on HRCT.

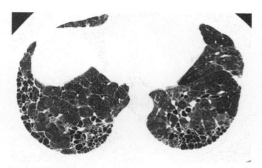

Figure 9.6

Idiopathic pulmonary fibrosis. A typical usual interstitial pneumonia pattern is present, manifested by patchy subpleural honeycombing. Idiopathic pulmonary fibrosis is the most common cause of this pattern.

A patient with idiopathic UIP has IPF. If a patient with a UIP pattern on HRCT has a disease or exposure that is known to be associated with this pattern (e.g., collagen disease and asbestos exposure), by definition, the diagnosis cannot be IPF. Also, there are fibrotic lung diseases, other than IPF, in which the clinical history may not be contributory. This is particularly true with other idiopathic disorders such

as sarcoidosis and diseases that may not have an identifiable exposure, such as HP. HRCT often allows the correct diagnosis is such cases.

IPF primarily affects patients over 50 years of age. It is progressive and patients have a poor prognosis, with a 50% 3-year survival. The disease is usually unresponsive to traditional immunosuppressive treatments. Clinical trials are underway to determine the efficacy of other drugs in arresting the progression of lung disease in patients with IPF.

The diagnosis of IPF, in many cases, is based solely upon a combination of clinical information and typical HRCT findings (i.e., a "UIP pattern"). Lung biopsy is not usually performed unless the HRCT findings are interpreted as "possible UIP" or "inconsistent with UIP" or the patient's clinical history suggests an alternative diagnosis.

In the absence of any clinical or radiographic findings to suggest an alternative diagnosis, a patient with a UIP pattern on HRCT will be given a presumptive diagnosis of IPF (Fig. 9.7). As a HRCT may be considered diagnostic of IPF without a biopsy, it is important to be conservative in diagnosing a definite UIP pattern.

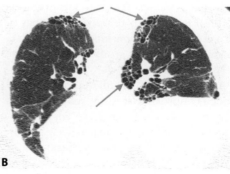

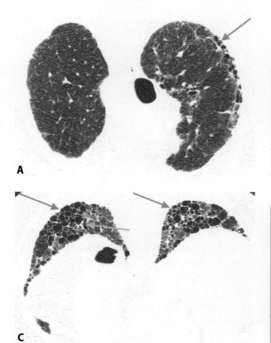

A

B

C

Figure 9.7

Idiopathic pulmonary fibrosis (IPF). HRCT images through the upper **(A)**, mid **(B)**, and lower **(C)** lungs show a subpleural and basilar predominance of honeycombing (*red arrows*) and traction bronchiectasis (*blue arrow*) compatible with usual interstitial pneumonia. In the absence of known diseases or exposures, this patient will be given a diagnosis of IPF.

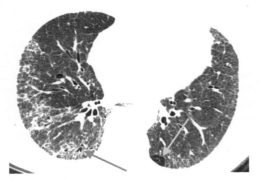

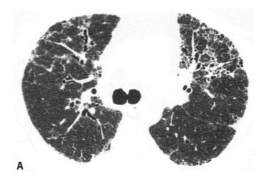

Figure 9.8

Nonspecific pattern of fibrosis. HRCT shows peripheral fibrosis with irregular reticulation and mild traction bronchiectasis (*red arrow*). Minimal mosaic perfusion is present (*yellow arrow*), but no honeycombing is seen. This pattern is not diagnostic of any particular disease and biopsy is required for definitive diagnosis.

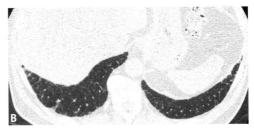

Figure 9.9

Idiopathic pulmonary fibrosis (IPF), atypical distribution. This patient with IPF and biopsy-proven usual interstitial pneumonia (UIP) shows atypical findings, with fibrosis that is not subpleural predominant and has significant involvement of the central lung regions **(A)**. Also, there is relative sparing of the costophrenic angles **(B)**. Atypical manifestations of IPF are not uncommon. On the basis of HRCT, this case would be read as "inconsistent" with UIP.

Keep in mind that not all cases of IPF show typical HRCT findings. Despite that, however, HRCT remains extremely important in making this diagnosis. Even if lung biopsy is interpreted as "UIP," a clinical diagnosis of UIP cannot be made with certainty if HRCT is interpreted as inconsistent with this diagnosis (Fig. 9.8). It has been recommended that in such a case, a careful consideration of all data by a multidisciplinary group of lung disease experts is necessary.

Atypical HRCT manifestations of IPF include (1) fibrosis that is not subpleural and basilar predominant (Fig. 9.9A, B), (2) predominant ground glass opacity (Fig. 9.10), and (3) focal areas of mosaic perfusion or air trapping (Fig. 9.11A, B).

Patients with IPF may show slow or rapid progression of their disease, with a progressive increase in findings of fibrosis. Patients with IPF also may present with an acute worsening of their symptoms. This is termed *acute exacerbation of IPF*. HRCT in such patients usually shows ground glass opacity involving areas previously affected by fibrosis or previously unaffected regions of lung (Fig. 9.12A–C). The ground glass opacity typically represents DAD.

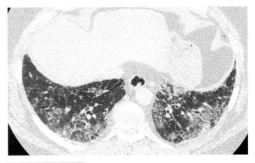

Figure 9.10

Idiopathic pulmonary fibrosis; presence of ground glass opacity (GGO). Rarely idiopathic pulmonary fibrosis may present with GGO as a predominant abnormality without definitive signs of fibrosis. In these cases, the GGO represents fibrosis below the resolution of HRCT and biopsy is required for definitive diagnosis.

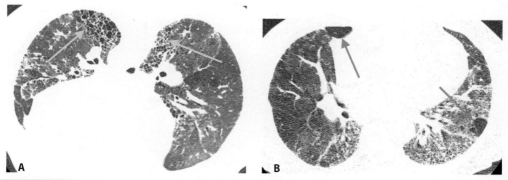

Figure 9.11

Idiopathic pulmonary fibrosis (IPF), mild air trapping. A. Prone HRCT through the mid-lung shows peripheral fibrosis with honeycombing (*yellow arrows*) characteristic of IPF. **B.** Mild air trapping (*red arrows*) is not uncommon in patients with IPF and should not suggest an alternative diagnosis if it is limited in severity and extent.

Differential Diagnosis

The lung abnormalities of IPF are typically indistinguishable on HRCT from other causes of a UIP pattern, including connective tissue disease, drug toxicity, and asbestosis. The distinction between IPF and these diseases is made primarily upon clinical grounds. Patients with connective tissue disease usually have additional clinical manifestations of a systemic disorder. The possibility of drug toxicity will be discovered by an investigation of a patient's medication list. Patients with asbestosis have long-term exposure in high-risk occupations.

Asbestosis shows associated pleural disease on HRCT in more than 80% of cases. Small centrilobular nodules in the peripheral lung, reflecting peribronchiolar fibrosis, have been described with asbestosis, but this is an uncommon finding and is typically seen in early disease.

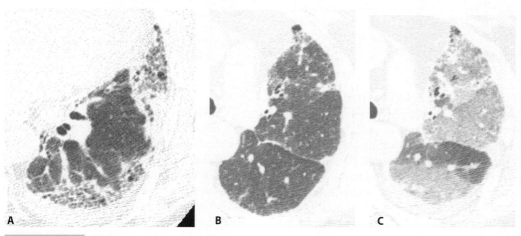

Figure 9.12

Acute exacerbation of idiopathic pulmonary fibrosis (IPF). A. HRCT through the left lung base shows peripheral reticulation in a patient with biopsy-proven IPF. **B.** HRCT through the mid-lung shows minimal abnormality. **C.** HRCT at the same level 3 months later shows development of diffuse ground glass opacity in a patient with an acute exacerbation of IPF.

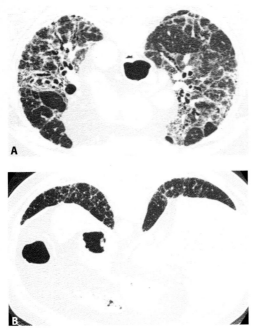

Figure 9.13

Hypersensitivity pneumonitis, distribution of fibrosis. While the interstitial pneumonias commonly have distribution that is peripheral and basilar, other causes of diffuse lung disease are characteristically diffuse or central in the axial plane **(A)**, with sparing of the costophrenic angles **(B)**. In this patient with hypersensitivity pneumonitis, prone scans show a central and mid-lung predominance of abnormalities. Because of the central and upper lobe distribution in this case, it would be read as inconsistent with usual interstitial pneumonia.

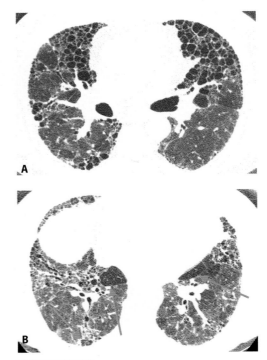

Figure 9.14

Hypersensitivity pneumonitis with honeycombing and air trapping. A. HRCT in a patent with hypersensitivity pneumonitis demonstrates extensive honeycombing with a mid-lung predominance. **B.** Expiratory image through the lung base shows patchy bilateral air trapping (*arrows*). Despite the presence of honeycombing, the HRCT does not suggest usual interstitial pneumonia (UIP). Because of the mid-lung distribution and air trapping in this case, it would be read as inconsistent with UIP.

Other diseases such as HP and sarcoidosis may show a UIP pattern pathologically if areas of severe fibrosis are sampled, but the HRCT usually shows distinguishing features.

HP typically does not predominate in the subpleural regions but involves the entire cross section of the lung and is most severe in the mid- or upper lungs (Fig. 9.13A, B). Additionally, HRCT in a patient with HP may show multiple areas of mosaic perfusion and/or air trapping (Fig. 9.14A, B). Sarcoidosis is often upper lobe predominant and central or peribronchovascular in distribution (Fig. 9.15). Perilymphatic nodules may be present in association with fibrosis.

NSIP may resemble UIP in some patients, as it often shows fibrosis in a subpleural and basilar distribution. However, fibrotic NSIP often shows a peribronchovascular predominance of reticulation or relative sparing of the subpleural lung; these findings are considered inconsistent with a UIP pattern. Furthermore, honeycombing is not a common finding in patients with NSIP, and when present, it tends to be mild and limited in extent (Fig. 9.16). As both UIP and fibrotic NSIP can show honeycombing, when mild honeycombing is present in the context of extensive fibrosis, the HRCT should not be considered typical for UIP.

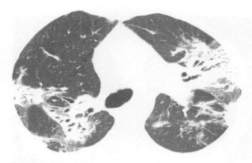

Figure 9.15

Sarcoidosis, distribution of fibrosis. An upper lung and peribronchovascular distribution of fibrosis is typical of chronic sarcoidosis. HRCT in this patient shows large consolidative areas of fibrosis and architectural distortion with a peribronchovascular distribution. This is in distinction to many of the interstitial pneumonias that are often peripheral and basilar predominant. Because of the central and upper lobe distribution in this case, it would be read as inconsistent with usual interstitial pneumonia.

Table 9.4	Features of nonspecific interstitial pneumonia
Frequency	Second most common IP; 25% of IP cases
HRCT findings	Subpleural, basilar predominant
	Ground glass opacity, irregular reticulation, traction bronchiectasis
	No or minimal honeycombing
	Subpleural sparing in 20–50%
Idiopathic syndrome	Idiopathic NSIP
Associated diseases	Connective tissue disease
	Drug toxicity
	Hypersensitivity pneumonitis

IP, interstitial pneumonia; NSIP, nonspecific interstitial pneumonia.

NONSPECIFIC INTERSTITIAL PNEUMONIA

The term NSIP was originally used to describe a pathological pattern that did not meet criteria for any of the other IPs. Over time, it has been recognized that cases classified as NSIP actually represent a specific entity with a characteristic pathologic appearance and clear associations with certain diseases.

NSIP (Table 9.4) is less common than UIP and tends to present in a younger patient population (peak 40 to 50 years) with symptoms that are not as severe. There are two subtypes of NSIP, cellular and fibrotic. The fibrotic subtype is more common.

In general, the prognosis of patients with NSIP is better than that of UIP (75% 5-year survival), although this survival difference is not as clear in patients with the fibrotic subtype of NSIP. Connective tissue disease is the most common systemic abnormality to be associated with a NSIP pattern, but NSIP may also be seen as a manifestation of drug toxicity, hypersensitivity pneumonitis or as an idiopathic disorder. Note that both connective tissue disease and drug toxicity may present with either a UIP or NSIP pattern.

Figure 9.16

Nonspecific interstitial pneumonia (NSIP), presence of honeycombing. Fibrotic NSIP may show honeycombing (*arrow*), but it is usually limited in severity such as in this patient with scleroderma. This is in contrast to usual interstitial pneumonia in which honeycombing is often a significant component of the abnormality present.

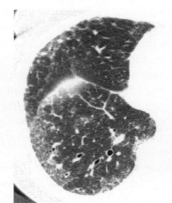
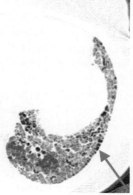

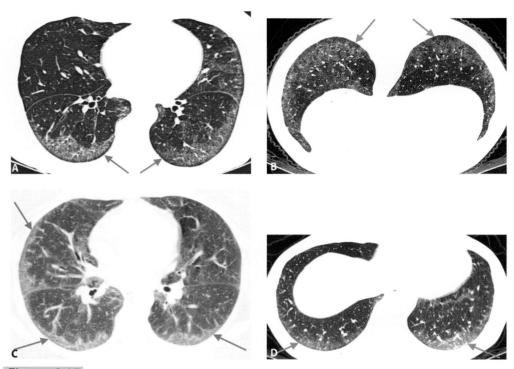

Figure 9.17

Cellular nonspecific interstitial pneumonia (NSIP). Four examples of cellular NSIP are shown. In each of these cases, ground glass opacity (*arrows*) is the most significant abnormality. Findings of fibrosis, such as traction bronchiectasis, are absent or mild in severity. Relative sparing of the immediate subpleural lung (**A–C**) is very suggestive of this diagnosis, but is absent in many cases of NSIP (**D**).

HRCT Findings

The HRCT findings in patients with NSIP depend upon whether the cellular or fibrotic subtype is present. Cellular NSIP presents with ground glass opacity as the predominant abnormality, although fine reticulation is often associated, and traction bronchiectasis may also be present (Fig. 9.17A–D). Fibrotic NSIP, in contrast, presents with traction bronchiectasis and irregular reticulation as the predominant findings (Fig. 9.18A–D). Ground glass opacity may also be present, but this may reflect superimposed cellular disease. Honeycombing is uncommon with fibrotic NSIP, seen in only a few percent of cases, and, when present, it is typically limited in severity and extent. Acute exacerbation of NSIP, similar to acute exacerbation in IPF, may occur.

The distribution of NSIP is similar to that of UIP, being subpleural and basilar predominant (Fig. 9.19). However, a peripheral, concentric distribution of abnormalities with relative sparing of the immediate subpleural lung is a finding that is highly predictive of NSIP; this finding is present in 20% to 50% of cases (Figs. 9.17A–C, 9.18A–C, 9.20A, B). NSIP may also show a peribronchovascular predominance.

Patients with connective tissue disease and suspected NSIP do not typically undergo lung biopsy for diagnosis, as the lung disease is assumed to be related to their systemic disorder. In the absence of a history of connective tissue disease, biopsy is usually performed when NSIP is suspected based on HRCT findings.

Differential Diagnosis

Differentiating fibrotic NSIP and UIP on HRCT may be difficult in some cases. When subpleural sparing is present and

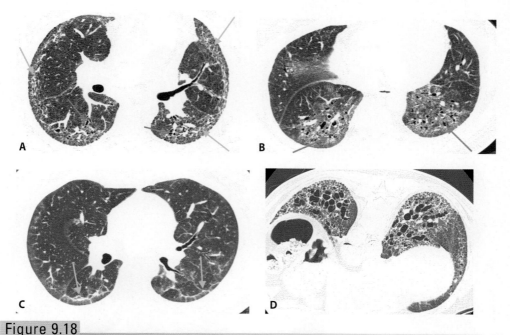

Figure 9.18

Fibrotic nonspecific interstitial pneumonia. Four examples of fibrotic nonspecific interstitial pneumonia are shown. In each of these cases, irregular reticulation (*blue arrows*) and traction bronchiectasis (*red arrows*) are the predominant findings. Sparing of the immediate subpleural lung (**A–C**) is suggestive of this diagnosis, but may be absent (**D**). Honeycombing is absent or inconspicuous.

honeycombing is absent or minimal, NSIP is very likely. When there is fibrosis with minimal or no honeycombing and no subpleural sparing is present, both UIP and NSIP are possible (Fig. 9.21A, B). The greater the severity of fibrosis without honeycombing, the more likely NSIP is as a diagnosis. The presence of significant honeycombing suggests UIP. Also, NSIP tends to appear concentric in distribution; UIP is often patchy.

DESQUAMATIVE INTERSTITIAL PNEUMONIA

DIP (Table 9.5) is a pattern of lung injury associated with cigarette smoking and will be discussed in greater detail in Chapter 11. Rarely, DIP is seen as a reaction in connective tissue disease, drug toxicity, toxic inhalations, and surfactant protein C mutations and as an idiopathic disorder. The name DIP is a misnomer as the primary pathologic abnormality is the presence of numerous intra-alveolar macrophages. DIP presents in younger patients (peak age 30 to 40 years) than NSIP or UIP and is typically more responsive to treatment (70% to 95% 5-year survival).

DIP and RB are both histologic patterns associated with smoking and represent different points on a spectrum of the same alveolar macrophage abnormality. In RB, the macrophage infiltrate predominates around small airways, whereas in DIP, the abnormalities are more diffuse. RB is a common incidental histologic abnormality in smokers. If a patient shows RB on histologic examination and is symptomatic, the disease is termed RB-ILD.

HRCT Findings

On HRCT, typical examples of DIP show a distribution similar to that of UIP and NSIP, being subpleural and basilar predominant (Fig. 9.22A–D). Ground glass opacity is present in most cases (Fig. 9.23). The ground glass opacity may be diffuse or have a basal predominance. Findings of fibrosis (reticulation, traction bronchiectasis,

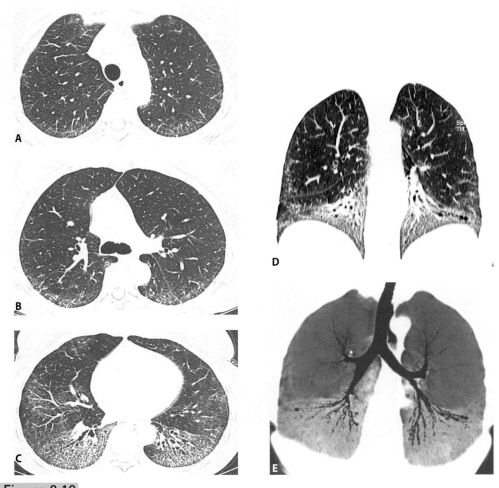

Figure 9.19

Nonspecific interstitial pneumonia, distribution. HRCT images through the upper **(A)**, mid **(B)**, and lower **(C)** lungs show a subpleural and basilar distribution of irregular reticulation and traction bronchiectasis. Coronal reformatted image **(D)** and coronal minimum intensity projection **(E)** confirm the basilar distribution of findings.

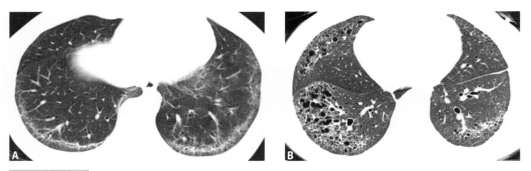

Figure 9.20

Nonspecific interstitial pneumonia (NSIP), subpleural sparing. A peripheral distribution of findings with relative sparing of the immediate subpleural interstitium is highly suggestive of NSIP. **A.** A rim of peripheral irregular reticulation is present with relative sparing of the immediate subpleural interstitium in a patient with NSIP related to rheumatoid arthritis. **B.** More severe traction bronchiectasis and irregular reticulation is present in a patient with scleroderma. The findings are peripheral; however, the subpleural lung is relatively spared. The immediate subpleural lung is less abnormal than lung 1 cm away from the pleura.

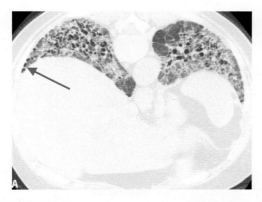

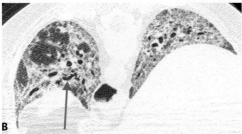

Figure 9.21

Fibrotic nonspecific interstitial pneumonia (NSIP) versus usual interstitial pneumonia (UIP). A. Prone HRCT shows mild honeycombing (*arrow*) in a patient with NSIP. This finding is not uncommon with fibrotic NSIP, but it is typically limited in severity compared with UIP. **B.** Prone HRCT shows peripheral and basilar predominant traction bronchiectasis (*arrow*) and irregular reticulation in a patient with idiopathic pulmonary fibrosis. The lack of honeycombing favors NSIP, but UIP can present with severe fibrosis in the absence of honeycombing. If the patient has a history of connective tissue disease, this appearance is assumed to represent NSIP, otherwise a biopsy is required for diagnosis.

Table 9.5	Features of desquamative interstitial pneumonia
Frequency	Uncommon; 15% of IP cases
HRCT findings	Subpleural, basilar predominant
	Ground glass opacity
	Cysts or emphysema
	Fibrosis may develop over time
Idiopathic syndrome	Idiopathic DIP (rare)
Associated diseases	Cigarette smoking
	Connective tissue disease (rare)
	Drug toxicity (rare)
	Toxic inhalations (rare)
	Surfactant protein C mutations (rare)
Related diseases	RB and RB-ILD

IP, interstitial pneumonia; DIP, desquamative interstitial pneumonia; RB, respiratory bronchiolitis; ILD, interstitial lung disease.

and honeycombing) tend to be absent or mild in severity, although DIP may progress to a fibrotic pattern in occasional cases. Scattered cysts and/or emphysema may be seen in affected regions (Fig. 9.24). These cysts can be a clue to diagnosis.

The most typical HRCT finding of RB is centrilobular nodules of ground glass opacity. The nodules are usually most severe in the central portions of the upper lungs. Mosaic perfusion and/or air trapping may also be present, although this tends to be mild.

As RB and DIP are part of the spectrum of the same disease, an overlap of findings may be present. Thus, DIP may show centrilobular ground glass opacity nodules, mosaic perfusion, and air trapping. The distribution of findings may not be subpleural and basilar predominant, particularly when there is an overlap of DIP and RB.

ORGANIZING PNEUMONIA

OP (Table 9.6) is an inflammatory, noninfectious abnormality associated with a wide variety of etiologies and diseases. It is a relatively common pattern seen both pathologically and on HRCT. It was previously known as bronchiolitis obliterans with organizing pneumonia, but this term has been dropped for several reasons. First, "OP" is a more accurate reflection of the pathologic appearance of this disorder. Second, this term avoids confusion with airways diseases, namely bronchiolitis obliterans.

Patients with OP commonly present with chronic symptoms of low-grade fever, dyspnea, and cough, but acute presentations are also possible. Symptoms are usually less severe than those of UIP and the disease is responsive

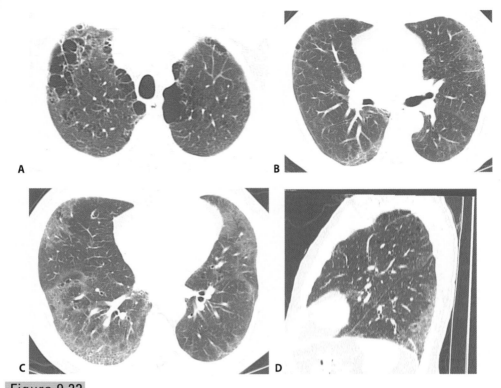

Figure 9.22

Desquamative interstitial pneumonia (DIP), distribution. HRCT through the upper **(A)**, mid **(B)**, and lower **(C)** lungs shows a peripheral and basilar distribution of ground glass opacity. This is also shown on a sagittal reformatted image **(D)**. Note emphysema in the upper lobes **(A)** in this patient with a history of smoking.

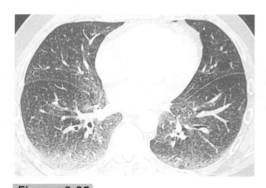

Figure 9.23

Desquamative interstitial pneumonia (DIP). HRCT shows peripheral ground glass opacity as an isolated abnormality. This is a nonspecific finding, but in a smoker with chronic symptoms, desquamative interstitial pneumonia is the favored diagnosis.

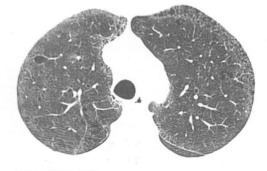

Figure 9.24

Desquamative interstitial pneumonia (DIP). The combination of ground glass opacity and cysts or emphysema in the same lung regions suggests DIP. When present in a patient with a smoking history, this combination is usually taken as sufficient evidence for DIP without the need for a biopsy.

Table 9.6 Features of organizing pneumonia

Frequency	10% of IP cases
HRCT findings	Peribronchovascular and subpleural predominant
	Consolidation (often nodular or mass-like)
	Irregular borders
	Small centrilobular nodules (rare)
	Lower lobe predominance
	Development of fibrosis after treatment
Idiopathic syndrome	COP
Associated diseases	Connective tissue disease
	Drug toxicity
	Infection
	Toxic inhalations
	Immunologic disorders
	Graft vs. host disease
	Secondary reaction to another disorder (chronic eosinophilic pneumonia, hypersensitivity pneumonitis, Wegener's granulomatosis, diffuse alveolar damage)

IP, interstitial pneumonia; NSIP, nonspecific interstitial pneumonia; COP, cryptogenic organizing pneumonia.

to steroids, although not uncommonly it recurs after treatment.

HRCT Findings

The most typical HRCT finding of OP is that of focal areas of consolidation, often nodular or mass-like, that predominate in the peribronchovascular and subpleural regions and may be irregular in contour (Fig. 9.25). The areas

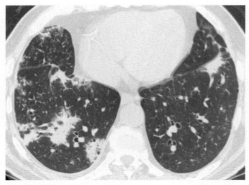

Figure 9.25

Organizing pneumonia (OP). The classic HRCT findings of OP are depicted in this patient. Peripheral and peribronchovascular consolidation, often with a nodular or mass-like appearance, and irregular margins, is seen bilaterally. Note significant unaffected lung intermixed with areas of OP.

of consolidation are intermixed with regions of normal lung. These findings are often most severe in the lower lobes (Fig. 9.26).

Ground glass opacity is rarely a predominant abnormality, but may be seen as the primary manifestation of OP in immunocompromised patients (Fig. 9.27). Centrilobular nodules are an infrequent finding in OP, but may be seen. While OP may eventually lead to lung scarring, significant fibrosis is not a typical feature.

One finding that is highly suggestive of OP is the *atoll sign* or *reversed halo sign*. This manifests as a ring or partial ring of consolidation surrounding a central region of clearing or ground glass opacity (Fig. 9.28). When the atoll sign is present, one can be quite confident that OP is present, either as the predominant abnormality or as a secondary reaction to a diffuse lung disease.

The multiple causes of OP include connective tissue disease, infection, drugs (Fig. 9.29), toxic inhalations, immunological disorders, and graft versus host disease. OP may also be seen as a secondary process in association with other diseases including infections, chronic eosinophilic pneumonia (Fig. 9.30), HP, Wegener's granulomatosis (granulomatosis with polyangiitis) (Fig. 9.31), and DAD. The HRCT in these cases may be indistinguishable

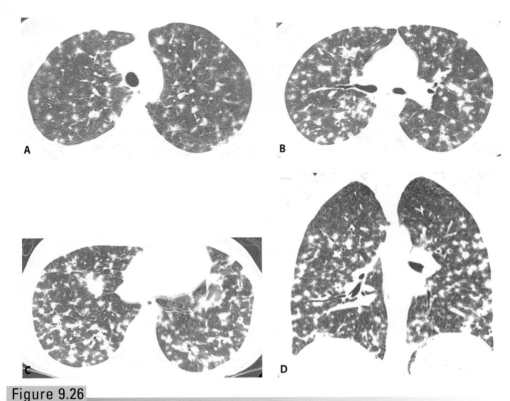

Figure 9.26

Organizing pneumonia, distribution. HRCT images through the upper **(A)**, mid **(B)**, and lower **(C)** lungs show nodular areas of subpleural and peribronchovascular consolidation. Coronal reformatted image **(D)** shows the lower lobe predominance of disease.

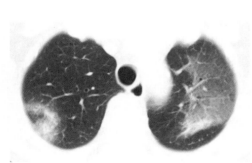

Figure 9.27

Organizing pneumonia, ground glass opacity. Organizing pneumonia typically presents with consolidation as the predominant abnormality. Rarely, ground glass opacity is the predominant HRCT finding, particularly in patients with a history of immunosuppression.

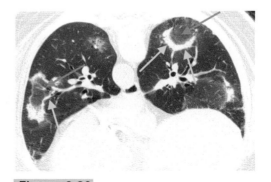

Figure 9.28

"Atoll sign" or "reversed halo sign" in organizing pneumonia (OP). A peripheral rim of consolidation (*yellow arrows*) surrounding a central area of clearing or ground glass opacity (*red arrows*) is called the atoll or reversed halo sign. This finding is highly suggestive of OP, but is not specific with respect to the cause of OP.

Figure 9.29

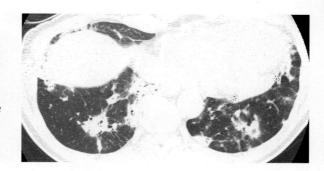

Organizing pneumonia, amiodarone toxicity. Patchy subpleural and peribronchovascular mass-like regions of irregular consolidation are present. This combination of findings is most suggestive of organizing pneumonia. There are multiple possible causes of organizing pneumonia, one of which is drug toxicity.

from those in which OP is the predominant abnormality. Approximately 50% of cases of OP are idiopathic; this is termed cryptogenic organizing pneumonia (Fig. 9.32).

The differential diagnosis of OP includes other causes of patchy and chronic consolidation, including chronic eosinophilic pneumonia, invasive mucinous adenocarcinoma, lymphoma, sarcoidosis, and lipoid pneumonia.

ACUTE INTERSTITIAL PNEUMONIA

AIP (Table 9.7) is the idiopathic IP associated with the histologic pattern of DAD. It usually presents as acute respiratory distress syndrome (ARDS) without an identifiable cause. It has also been called Hamman-Rich syndrome. The clinical presentation is different from the other

IPs and is similar to ARDS associated with a known etiology. Early mortality is high, similar to other causes of ARDS.

HRCT Findings

The HRCT findings of AIP are usually indistinguishable from other causes of DAD and ARDS (see Chapter 8). Extensive or diffuse ground glass opacity and consolidation are present (Fig. 9.33). If imaged early in its course, the abnormalities may have a peripheral distribution, but then quickly become diffuse in nature. Over time, the HRCT of patients who survive shows interval decrease in ground glass opacity

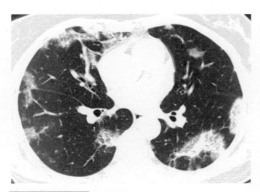

Figure 9.30

Chronic eosinophilic pneumonia with organizing pneumonia (OP). Patchy bilateral focal areas of consolidation are seen, most suggestive of OP. OP may be seen as a primary abnormality or as a secondary reaction to another diffuse lung disease, such as chronic eosinophilic pneumonia.

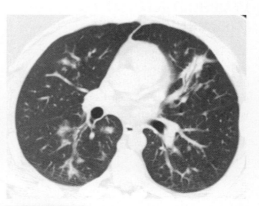

Figure 9.31

Wegener's granulomatosis with organizing pneumonia (OP). There are several diseases that may be associated with an OP pattern on pathology and HRCT. These include chronic eosinophilic pneumonia, infection, hypersensitivity pneumonitis, and Wegener's granulomatosis. Focal patchy peribronchovascular consolidation in this patient with Wegener's granulomatosis corresponded to OP seen on pathology.

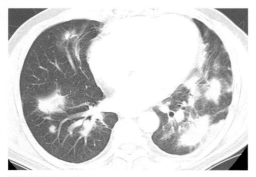

Figure 9.32

Cryptogenic organizing pneumonia (COP).
Patchy, bilateral mass-like regions of consolidation
and ground glass opacity are seen in a patient with
chronic symptoms and no contributing history or
exposures. COP accounts for approximately 50% of
cases of organizing pneumonia.

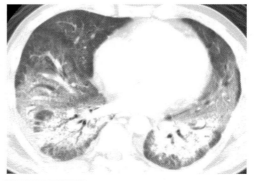

Figure 9.33

Acute interstitial pneumonia. Extensive bilateral
ground glass opacity and consolidation in a patient
with acute symptoms may represent edema, diffuse
alveolar damage, infection, and/or hemorrhage. This
patient had a clinical diagnosis of acute respiratory
distress syndrome (ARDS) and lung biopsy showed
diffuse alveolar damage. No cause for ARDS was
identified, and a diagnosis of acute interstitial
pneumonia was made.

and consolidation. Often irregular reticulation
and other signs of fibrosis develop. Eventually,
fibrosis may be the only sequela of AIP. This
fibrosis commonly has a peripheral and anterior distribution (Fig. 9.34).

LYMPHOID INTERSTITIAL PNEUMONIA

LIP is a lymphoproliferative disorder associated with connective tissue disease and
immunodeficiency disorders such as human
immunodeficiency virus infection or common
variable immunodeficiency. In some patients,
it is idiopathic. It will be discussed in more
detail in Chapter 17.

The clinical presentation is usually that
of the underlying systemic disorder, although
chronic dyspnea and dry cough may be
present. LIP tends to be steroid responsive,
although up to a third of patients may progress to fibrosis.

Table 9.7	Features of acute interstitial pneumonia
Frequency	Rare; <2% of cases
Histologic pattern	DAD
HRCT findings	Diffuse
	Ground glass opacity and consolidation
	Fibrosis may develop over time (anterior distribution)
Differential diagnosis	Other causes of DAD and ARDS

DAD, diffuse alveolar damage; ARDS, acute respiratory
distress syndrome.

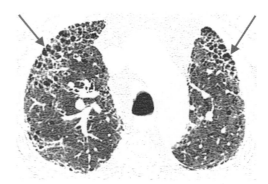

Figure 9.34

Acute interstitial pneumonia, fibrosis. One year
after a diagnosis of acute interstitial pneumonia
(AIP), this patient showed subpleural fibrosis with
honeycombing (*arrows*) that has a striking anterior
distribution. This is a typical appearance of post–AIP
fibrosis.

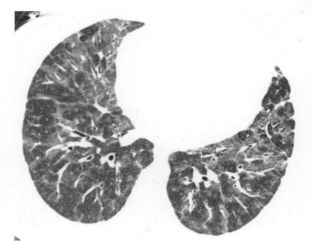

Figure 9.35

Lymphocytic interstitial pneumonia. HRCT shows patchy bilateral ground glass opacity in a patient with connective tissue disease. Although this appearance is nonspecific, in this clinical setting, lymphocytic interstitial pneumonia is a possible diagnosis.

HRCT Findings

The most common HRCT finding of LIP is patchy ground glass opacity (Fig. 9.35). Consolidation may also be present. These findings are quite nonspecific, and thus, the clinical history is important in diagnosis. Nodules, when present, may be more suggestive of the diagnosis in the appropriate clinical setting and are usually centrilobular or perilymphatic in distribution. Centrilobular nodules in LIP reflect the presence of follicular bronchiolitis. Cysts may be present in association with other abnormalities or may be the only manifestation of LIP, particularly in the setting of Sjögren's disease or other connective tissue diseases.

FURTHER READING

Akira M, Yamamoto S, Sakatani M. Bronchiolitis obliterans organizing pneumonia manifesting as multiple large nodules or masses. *AJR Am J Roentgenol.* 1998;170:291-295.

American Thoracic Society/European Respiratory Society International Multidisciplinary Consensus Classification of the Idiopathic Interstitial Pneumonias. *Am J Respir Crit Care Med.* 2002;165:277-304.

Colby TV, Myers JL. The clinical and histologic spectrum of bronchiolitis obliterans including bronchiolitis obliterans organizing pneumonia (BOOP). *Semin Respir Dis.* 1992;13:119-133.

Hartman TE, Primack SL, Swensen SJ, et al. Desquamative interstitial pneumonia: thin-section CT findings in 22 patients. *Radiology.* 1993;187:787-790.

Hartman TE, Swensen SJ, Hansell DM, et al. Nonspecific interstitial pneumonia: variable appearance at high-resolution chest CT. *Radiology.* 2000;217:701-705.

Heyneman LE, Ward S, Lynch DA, et al. Respiratory bronchiolitis, respiratory bronchiolitis-associated interstitial lung disease, and desquamative interstitial pneumonia: different entities or part of the spectrum of the same disease process? *AJR Am J Roentgenol.* 1999;173:1617-1622.

Johkoh T, Müller NL, Cartier Y, et al. Idiopathic interstitial pneumonias: diagnostic accuracy of thin-section CT in 129 patients. *Radiology.* 1999;211:555-560.

Johkoh T, Müller NL, Colby TV, et al. Nonspecific interstitial pneumonia: correlation between thin-section CT findings and pathologic subgroups in 55 patients. *Radiology.* 2002;225:199-204.

Johkoh T, Müller NL, Pickford HA, et al. Lymphocytic interstitial pneumonia: thin-section CT findings in 22 patients. *Radiology.* 1999;212:567-572.

Johkoh T, Müller NL, Taniguchi H, et al. Acute interstitial pneumonia: thin-section CT findings in 36 patients. *Radiology.* 1999; 211:859-863.

Katzenstein AL, Myers JL. Idiopathic pulmonary fibrosis: clinical relevance of pathologic classification. *Am J Respir Crit Care Med.* 1998;157:1301-1315.

Kim SJ, Lee KS, Ryu YH, et al. Reversed halo sign on high-resolution CT of cryptogenic organizing pneumonia: diagnostic implications. *AJR Am J Roentgenol.* 2003;180:1251-1254.

Lee KS, Kullnig P, Hartman TE, Müller NL. Cryptogenic organizing pneumonia: CT findings in 43 patients. *AJR Am J Roentgenol.* 1994;162:543-546.

Lynch DA, Travis WD, Müller NL, et al. Idiopathic interstitial pneumonias: CT features. *Radiology.* 2005;236:10-21.

Müller NL, Colby TV. Idiopathic interstitial pneumonias: high-resolution CT and histologic findings. *Radiographics.* 1997;17:1016-1022.

Park JS, Lee KS, Kim JS, et al. Nonspecific interstitial pneumonia with fibrosis: radiographic and CT findings in seven patients. *Radiology.* 1995;195:645-648.

Primack SL, Hartman TE, Ikezoe J, et al. Acute interstitial pneumonia: radiographic and CT findings in nine patients. *Radiology.* 1993;188:817-820.

Raghu G, Collard HR, Egan JJ, et al. An official ATS/ERS/JRS/ALAT statement: idiopathic pulmonary fibrosis: evidence-based guidelines for diagnosis and management. *Am J Respir Crit Care Med.* 2011;183:788-824.

Travis WD, Hunninghake G, King TE, et al. Idiopathic nonspecific interstitial pneumonia: report of an American Thoracic Society project. *Am J Respir Crit Care Med.* 2008;177:1338-1347.

10

Connective Tissue Diseases

Connective tissue diseases (CTDs) may be associated with a variety of lung abnormalities. Most patients with CTD have extra-pulmonary manifestations but in some cases, lung abnormalities are seen in isolation or as the first manifestation of disease.

This chapter provides an overview of the approach to diagnosis of lung disease in these patients, followed by a discussion of the most common lung manifestations of specific CTDs.

A GENERAL APPROACH TO DIAGNOSIS

CTDs may be manifested by a number of pulmonary abnormalities that reflect the various ways the lung reacts to injury (Table 10.1). The interstitial pneumonias (IPs) are common in patients with CTD, including usual interstitial pneumonia (UIP), nonspecific interstitial pneumonia (NSIP), lymphoid interstitial pneumonia (LIP) and follicular bronchiolitis, organizing pneumonia (OP), and diffuse alveolar damage (DAD). While patients tend to present with a single pattern, an overlap of more than one pattern is sometimes seen. The IPs are described in detail in the preceding chapter.

In addition, patients with CTD may show intrathoracic abnormalities not related to an IP. These may be specific to the individual CTD. These include pulmonary edema, vasculitis, pulmonary hypertension, pulmonary hemorrhage, pleural or pericardial effusion, lung nodules, bronchiectasis, constrictive bronchiolitis, and esophageal dilatation.

The initial presentation of diffuse lung disease may precede the diagnosis of CTD. HRCT plays a major role in suggesting the presence of a pattern of lung disease (e.g., NSIP) consistent with CTD, and excluding alternative diagnoses. In some patients, HRCT findings precipitate a workup for CTD.

HRCT may also be used to categorize the pattern of lung disease present in patients with known CTD. This is important for treatment and determining prognosis. Serologies are also commonly obtained to suggest etiology in a patient with undiagnosed diffuse lung disease or for further classification of the CTD present. The most useful serologies are those that are relatively specific for a particular CTD, although no serology is diagnostic

Table 10.1	Abnormalities that may be seen in patients with connective tissue disease
Usual interstitial pneumonia	
Nonspecific interstitial pneumonia	
Lymphoid interstitial pneumonia	
Follicular bronchiolitis	
Organizing pneumonia	
Diffuse alveolar damage	
Constrictive bronchiolitis	
Pulmonary edema	
Pulmonary hemorrhage	
Pulmonary hypertension	
Serositis (pleural or pericardial effusion)	
Miscellaneous (nodules, bronchiectasis, esophageal dilatation)	

of a single disease. For instance, the serology Scl-70 is relatively specific for a diagnosis of scleroderma.

Any CTD may be present with any of the HRCT patterns listed above; however, some general trends exist. When diffuse lung disease is present in a patient whose diagnosis of CTD is established, it is usually assumed to be a manifestation of that systemic disorder unless there is convincing evidence to the contrary. For this reason, patients with CTD uncommonly undergo biopsy and HRCT is often the primary diagnostic examination that determines the pattern of lung disease.

PATTERNS OF DIFFUSE LUNG DISEASE

As HRCT is the primary method of characterizing diffuse lung disease in patients with CTD, an in-depth knowledge of their manifestations and differentiating features is important.

UIP and NSIP

UIP and NSIP are the most common causes of diffuse lung disease and fibrosis in patients with CTD. Typical findings (Table 10.2) include honeycombing, traction bronchiectasis, and irregular reticulation. Ground glass opacity is less common, but may be seen in NSIP,

particularly the cellular subtype. Fibrosis is only rarely seen with LIP and follicular bronchiolitis, OP, and constrictive bronchiolitis.

In general, NSIP is the most common pattern seen in patients with CTD. It is most typical of scleroderma, polymyositis, dermatomyositis, and mixed CTD. UIP is seen most frequently in patients with rheumatoid lung disease.

UIP and NSIP may be difficult to differentiate radiographically, unless ground glass opacity or subpleural sparing is present. In particular, the fibrotic subtype of NSIP can closely resemble UIP, although the clinical significance of this distinction is uncertain. In UIP, honeycombing is a significant finding (Fig. 10.1), whereas in NSIP, it is either absent or minimal in extent (Fig. 10.2). The greater the severity of fibrosis in the absence of honeycombing, the more likely NSIP becomes. Subpleural sparing strongly suggests NSIP over UIP (Fig. 10.3).

LIP and Follicular Bronchiolitis

LIP and follicular bronchiolitis are thought to represent different points on a spectrum of the lymphocytic lung infiltration; thus, their findings may overlap. The typical findings of

Table 10.2	HRCT findings of usual and nonspecific interstitial pneumonia
Usual interstitial pneumonia	Subpleural, basilar predominant
	Honeycombing
	Other signs of fibrosis (traction bronchiectasis, irregular reticulation)
Nonspecific interstitial pneumonia	Subpleural, basilar predominant
	Ground glass opacity
	Fibrosis (traction bronchiectasis, irregular reticulation)
	No or mild honeycombing
	Subpleural sparing

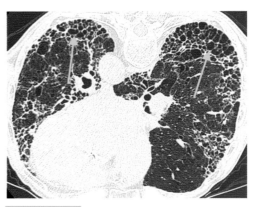

Figure 10.1

Usual interstitial pneumonia in rheumatoid arthritis. Prone HRCT shows peripheral and basilar fibrosis with extensive honeycombing (*arrows*) typical of usual interstitial pneumonia. While this may be seen with any connective tissue disease, it is most common with rheumatoid lung disease.

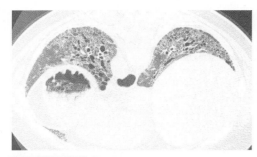

Figure 10.2

Nonspecific interstitial pneumonia (NSIP) in scleroderma. Basilar predominant fibrosis is present with irregular reticulation and traction bronchiectasis. No honeycombing is seen. In the setting of known connective tissue disease, this is compatible with fibrotic NSIP, and a biopsy is not usually required for diagnosis.

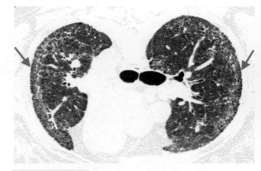

Figure 10.3

Nonspecific interstitial pneumonia (NSIP) with subpleural sparing. Prone HRCT shows irregular reticulation and traction bronchiolectasis in the peripheral lung, without significant honeycombing. Sparing of the immediate subpleural lung (*arrows*) is highly suggestive of NSIP. While the irregular reticulation likely represents irreversible disease (fibrotic NSIP), some of these abnormalities may resolve with treatment.

LIP (Table 10.3) include patchy ground glass opacity, centrilobular or perilymphatic nodules, and, to a lesser extent, consolidation. Lung cysts may be seen in association with other findings (Fig. 10.4) or as an isolated abnormality. Cysts are typically thin walled and limited in number and vessels may be seen in association with their walls.

Follicular bronchiolitis represents localized lymphoid infiltration of bronchioles. It commonly presents with centrilobular nodules of ground glass opacity (Fig. 10.5). Air trapping and mosaic perfusion may also be present. Lung cysts are thought to reflect the presence of air trapping associated with follicular bronchiolitis.

Table 10.3	HRCT findings of lymphoid interstitial pneumonia and follicular bronchiolitis

Centrilobular nodules of ground glass opacity
Perilymphatic nodules
Patchy, bilateral ground glass opacity
Patchy, bilateral consolidation
Lung cysts (thin walled, limited in number)

Figure 10.4

Lymphoid interstitial pneumonia. Cysts are seen in association with ground glass opacity in a patient with polymyositis. Small areas of ground glass opacity appear to have a centrilobular distribution (*arrow*).

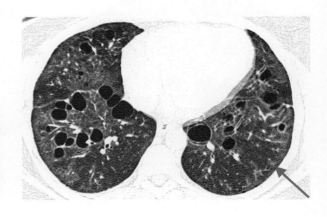

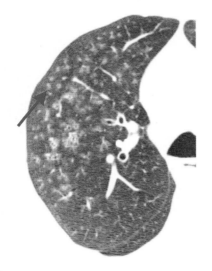

Figure 10.5

Follicular bronchiolitis. Centrilobular nodules of ground glass opacity are noted, associated with mild bronchial dilatation. Note that the nodules are located at a distance from the pleural surfaces (*arrow*) and are evenly spaced from one another. This is typical of a centrilobular distribution.

Among the CTDs, LIP and follicular bronchiolitis are most commonly seen in patients with Sjögren's disease. Isolated cysts in the setting of Sjögren's disease are highly suggestive of LIP. LIP and follicular bronchiolitis may also be seen in combination with other patterns of lung disease. For instance, patients with NSIP may have centrilobular nodules

Table 10.4	HRCT findings of organizing pneumonia

Consolidation, focal, irregular borders, often nodular or mass-like
Ground glass opacity (uncommon)
Centrilobular nodules (rare)
Peribronchovascular/subpleural predominant
Atoll or reversed halo sign

in the peripheral lung representing follicular bronchiolitis.

In the absence of signs of fibrosis, ground glass opacity is not commonly seen with the other patterns of chronic lung disease in CTD, with the exception of NSIP. NSIP is typically peripheral and basilar in distribution, whereas LIP and follicular bronchiolitis usually show involvement of the central lung regions. Chronic ground glass and centrilobular nodules may be seen with diseases unrelated to CTD such as hypersensitivity pneumonitis and smoking-related lung disease.

Organizing Pneumonia

OP typically presents with focal areas of consolidation with irregular borders that often appear nodular or mass-like (Table 10.4). The distribution of consolidation is typically peribronchovascular and/or subpleural (Fig. 10.6A, B). Ground glass opacity is less common and typically seen in immunosuppressed patients. Centrilobular nodules are a rare finding. Architectural distortion and mild

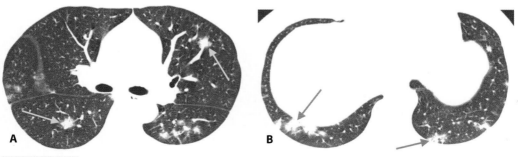

Figure 10.6

Organizing pneumonia. Patchy peribronchovascular (**A**, *arrows*) and subpleural (**B**, *arrows*) consolidation is seen in a patient with organizing pneumonia due to systemic lupus erythematosus–associated lung disease.

10

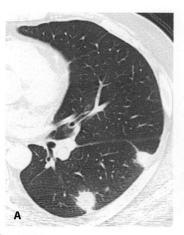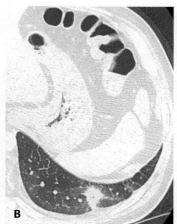

Figure 10.7

Fungal infection resembling organizing pneumonia in a patient with connective tissue disease. HRCT images through the mid-lung **(A)** and lung base **(B)** show large ill-defined nodules from fungal infection that have an appearance similar to organizing pneumonia.

bronchial dilatation may be seen associated with these opacities. After treatment, OP may result in mild scarring; however, extensive fibrosis resembling NSIP or UIP is rare.

OP is one of the least common patterns seen in CTD, but is most closely associated with polymyositis and dermatomyositis. While it may be seen as the primary abnormality, it is commonly associated with other patterns such as NSIP.

Consolidation is uncommon with other causes of chronic CTD-related diffuse lung disease, although it may occasionally be seen with LIP. Patients on immunosuppressive medications are predisposed to developing infections that may closely resemble OP, particularly fungal and mycobacterial disease (Fig. 10.7). Patients with fibrotic lung disease are at increased risk for malignancies whose findings occasionally overlap with those of OP.

Pulmonary Edema, Pulmonary Hemorrhage, and DAD

Pulmonary edema, pulmonary hemorrhage, and DAD are uncommon patterns in CTD. They are most closely associated with systemic lupus erythematosus (SLE). Patients present with a single or multiple acute episodes.

These three patterns share many HRCT features. They all commonly present with diffuse or symmetric ground glass opacity. Consolidation may also be present. Smooth interlobular septal thickening as an isolated finding suggests pulmonary edema. The combination of ground glass opacity and interlobular septal thickening, the crazy paving pattern, may be seen with any of these patterns.

Constrictive Bronchiolitis

Constrictive bronchiolitis (Table 10.5) is associated with mosaic perfusion and/or air trapping on HRCT, with or without associated bronchiectasis (Fig. 10.8). The severity of constrictive bronchiolitis may vary from patchy and lobular to diffuse lung involvement. Consolidation, ground glass opacity, nodules, and tree-in-bud opacities are typically absent.

Table 10.5	HRCT findings of constrictive bronchiolitis

Mosaic perfusion
Air trapping
Bronchiectasis
Absence of nodules, tree-in bud unless complicated by infection

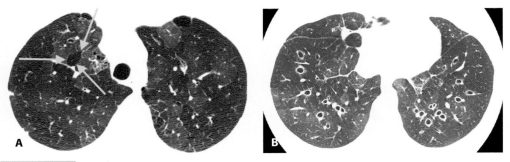

Figure 10.8

Constrictive bronchiolitis in rheumatoid arthritis. HRCT image through the apex **(A)** demonstrates patchy mosaic perfusion with sharply demarcated lobules of decreased attenuation (*arrows*). Image through the lung bases **(B)** shows bronchiectasis in association with mosaic perfusion.

Constrictive bronchiolitis is not a common manifestation of CTD. It is most commonly associated with rheumatoid arthritis (RA), SLE, and rarely scleroderma.

Isolated mosaic perfusion on HRCT may also be seen with asthma, hypersensitivity pneumonitis, and chronic vascular diseases. In the setting of CTD, chronic vascular disease may be associated with pulmonary arterial hypertension and/or pulmonary arterial thromboembolic disease. Airways and vascular causes of mosaic perfusion are often distinguishable by their morphology (Fig. 10.9). The mosaic perfusion associated with airways disease often involves smaller lung regions, is patchy in distribution, and may show lobular regions of decreased lung attenuation. Mosaic perfusion from vascular disease is typically more extensive, peripheral, and non-lobular in appearance. The presence of air trapping confirms airways disease.

Bronchiectasis

Bronchiectasis in the absence of fibrosis is most commonly seen in patients with RA and Sjögren's disease. This finding may be due to chronic infection or constrictive bronchiolitis. Bronchiectasis may be seen as an isolated finding or in association with bronchial wall thickening, mosaic perfusion,

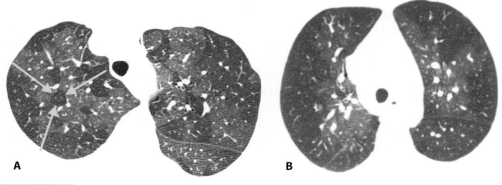

Figure 10.9

Mosaic perfusion from airways vs. vascular disease. Mosaic perfusion from airways disease **(A)** appears as sharply demarcated, lobular areas of decreased lung attenuation (*arrows*). Vascular disease, such as chronic pulmonary embolism **(B)** appears as larger, peripheral, non-lobular areas of decreased lung attenuation.

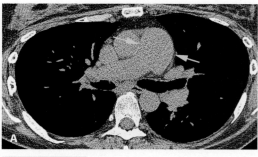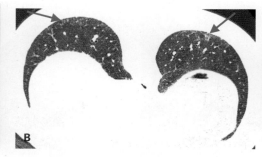

Figure 10.10

Pulmonary hypertension with mild-lung fibrosis. A. Enlargement of the main pulmonary artery (*yellow arrows*) is present in a scleroderma patient with pulmonary hypertension. **B.** Prone HRCT shows minimal subpleural reticulation and ground glass opacity (*red arrows*) likely due to nonspecific interstitial pneumonia. The degree of pulmonary hypertension is out of proportion to the severity of lung findings, suggesting vasculitis.

or air trapping. When infection is present, it is usually associated with centrilobular nodules, tree-in-bud opacities, and/or consolidation.

Pulmonary Hypertension

Pulmonary hypertension is a relatively common manifestation of collagen vascular disease. It is most closely associated with scleroderma, SLE, and mixed CTD. Pulmonary hypertension may be due to parenchymal lung fibrosis or pulmonary vascular disease. The vascular disease may be due to vasculitis, arterial fibrosis, chronic pulmonary emboli, or in situ thrombus. Primary vascular disease should be considered when the HRCT shows main pulmonary artery or right heart dilatation in the presence of mild or no parenchymal lung disease (Fig. 10.10).

Serositis

Inflammation of the pleura and pericardium is a common occurrence in patients with CTD. This may be manifested as pleural/pericardial effusions or thickening on CT. These effusions are commonly exudative; thus, pleural thickening and enhancement may be present. Effusions are not typical of other causes of diffuse lung disease such as idiopathic pulmonary fibrosis and hypersensitivity pneumonitis. The combination of diffuse lung disease and pleural or pericardial abnormalities increases the likelihood of CTD as a cause. Serositis is most closely associated with SLE and RA.

Overlap of Patterns

While one of the above patterns often predominates in patients with CTD, it is not uncommon for two or more of these patterns to be present simultaneously. In fact, an overlap of patterns seen pathologically is specifically suggestive of CTD compared with other causes of diffuse lung disease. In this context, HRCT in a patient with CTD may have findings of more than one pattern (Fig. 10.11). The most common patterns to overlap include NSIP, LIP/follicular bronchiolitis, and OP.

HRCT FINDINGS IN SPECIFIC CTDs

Any type of CTD may present with any of the abnormalities listed above, but specific diseases tend to be associated with specific abnormalities (Table 10.6). It is important for the radiologist to be able to recognize the pattern present on HRCT and the connective tissues with which it is most commonly associated. This is particularly true during the initial presentation of a patient with diffuse lung disease. Initially, patients may not meet all the criteria for a specific CTD, and imaging may be helpful in elucidating the nature of the patient's systemic disorder.

Progressive Systemic Sclerosis (Scleroderma)

Progressive systemic sclerosis, or scleroderma, is a systemic disorder with primary manifestations of skin thickening and tightening. Other

10

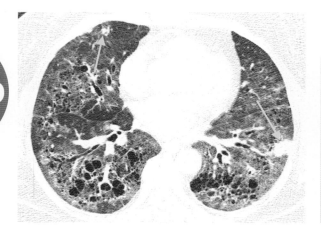

Figure 10.11

Overlap of patterns in connective tissue disease. Pathologically this patient with mixed connective tissue disease had more than one interstitial pneumonia pattern present. Patchy, bilateral ground glass opacity and cysts correspond to lymphoid interstitial pneumonia. Focal areas of nodular consolidation (*arrows*) correspond to organizing pneumonia.

common abnormalities include Raynaud's phenomenon and esophageal dysmotility. Lung disease is present in up to 80% of patients. Scl-70 and Anti-U3 RNP antibodies are specific for scleroderma.

The majority of patients with scleroderma-related lung disease show a NSIP pattern on HRCT (Fig. 10.12A–D), manifested as

Table 10.6	Common patterns associated with specific connective tissue diseases
Scleroderma	NSIP
	UIP
	Pulmonary hypertension (particularly in CREST)
Rheumatoid arthritis	UIP
	NSIP
	Bronchiectasis
Systemic lupus erythematosus	Diffuse alveolar damage
	Hemorrhage
	Edema
	Pleural/pericardial effusions
Poly/dermatomyositis	NSIP
	OP
	Diffuse alveolar damage
Sjögren's syndrome	NSIP
	LIP
Mixed connective tissue disease	NSIP
	UIP

NSIP, nonspecific interstitial pneumonia; UIP, usual interstitial pneumonia; OP, organizing pneumonia; LIP, lymphoid interstitial pneumonia; CREST, calcinosis, Raynaud's phenomena, esophageal dysmotility, sclerodactyly, and telangiectasia.

subpleural and basilar predominant traction bronchiectasis, irregular reticulation, and/or ground glass opacity. Sparing of the immediate subpleural lung is not uncommon and supports a diagnosis of NSIP.

When significant honeycombing is present, UIP is more likely, the second most common pattern seen with scleroderma (Fig. 10.13). Pulmonary hypertension may also be seen in scleroderma patients due to either the parenchymal lung disease or vascular disease.

CREST

The CREST syndrome is a form of limited cutaneous scleroderma. CREST is an acronym for Calcinosis, Raynaud's phenomena, Esophageal dysmotility, Sclerodactyly, and Telangiectasia. Patients with CREST show a higher incidence of pulmonary vascular disease and a lower incidence of fibrotic lung disease than other patients with scleroderma.

Rheumatoid Arthritis

RA is characterized by an arthritis that has a predilection for the hands, particularly the proximal interphalangeal and metacarpophalangeal joints. Rheumatoid factor is commonly positive in patients with RA. Approximately 40% of patients with RA will have lung disease.

The most common pattern present on HRCT is UIP with a peripheral and basilar predominance of fibrosis with honeycombing, indistinguishable from idiopathic pulmonary fibrosis (Fig. 10.14A, B). NSIP is the

10

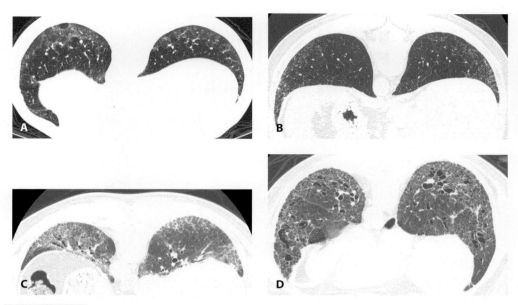

Figure 10.12

Spectrum of nonspecific interstitial pneumonia (NSIP) abnormalities in scleroderma. Four patients with scleroderma-related NSIP are shown on prone HRCT. **A.** Prone HRCT shows peripheral and basilar ground glass opacity without evidence of fibrosis in a patient with cellular NSIP. **B.** Prone HRCT shows very early irregular reticulation without traction bronchiectasis or honeycombing. This could represent either fibrotic or cellular NSIP. **C.** The irregular reticulation in this case is more severe and associated with traction bronchiectasis, compatible with fibrotic NSIP. **D.** Late disease with severe fibrosis shows extensive traction bronchiectasis and irregular reticulation.

second most common pattern. Uncommon patterns seen in patients with RA include OP and follicular bronchiolitis.

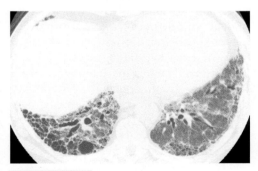

Figure 10.13

Usual interstitial pneumonia (UIP) in scleroderma. Peripheral, basilar fibrosis with honeycombing is compatible with a pattern of UIP in a patient with scleroderma. This appearance is indistinguishable from idiopathic pulmonary fibrosis and other causes of a UIP pattern.

Bronchiectasis is a frequent finding on HRCT in patients with RA, including those without fibrotic lung disease. Bronchiolitis may be due to chronic infection or constrictive bronchiolitis.

Rheumatoid nodules are a rare manifestation and patients are typically asymptomatic. They may be single or multiple, can become large, and may cavitate. As with any cause of cavitary nodules, rheumatoid nodules may be complicated by bronchopleural fistula.

Systemic Lupus Erythematosus

SLE has a variety of possible clinical manifestations including rash, oral ulcers, photosensitivity, arthritis, and serositis. Disorders involving the renal, neurologic, and hematological systems are common as well. Multiple serologies may be positive, including antinuclear antibody, antiphospholipid antibodies, anti–double-stranded DNA antibodies, and

10

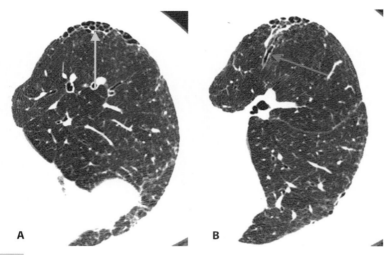

A   B

Figure 10.14

Usual interstitial pneumonia (UIP) in rheumatoid arthritis. Honeycombing (**A**, *yellow arrow*) and mild traction bronchiectasis (**B**, *red arrow*) are seen in the subpleural lung regions. UIP is the most common pattern seen in patients with rheumatoid arthritis–related interstitial lung disease.

anti-Smith antibodies. Anti–double-stranded DNA antibodies are specific for SLE.

The lung disease associated with SLE differs somewhat from that of other CTDs. DAD, diffuse alveolar hemorrhage, and pulmonary edema are the most common manifestations (Fig. 10.15). A combination of these is seen in patients with lupus pneumonitis. These patterns manifest in a similar manner on HRCT with extensive or diffuse areas of ground glass opacity and/or

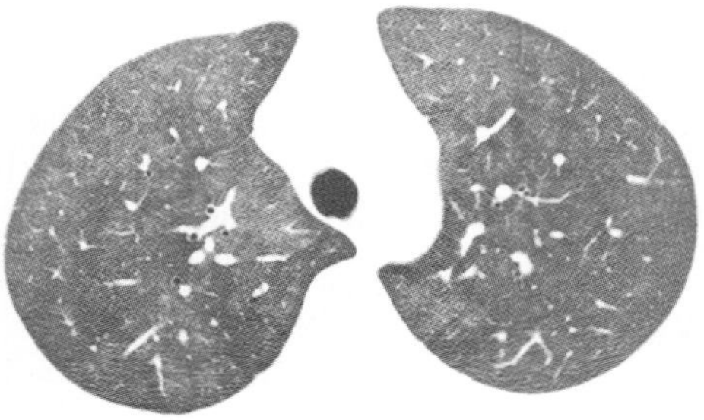

Figure 10.15

Pulmonary hemorrhage in systemic lupus erythematosus. Symmetric bilateral ground glass opacity in the setting of systemic lupus erythematosus is a nonspecific finding and could represent edema, DAD, atypical infection, or hemorrhage.

consolidation. Patients with multiple episodes of pulmonary hemorrhage may eventually develop fibrosis.

Serositis is a common sequela of SLE. Pleural or pericardial effusions may be seen in isolation or associated with lung disease. Pleural/pericardial thickening or enhancement may also be present, reflecting the presence of an exudative effusion.

Vanishing or *shrinking lung syndrome* is a rare manifestation of SLE, in which patients present with dyspnea and restrictive defects on pulmonary function tests, but have no evidence of parenchymal lung disease on HRCT. The primary radiographic finding is elevation of the hemidiaphragms. This may be due to muscular weakness or phrenic nerve dysfunction.

IPs and pulmonary fibrosis are uncommon manifestations of SLE, but UIP, NSIP, and OP may be seen.

Polymyositis and Dermatomyositis

The features of myositis include muscle weakness, arthritis, and constitutional symptoms. Dermatomyositis also shows skin changes. Anti-Jo-1 antibodies are frequently positive and specific for an inflammatory myositis. Pulmonary symptoms are often due to chronic

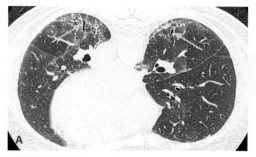
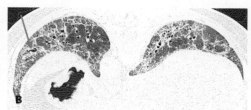

Figure 10.16

Polymyositis with nonspecific interstitial pneumonia. Prone HRCT through the mid **(A)** and lower **(B)** lungs demonstrates peripheral and basilar predominant irregular reticulation and traction bronchiectasis (*arrows*). There is relative sparing of the immediate subpleural interstitium.

interstitial lung disease, but weakness of the respiratory muscles and recurrent aspiration from pharyngeal muscle weakness may also be responsible.

NSIP is the most common diffuse lung disease associated with myositis (Fig. 10.16). HRCT often shows basilar, subpleural predominant ground glass, irregular reticulation, and/or traction bronchiectasis with or without subpleural sparing. OP is another common pattern, manifesting by patchy consolidation. An overlap of NSIP and OP may be present with consolidation involving the subpleural and basilar lung regions (Fig. 10.17).

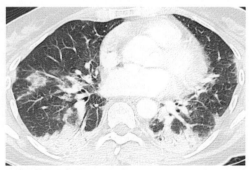

Figure 10.17

Polymyositis with overlap of nonspecific interstitial pneumonia (NSIP) and organizing pneumonia. HRCT shows subpleural and posterior consolidation. The distribution is typical of NSIP, but consolidation is not a typical NSIP finding. Pathologically there were components of both NSIP and organizing pneumonia present. Consolidation on HRCT is more typical of organizing pneumonia.

An acute presentation of DAD is not uncommon with a rapid development of extensive ground glass opacity on HRCT. UIP is an uncommon manifestation of myositis. Rare associated patterns include LIP.

Sjögren's Disease

Sjögren's disease is a CTD that shows prominent ocular and oral involvement. Dysfunction of the lacrimal and salivary glands produces dry eyes and dry mouth. Patients often show the positive autoantibodies anti-SSA and anti-SSB.

The most common patterns of lung disease in patients with Sjögren's disease are NSIP and LIP. The HRCT findings of NSIP are similar to those of scleroderma. OP and UIP may be seen in Sjögren's disease, but are relatively uncommon.

LIP commonly shows multiple lung cysts as an isolated abnormality (Fig. 10.18). Cysts are usually round and thin walled. They involve all lung regions and are less numerous than cysts seen in lymphangioleiomyomatosis and Langerhans cell histiocytosis; usually cysts number a few dozen or less. Ground glass opacity and centrilobular ground glass opacity nodules may also be associated with LIP or follicular bronchiolitis, but this is less common than isolated cysts.

Other lymphoproliferative diseases may be present in patients with Sjögren's disease. Focal lymphoid hyperplasia represents a benign, reactive collection of lymphoid cells. Its most common HRCT manifestation is a solitary pulmonary nodule or focal region of consolidation. Multiple nodules have also been

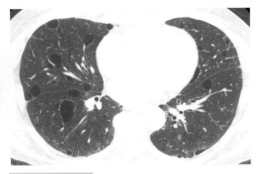

Figure 10.18

Lymphoid interstitial pneumonia in Sjögren's disease. Lung cysts may be seen as an isolated abnormality in lymphoid interstitial pneumonia, particularly in the setting of Sjögren's disease. They are round and thin walled and limited in number.

described. Lymphoma is seen with a much greater incidence in patients with Sjögren's disease compared with the population as a whole and may resemble focal lymphoid hyperplasia. Biopsy of suspicious abnormalities is generally performed to distinguish these two entities.

Mixed CTD

As the name suggests, mixed CTD shows overlapping features of other CTDs, primarily scleroderma, SLE, and myosytis. Anti-RNP antibodies are often present and may precede the development of symptoms. Lung disease is present in approximately 60% of patients.

NSIP and UIP are the most common patterns seen. Other less common patterns include LIP, OP, and pulmonary vascular disease.

FURTHER READING

Aquino SL, Webb WR, Golden J. Bronchiolitis obliterans associated with rheumatoid arthritis: findings on HRCT and dynamic expiratory CT. *J Comput Assist Tomogr.* 1994;18:555-558.

Bankier AA, Kiener HP, Wiesmayr MN, et al. Discrete lung involvement in systemic lupus erythematosus: CT assessment. *Radiology.* 1995;196:835-840.

Bhalla M, Silver RM, Shepard JO, McLoud TC. Chest CT in patients with scleroderma: prevalence of asymptomatic esophageal dilatation and mediastinal lymphadenopathy. *AJR Am J Roentgenol.* 1993;161:269-272.

Fenlon HM, Doran M, Sant SM, Breatnach E. High-resolution chest CT in systemic lupus erythematosus. *AJR Am J Roentgenol.* 1996;166:301-307.

Franquet T, Giménez A, Monill JM, et al. Primary Sjögren's syndrome and associated lung disease: CT findings in 50 patients. *AJR Am J Roentgenol.* 1997;169:655-658.

Fujii M, Adachi S, Shimizu T, et al. Interstitial lung disease in rheumatoid arthritis: assessment with high-resolution computed tomography. *J Thorac Imaging.* 1993;8:54-62.

Kim EJ, Elicker BM, Maldonado F, et al. Usual interstitial pneumonia in rheumatoid arthritis-associated interstitial lung disease. *Eur Respir J.* 2010;35:1322-1328.

Kim JS, Lee KS, Koh EM, et al. Thoracic involvement of systemic lupus erythematosus: clinical, pathologic, and radiologic findings. *J Comput Assist Tomogr.* 2000;24:9-18.

Lee HK, Kim DS, Yoo B, et al. Histopathologic pattern and clinical features of rheumatoid arthritis-associated interstitial lung disease. *Chest.* 2005;127:2019-2027.

Mino M, Noma S, Taguchi Y, et al. Pulmonary involvement in polymyositis and dermatomyositis: sequential evaluation with CT. *AJR Am J Roentgenol.* 1997;169:83-87.

Primack SL, Müller NL. Radiologic manifestations of the systemic autoimmune diseases. *Clin Chest Med.* 1998;19:573-586.

Remy-Jardin M, Remy J, Cortet B, et al. Lung changes in rheumatoid arthritis: CT findings. *Radiology.* 1994;193:375-382.

Remy-Jardin M, Remy J, Wallaert B, et al. Pulmonary involvement in progressive systemic sclerosis: sequential evaluation with CT, pulmonary function tests, and bronchoalveolar lavage. *Radiology.* 1993;188:499-506.

Schurawitzki H, Stiglbauer R, Graninger W, et al. Interstitial lung disease in progressive systemic sclerosis: high-resolution CT versus radiography. *Radiology.* 1990;176:755-759.

Souza AS Jr, Müller NL, Marchiori E, Soares-Souza LV, de Souza Rocha M. Pulmonary abnormalities in ankylosing spondylitis: inspiratory and expiratory high-resolution CT findings in 17 patients. *J Thorac Imaging.* 2004;19:259-263.

Tanaka N, Kim JS, Newell JD, et al. Rheumatoid arthritis-related lung diseases: CT findings. *Radiology.* 2004;232:81-91.

Tanaka N, Newell JD, Brown KK, Cool CD, Lynch DA. Collagen vascular disease-related lung disease: high-resolution computed tomography findings based on the pathologic classification. *J Comput Assist Tomogr.* 2004;28:351-360.

Tanoue LT. Pulmonary involvement in collage vascular disease: a review of the pulmonary manifestations of the Marfan syndrome, ankylosing spondylitis, Sjögren's syndrome, and relapsing polychondritis. *J Thorac Imaging.* 1992;7:62-77.

Taorimina VJ, Miller WT, Gefter WB, Epstein DM. Progressive systemic sclerosis subgroups: variable pulmonary features. *AJR Am J Roentgenol.* 1981;137:277-285.

Tazelaar HD, Viggiano RW, Pickersgill J, Colby TV. Interstitial lung disease in polymyositis and dermatomyositis. clinical features and prognosis as correlated with histologic findings. *Am Rev Respir Dis.* 1990;141:727-733.

11

Smoking-Related Lung Disease

Cigarette smoking is well known for its association with lung cancer, but diffuse lung disease is also an established cause of smoking-related morbidity. There are a variety of different manifestations of smoking-related diffuse lung disease with different treatments and prognoses. This chapter focuses on respiratory bronchiolitis (RB), desquamative interstitial pneumonia (DIP), emphysema, and Langerhans cell histiocytosis (LCH) as the primary manifestations of diffuse lung disease related to cigarette smoke inhalation. Idiopathic pulmonary fibrosis (IPF) is also associated with cigarette smoking.

RB AND DIP

RB and *DIP* represent a similar reaction of lung to inhaled cigarette smoke, although they differ in their incidence, the severity of the specific abnormality present, and their association with symptoms. In the case of RB, cigarette smoke inhalation induces reactive changes in and around small airways, characterized by focal areas of alveolar macrophage infiltrate and mild interstitial inflammation. In DIP, there is more generalized intra-alveolar macrophage accumulation and inflammation. DIP is more commonly symptomatic than RB.

Pathologically, RB is seen in virtually all smokers, but it is responsible for symptoms in only a small minority of patients. RB is thought to represent a factor in the development of centrilobular emphysema. Chronic cellular infiltration and inflammation associated with

RB, it is hypothesized, eventually leads to lung destruction and emphysema.

When RB is a cause of symptoms, the disease is termed *respiratory bronchiolitis interstitial lung disease (RB-ILD)*.

Both RB-ILD and DIP typically present in young patients (peak age 30 to 40 years) and have a significantly better prognosis than most other interstitial lung diseases, with a good response to smoking cessation and/or treatment with steroids. Up to 25% of patients with DIP may eventually develop lung fibrosis in the absence of appropriate treatment.

HRCT Findings in RB and DIP

The HRCT findings of RB and DIP differ (Tables 11.1 and 11.2), but commonly coexist, given the overlap between these two entities. Typically, HRCT in RB/RB-ILD shows centrilobular ground glass opacity (GGO) nodules, reflecting the bronchiolar and peribronchiolar macrophage infiltrate typical of this disease (Fig. 11.1A, B). These nodules tend to predominate in the upper lobes and in central lung regions, similar to the distribution of centrilobular emphysema. There may be

Table 11.1	HRCT findings of respiratory bronchiolitis

HRCT finding
Centrilobular nodules of ground glass opacity
Mild mosaic perfusion/air trapping
Central, upper lobe distribution

Table 11.2	HRCT findings of desquamative interstitial pneumonia

HRCT finding

Ground glass opacity
Focal air-density lucencies (cysts or emphysema)
Subpleural and basilar distribution

associated mosaic perfusion or air trapping, but this tends to be mild (Fig. 11.2A, B).

DIP almost always presents with GGO as the predominant finding. The GGO is typically subpleural and basal in distribution (Fig. 11.3), similar to the distribution of usual interstitial pneumonia and nonspecific interstitial pneumonia (NSIP). Scattered cysts or patchy emphysema may be associated with the areas of GGO (Fig. 11.4). The combination of GGO with associated cysts or emphysema in a

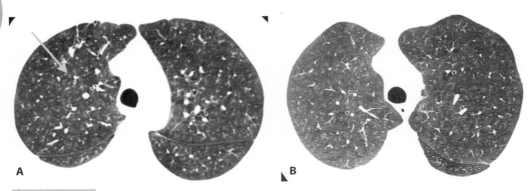

A   B

Figure 11.1

Respiratory bronchiolitis and respiratory bronchiolitis interstitial lung disease. A. An asymptomatic smoker shows centrilobular nodules of ground glass opacity (*arrow*) on HRCT, typical of the peribronchiolar cellular infiltration and inflammation seen in respiratory bronchiolitis (RB). **B.** HRCT in a patient with mild dyspnea shows more extensive and larger centrilobular nodules of ground glass opacity, reflecting respiratory bronchiolitis. Because RB is associated with symptoms in this patient, it is termed respiratory bronchiolitis interstitial lung disease.

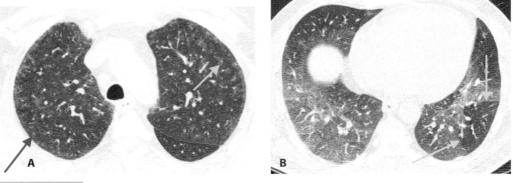

A   B

Figure 11.2

Respiratory bronchiolitis with mild air trapping. HRCT through the upper lobes **(A)** shows centrilobular nodules of ground glass opacity (*arrows*). Expiratory HRCT through the lower lungs **(B)** shows patchy air trapping (*arrows*).

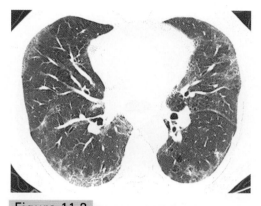

Figure 11.3

Desquamative interstitial pneumonia. HRCT shows peripheral areas of ground glass opacity in this smoker with desquamative interstitial pneumonia.

smoker is strongly suggestive of this diagnosis. In a minority of patients, fibrosis develops in areas previously affected by GGO. This is manifested by irregular reticulation and traction bronchiectasis (Fig. 11.5). Honeycombing is rare.

As RB and DIP represent a spectrum of abnormalities, an overlap of their typical findings may be present on HRCT in smokers (Fig. 11.6A, B). GGO may have a variable distribution from subpleural/basilar predominant to central/upper lobe predominant. Patchy GGO may be seen in combination with GGO centrilobular nodules. Cysts or emphysema, mosaic perfusion, and air trapping may be associated with any of these abnormalities.

Differential Diagnosis

The differential diagnosis of RB and DIP in a patient with chronic symptoms includes

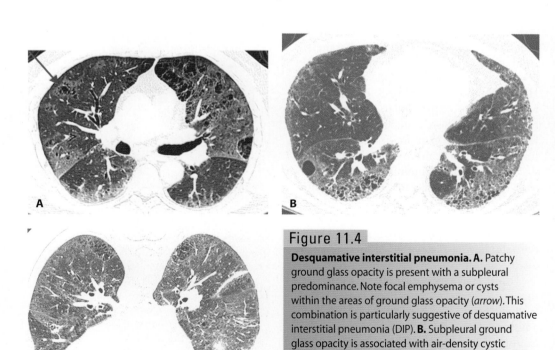

Figure 11.4

Desquamative interstitial pneumonia. A. Patchy ground glass opacity is present with a subpleural predominance. Note focal emphysema or cysts within the areas of ground glass opacity (*arrow*). This combination is particularly suggestive of desquamative interstitial pneumonia (DIP). **B.** Subpleural ground glass opacity is associated with air-density cystic lucencies. The cystic lucencies can be distinguished from honeycombing by the fact that many are not subpleural and there is no evidence of fibrosis such as traction bronchiectasis. **C.** Prone computed tomography shows predominantly peripheral ground glass opacity and cystic lucencies in a smoker with DIP.

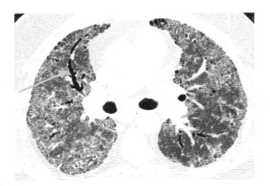

Figure 11.5

Desquamative interstitial pneumonia with fibrosis. Fibrosis is an uncommon sequela of desquamative interstitial pneumonia and typically is manifested by traction bronchiectasis (*arrow*) and/or irregular reticulation superimposed upon ground glass opacity. Honeycombing is distinctly rare.

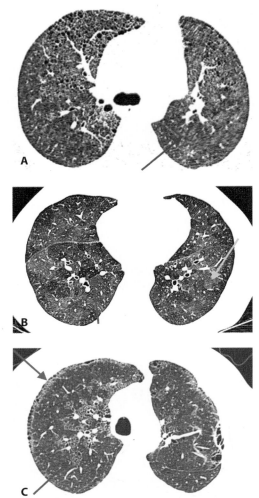

Figure 11.6

Respiratory bronchiolitis and desquamative interstitial pneumonia overlap in three patients. A. A combination of centrilobular nodules of ground glass opacity (*arrow*) and more diffuse patchy ground glass opacity and emphysema are present. **B.** High-resolution computed tomography shows a combination of ground glass opacity (*yellow arrow*) and lobular mosaic perfusion (*red arrow*). This represents the "headcheese" sign. **C.** Patchy glass opacity is associated with cystic lucencies. The more peripheral areas of ground glass (*blue arrow*) are more typical of desquamative interstitial pneumonia, whereas the central lobular areas of ground glass (*red arrow*) are more typical of respiratory bronchiolitis.

other disorders that produce GGO, ground glass centrilobular nodules, cysts, and mosaic perfusion. Hypersensitivity pneumonitis (HP) is a common cause of these findings (Fig. 11.7). Although it is thought that there is a reduced likelihood of HP in cigarette smokers, smoking does not preclude a diagnosis of HP. The presence of fibrosis in association with GGO or centrilobular nodules favors HP, because fibrosis is uncommon with RB/DIP (Fig. 11.8). Also, mosaic perfusion and air trapping tend to be more severe in HP.

Follicular bronchiolitis/lymphoid interstitial pneumonia (FB/LIP) is another abnormality that may show centrilobular ground glass nodules, GGO, and mild mosaic perfusion/air trapping. Patients with FB/LIP typically have a history of connective tissue disease or immunocompromise.

NSIP may have a distribution identical to that of DIP, with subpleural and basilar abnormalities (Fig. 11.9). These patients usually have a history of connective tissue disease or a drug exposure. The presence of fibrosis suggests NSIP.

EMPHYSEMA

Chronic cellular infiltration and inflammation due to smoke inhalation may eventually lead to lung destruction and emphysema.

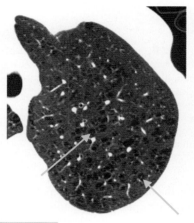

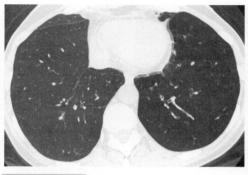

Figure 11.7

Centrilobular emphysema. Magnified HRCT of the left lung shows the typical morphology of centrilobular emphysema. Focal air-attenuation lucencies are present in the central lung regions, without visible walls. A centrilobular artery is seen in the center of some of these lucencies (*arrows*).

Figure 11.8

Panlobular emphysema associated with smoking. When extensive, smoking-related emphysema may be panlobular in distribution. This manifests as diffuse lung lucency associated with small vessels.

The HRCT appearances are reviewed briefly here (Table 11.3) and described in detail in Chapter 5.

Centrilobular Emphysema

Centrilobular emphysema is most closely associated with smoking. The HRCT findings of centrilobular emphysema are usually diagnostic and do not require lung biopsy. HRCT may be more sensitive than pulmonary function tests in patients with early disease.

The HRCT findings of centrilobular emphysema include focal air-attenuation lucencies without well-defined walls (i.e., black holes), which involve the central and upper lung regions (Fig. 11.7). Small vessels, representing the centrilobular artery or arteries, may be seen in the center of these focal lucencies. Bullae may be seen.

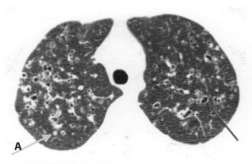

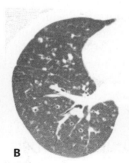

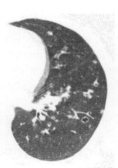

Figure 11.9

Langerhans cell histiocytosis, early stage. HRCT shows a combination of soft tissue attenuation nodules (*yellow arrow*) and cavitary nodules or cysts (*red arrow*). The cysts are irregularly shaped and have variable thickness of their walls. These show much greater involvement of the upper lungs **(A)** compared with the lower lungs **(B).** Nodules are typical of early disease.

Table 11.3	HRCT findings of emphysema
Centrilobular	Upper, central lung distribution Focal air-density lucencies Walls not typically seen Centrilobular arteries (dots) at the center of the lucencies
Paraseptal	Subpleural distribution Focal air-density lucencies Lucencies have discrete, thin walls Cysts in single layer Associated centrilobular emphysema may be present
Panlobular	Lower lung, diffuse distribution Increased lung lucency, abnormality not usually focal Small vessels in affected regions

Table 11.4	HRCT findings of Langerhans cell histiocytosis
Centrilobular nodules of soft tissue attenuation Cavitation of nodules with progression to thick-walled cysts Irregular, bizarre-shaped cysts Upper lobe predominance; sparing of the costophrenic angles Spontaneous pneumothorax	

Paraseptal Emphysema

Paraseptal emphysema may be seen in association with centrilobular emphysema. It is related to smoking in many patients. This form of emphysema appears as a single layer of subpleural air-attenuation cysts with paper-thin walls. When large, areas of paraseptal emphysema represent bullae.

Panlobular Emphysema

Panlobular emphysema is often associated with alpha-1-antitrypsin deficiency, but may also be seen in severe cases of smoking-related emphysema (Fig. 11.8). As areas of lung destruction typical of centrilobular emphysema become larger and confluent, they may involve the entire pulmonary lobule. Panlobular emphysema on HRCT shows diffuse lung lucency with attenuated vessels. The distribution is usually lower lobe predominant in alpha-1-antitrypsin deficiency. In smokers, it may be more severe in the upper lobes.

LANGERHANS CELL HISTIOCYTOSIS

In adults, pulmonary LCH occurs primarily in smokers. As with RB and DIP, the peak age at presentation for adult LCH is approximately 30 to 40 years. Symptoms vary widely. Patients may be asymptomatic or may have severe dyspnea. Lung transplantation may be necessary in some patients. As with any cystic lung

disease, the initial clinical presentation may be the development of a pneumothorax.

HRCT Findings

On HRCT, the appearance of LCH (Table 11.4) varies with the stage of disease. In early cases, small scattered lung nodules are typically seen; over time, these may cavitate (Fig. 11.9A, B). Nodules in LCH are commonly of soft tissue attenuation, although rarely centrilobular ground glass nodules may be the primary manifestation.

With further progression, thick-walled lung cysts develop, and a combination of nodules, cavitary nodules, and cysts may be seen. Cysts tend to be irregular, having bizarre, branching, and clover-leaf shapes (Fig. 11.10). Late disease may present with cysts that nearly replace the normal lung (Fig. 11.11). Cysts eventually become thin walled, and differentiation from centrilobular emphysema may be difficult.

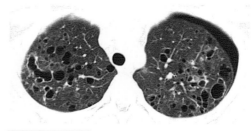

Figure 11.10

Langerhans cell histiocytosis, cysts. There is a predominance of cysts in this smoker. The cysts are irregular in shape. Some have thin walls and others are thick walled. A left pneumothorax is also present. Except for acute symptoms associated with the pneumothorax, the patient was asymptomatic.

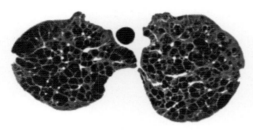

Figure 11.11

Langerhans cell histiocytosis, cysts. When severe, the cysts of Langerhans cell histiocytosis are extensive and may show near-complete replacement of the lung parenchyma. Usually nodules are not present at this stage. This pattern may be difficult to distinguish from extensive emphysema.

Abnormalities in LCH show a distinct upper lobe predominance, with relative sparing of the lung bases and costophrenic angles. Associated pleural effusions are uncommon.

Differential Diagnosis

The differential diagnosis of LCH includes other cystic lung diseases (Fig. 11.12A, B), particularly lymphangioleiomyomatosis (LAM). Both of these diseases may produce extensive cystic lung disease. However, differentiation is often possible. In LCH, cysts have bizarre shapes and upper lobe predominance and may be thick walled. The cysts of LAM, in contrast, are usually round, thin walled, and diffuse in distribution. Furthermore, LAM occurs almost entirely in women. A man with cystic lung disease is not likely to have LAM. Other cystic lung diseases, such as LIP, usually show fewer cysts.

The presence of nodules favors LCH, whereas the presence of pleural effusions favors LAM. Other causes of cavitary nodules, such as septic emboli, fungal infection, Wegener's granulomatosis, cystic metastases (e.g., endometrial carcinoma), and tracheobronchial papillomatosis, may resemble LCH, but nodules in these diseases are often larger.

FIBROTIC LUNG DISEASE

Lung fibrosis is a common pathologic finding in smokers, but is infrequently seen on HRCT. As discussed previously, a subset of patients with

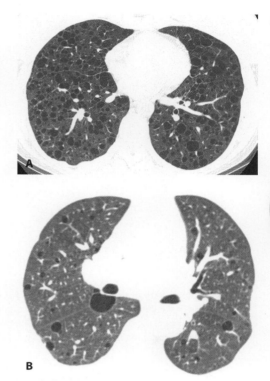

A

B

Figure 11.12

Differential diagnosis of Langerhans cell histiocytosis (LCH). Both LCH and lymphangioleiomyomatosis (LAM) can produce extensive cystic lung disease. **A.** The cysts of LAM differ from those of LCH in that they have a round and regular shape. Nodules are not common in LAM and the disease does not show sparing of the lung bases. **B.** Lung cysts in neurofibromatosis. Cysts are less numerous than in LCH and are round in shape.

DIP may progress to fibrosis. There is also an association between cigarette smoking and IPF.

Forty to 80% of patients with IPF have a smoking history. Patients with a combination of emphysema and IPF (Fig. 11.13) may have relatively normal pulmonary function tests, but have a higher incidence of pulmonary hypertension than other patients with IPF.

The presence of emphysema can complicate the diagnosis of fibrotic lung disease on HRCT. Centrilobular or paraseptal emphysema in the peripheral lung may be mistaken for honeycombing, particularly when there is adjacent GGO or reticulation. In such cases,

11

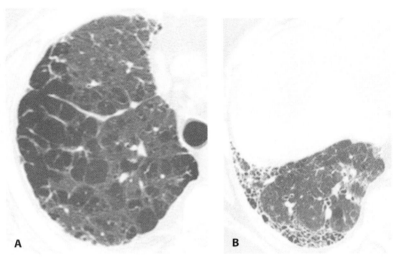

A   **B**

Figure 11.13

Combined pulmonary fibrosis and emphysema. A. Centrilobular emphysema is seen in the upper lobes. **B.** Fibrosis is present in the lower lobes, resulting in peripheral honeycombing, compatible with usual interstitial pneumonia. This combination is associated with relatively normal pulmonary function tests and a higher incidence of pulmonary hypertension.

abnormalities in the lower lungs on HRCT may be more diagnostic of fibrosis, as emphysema tends to be an upper lobe process. There should be a higher threshold for describing the pattern of usual interstitial pneumonia on HRCT when significant emphysema is present.

FURTHER READING

Abbott GF, Rosado-de-Christenson ML, Franks TJ, et al. Pulmonary Langerhans cell histiocytosis. *Radiographics*. 2004;24:821-841.

Brauner MW, Grenier P, Mouelhi MM, et al. Pulmonary histiocytosis X: evaluation with high resolution CT. *Radiology*. 1989;172:255-258.

Brauner MW, Grenier P, Tijani K, et al. Pulmonary Langerhans cell histiocytosis: evolution of lesions on CT scans. *Radiology*. 1997;204:497-502.

Foster WL Jr, Gimenez EI, Roubidoux MA, et al. The emphysemas: radiologic-pathologic correlations. *Radiographics*. 1993;13:311-328.

Goldin JG. Imaging the lungs in patients with pulmonary emphysema. *J Thorac Imaging*. 2009;24:163-170.

Hartman TE, Primack SL, Swensen SJ, et al. Desquamative interstitial pneumonia: thin-section CT findings in 22 patients. *Radiology*. 1993;187:787-790.

Heyneman LE, Ward S, Lynch DA, et al. Respiratory bronchiolitis, respiratory bronchiolitis-associated interstitial lung disease, and desquamative interstitial pneumonia: different entities or part of the spectrum of the same disease process? *AJR Am J Roentgenol*. 1999;173:1617-1622.

Hidalgo A, Franquet T, Gimenez A, et al. Smoking-related interstitial lung disease: radiologic-pathologic correlation. *Eur Radiol*. 2006;16:2463-2470.

Nakanishi M, Demura Y, Mizuno S, et al. Changes in HRCT findings in patients with respiratory bronchiolitis-associated interstitial lung disease after smoking cessation. *Eur Respir J*. 2007;29:453-461.

Park JS, Brown KK, Tuder RM, Hale VA, King TE Jr, Lynch DA. Respiratory bronchiolitis-associated interstitial lung disease: radiologic features with clinical and pathologic correlation. *J Comput Assist Tomogr*. 2002;26:13-20.

Remy-Jardin M, Edme JL, Boulenguez C, Remy J, Mastora I, Sobaszek A. Longitudinal follow-up study of smoker's lung with thin-section CT in correlation with pulmonary function tests. *Radiology*. 2002;222:261-270.

Remy-Jardin M, Remy J, Gosselin B, Becette V, Edme JL. Lung parenchymal changes secondary to cigarette smoking: pathologic-CT correlations. *Radiology*. 1993;186:643-651.

Ryu JH, Myers JL, Capizzi SA, Douglas WW, Vassallo R, Decker PA. Desquamative interstitial pneumonia and respiratory bronchiolitis-associated interstitial lung disease. *Chest*. 2005;127:178-184.

Tazi A, Soler P, Hance AJ. Adult pulmonary Langerhans cell histiocytosis. *Thorax*. 2000;55:405-416.

Thurlbeck WM, Müller NL. Emphysema: definition, imaging, and quantification. *AJR Am J Roentgenol*. 1994;163:1017-1025.

12

Sarcoidosis

Sarcoidosis is an idiopathic disorder characterized by the presence of noncaseating granulomas, often found in relation to lymphatics, and involving many organs. It typically presents in patients less than 50 years of age, but may rarely be first diagnosed in older patients. While sarcoidosis is a systemic disease, it affects the thorax in at least 90% of cases. For this reason, HRCT is often the initial diagnostic examination obtained in patients suspected of having sarcoidosis.

Sarcoidosis demonstrates striking demographic differences, with the highest prevalence seen in people of Scandinavian descent and African Americans. Sarcoidosis is much less common in Asia and in countries close to the equator than in the United States.

Up to one-half of patients with sarcoidosis are asymptomatic and diagnosed by incidental findings on radiological examinations performed for other purposes. Mortality from sarcoidosis, approximately 1% to 5%, is low compared with other diffuse lung diseases.

STAGING OF SARCOIDOSIS

Staging of sarcoidosis is based upon plain radiography and has not been validated using HRCT. Subtle parenchymal lung changes or lymphadenopathy on HRCT may not be seen on chest radiographs.

The stages based upon chest radiographs are as follows:

Stage 0: normal
Stage I: hilar lymphadenopathy only

Stage II: hilar lymphadenopathy + parenchymal lung disease
Stage III: parenchymal lung disease only
Stage IV: fibrosis

This staging system is of some value in determining prognosis and predicting the likelihood of spontaneous regression of findings without treatment. Sixty to 90% of patients with Stage I disease show spontaneous regression, whereas only 10% to 20% of patients with Stage III disease will show spontaneous regression.

LUNG ABNORMALITIES IN SARCOIDOSIS

Pulmonary abnormalities in sarcoidosis are a manifestation of interstitial or airway granulomas and the subsequent development of pulmonary fibrosis or airway obstruction. The variety of abnormalities that may be seen on HRCT include perilymphatic nodules, consolidation and masses, ground glass opacity, mosaic perfusion, air trapping, irregular reticulation, traction bronchiectasis, cysts, and honeycombing (Table 12.1). Abnormalities typically have an upper lobe predominance, although this is not always the case.

Perilymphatic Nodules

The granulomas of sarcoidosis involve pulmonary lymphatics. Clusters of microscopic granulomas appear as small nodules having a *perilymphatic distribution*, described in detail in Chapter 3. Nodules tend to involve the lung

Table 12.1	Characteristic HRCT findings of sarcoidosis
Nodules	Perilymphatic distribution
	Peribronchovascular and subpleural predominance
	Nodules well defined
	Satellite nodules and the galaxy sign
Consolidation	Patchy, bilateral
	Peribronchovascular and subpleural distribution
Airways disease	Bronchostenosis or obstruction
	Atelectasis
	Mosaic perfusion
	Air trapping
Fibrosis	Irregular reticulation
	Traction bronchiectasis
	Parahilar fibrotic masses
	Cystic disease
	Honeycombing (rare)
	Upper lobe, peribronchovascular distribution

12

in a patchy fashion, with some areas of lung appearing abnormal and some areas appearing unaffected.

The following structures are typically involved by perilymphatic nodules in sarcoidosis:

1. Parahilar peribronchovascular interstitium
2. Centrilobular (peribronchovascular) interstitium
3. Subpleural interstitium
4. Interlobular septa

Nodules in sarcoidosis are typically well defined and have a preference for the parahilar peribronchovascular and subpleural interstitium (Figs. 12.1 to 12.3). Frequently, there are clusters of nodules within the interstitium surrounding central bronchi and pulmonary arteries. Mass-like conglomerates of nodules may be present in these locations. Nodules and clusters of nodules are also frequently seen in the subpleural interstitium, including the interstitium adjacent to fissures. Often in patients with sarcoidosis, nodules are limited to the peribronchovascular and subpleural regions, although the severity of involvement in these two locations may vary greatly (Figs. 12.1 to 12.3).

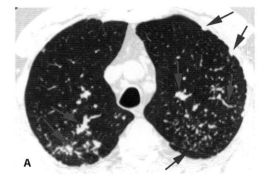

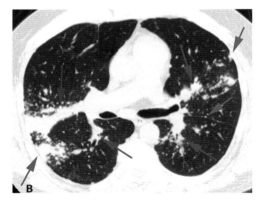

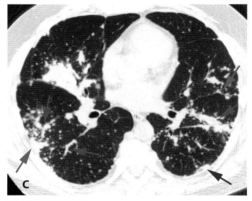

Figure 12.1

Typical sarcoidosis with peribronchovascular and subpleural nodules. A–C. In a patient with extensive lung involvement, HRCT shows clusters and masses of nodules that predominate in relation to the peribronchovascular interstitium surrounding parahilar arteries and bronchi (*red arrows,* **B**), more peripheral artery and bronchial branches (*red arrows* **A** and **C**), and the subpleural interstitium in the peripheral lung and adjacent to fissures (*blue arrows*). This patient has extensive lung involvement.

When peribronchovascular nodules are numerous, or when they involve the airway wall, they may cause narrowing or obstruction of central bronchi, occasionally producing lobar collapse (Fig. 12.4).

Rarely, the nodules of sarcoidosis show a centrilobular (Fig. 12.5) or interlobular septal predominance (Fig. 12.6). In such cases, nodules are usually also seen in the subpleural and peribronchovascular interstitium.

Sarcoidosis may occasionally have an appearance that mimics a random distribution of nodules. However, in such cases, there is often evidence that the pattern is perilymphatic. Nodules in these cases are usually not uniform, with a greater number of peribronchovascular

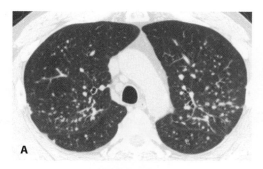
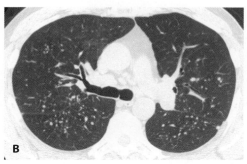

Figure 12.2

Typical sarcoidosis with peribronchovascular and subpleural nodules. A. HRCT shows scattered nodules in the parahilar regions, although a clear-cut relationship to airways and bronchi is more difficult to identify than in Fig. 12.1. Subpleural nodules are easily seen. **B.** At a lower level, the nodules are less numerous. An upper lobe predominance is typical of sarcoidosis.

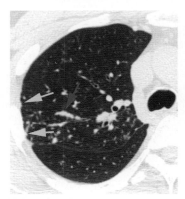

Figure 12.3

Typical sarcoidosis with peribronchovascular and subpleural nodules. In this patient with limited involvement of the right upper lobe, peribronchovascular (*red arrow*) and subpleural (*yellow arrows*) nodules are visible.

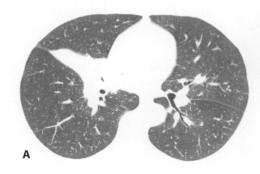
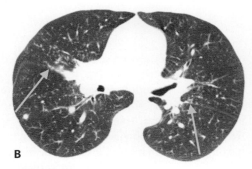

Figure 12.4

Sarcoidosis with right middle lobe collapse. Extensive peribronchovascular granulomas or endobronchial granulomas may cause bronchial narrowing or obstruction. **A.** In this patient, right middle lobe collapse is the result of bronchial involvement associated with hilar lymph node enlargement. **B.** At a different level, this patient shows scattered nodules with involvement of the fissures (*arrows*).

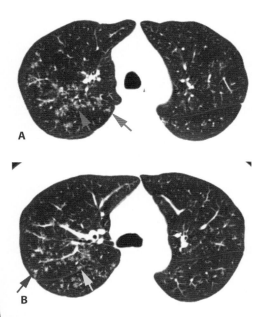

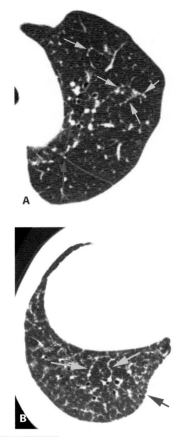

Figure 12.5

Centrilobular nodules in sarcoidosis. A and B. In this patient, nodules predominate in relation to centrilobular structures and appear ill-defined (*red arrows*). A few scattered subpleural nodules are also visible (*yellow arrow*, **B**). The peribronchovascular interstitium extends into the peripheral lung, in relation to centrilobular bronchioles and arteries. In some patients, granulomas in sarcoidosis predominate in relation to these structures, resulting in well-defined or ill-defined centrilobular nodules.

Figure 12.6

Interlobular septal thickening in two patients with sarcoidosis. Rarely sarcoidosis presents with nodular interlobular septal thickening as a predominant abnormality. **A.** In a patient with limited lung involvement, nodular septal thickening (*yellow arrows*) is visible in the left upper lobe. A few subpleural nodules are also seen (*red arrow*). **B.** In a different patient, nodular interlobular septal thickening predominates (*yellow arrows*) in the right lower lobe, and subpleural nodules are also visible (*red arrow*).

or subpleural nodules present than is expected for a random distribution (Fig. 12.7).

Because the nodules in sarcoidosis involve the interstitium around the central and peripheral airways, transbronchial biopsy is frequently able to obtain diagnostic tissue for histologic confirmation of disease. The biopsy results in these cases must be interpreted in the context of the HRCT findings and clinical presentation. Biopsies in patients with sarcoidosis show noncaseating granulomas, but these may be seen in other disorders as well. Thus the final diagnosis reflects a compilation of the pathology, radiology, and clinical factors.

Differential Diagnosis

The differential diagnosis of perilymphatic nodules (Table 12.2) includes lymphangitic spread of malignancy, lymphoid interstitial

pneumonia (LIP), pneumoconioses such as silicosis and coal worker's pneumoconiosis, and amyloidosis. Clinical history is important in suggesting one of these alternative diagnoses. For instance, patients with LIP usually have a history of connective tissue disease or immunocompromise. Lymphangitic spread of malignancy typically occurs in patients with a known tumor. Patients with pneumoconiosis have an extensive exposure history. Sarcoidosis tends to occur in a younger

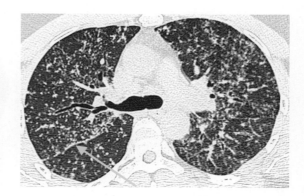

Figure 12.7

Sarcoidosis resembling a random distribution of nodules. Superficially the nodules appear random in distribution, with uniform lung involvement. A more detailed inspection reveals that the nodules are patchy in distribution, with more nodules along the fissures (*arrow*) than would be expected with a random pattern.

patient population than the other causes of perilymphatic nodules.

The morphology and distribution of nodules may also be helpful in suggesting sarcoidosis as the likely cause of perilymphatic nodules. Nodules in sarcoidosis often predominate in the peribronchovascular and subpleural interstitium. The nodules of lymphangitic spread of malignancy, the second most frequent cause of perilymphatic nodules, often predominate in relation to interlobular septa. Also lymphangitic spread of malignancy

Table 12.2	Differential diagnosis of sarcoidosis
Finding	**Differential diagnosis**
Perilymphatic nodules	Lymphangitic spread of malignancy
	Pneumoconioses
	Amyloid
	Lymphoid interstitial pneumonia
Patchy consolidation	Organizing pneumonia
	Eosinophilic pneumonia
	Invasive mucinous adenocarcinoma
	Lymphoma
	Lipoid pneumonia
Upper lobe fibrosis	Hypersensitivity pneumonitis
	Prior tuberculosis/fungal infection
	Pneumoconioses
	Radiation
	Ankylosing spondylitis
Symmetric hilar lymphadenopathy	Pneumoconioses
	Metastases
	Amyloid
	Castleman's disease

may be unilateral or basilar predominant, whereas sarcoidosis is typically bilateral, symmetric, and upper lobe predominant. Peribronchovascular nodules in lymphangitic spread of malignancy are usually associated with other evidence of tumor within the chest. Pneumoconioses may have a predominance of nodules in the centrilobular regions and typically involve the posterior upper lobes.

Consolidation and Masses

Sarcoidosis may present with mass-like consolidation representing confluent granulomatous disease. Because the masses of granulomas are often peribronchial, air bronchograms may be visible (Figs. 12.8 to 12.10). This appearance is sometimes termed "alveolar sarcoid," despite the fact that the granulomas do not involve the alveolar spaces.

Consolidation in sarcoidosis is often patchy, upper lobe predominant, and peribronchovascular in distribution. It may be mass-like in appearance. Discrete small nodules ("satellite nodules") may be seen at the periphery of areas of consolidation (Figs. 12.8 and 12.10), evidence that consolidation represents confluent granulomatous disease as opposed to an alveolar process. An area of mass-like consolidation with individual nodules at the periphery has been termed the *galaxy sign* and is most commonly seen with sarcoidosis.

The differential diagnosis of chronic consolidation includes organizing pneumonia, eosinophilic pneumonia, invasive mucinous adenocarcinoma, lymphoma, and lipoid pneumonia. The atoll or reversed halo sign or atoll sign is very suggestive of organizing pneumonia and only very rarely seen with sarcoidosis. Although

12

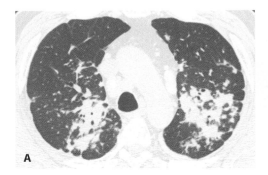

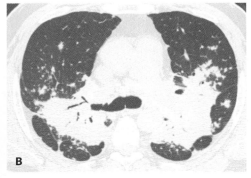

12

Figure 12.8

"Alveolar" sarcoidosis and the galaxy sign. A and **B.**
Confluent peribronchovascular granulomas result in
mass-like parahilar consolidation. Air bronchograms
are visible within the areas of consolidation. Small
nodules adjacent to the large masses are satellite
nodules. The combination of the large mass and
surrounding satellites is termed the "galaxy sign."

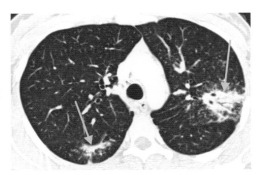

Figure 12.10

Consolidation in sarcoidosis. Patchy consolidation
is seen adjacent to bronchi and fissures (*yellow
arrows*), with an air bronchogram visible in the left
upper lobe. Small nodules are present at the edges
of the areas of consolidation (satellite nodules). This
feature may help distinguish sarcoidosis from other
causes of chronic consolidation and is termed the
galaxy sign.

the galaxy sign is common in sarcoidosis, it may
also be seen in silicosis and coal worker's pneumoconiosis, talcosis, other granulomatous diseases, and invasive mucinous adenocarcinoma.

Ground Glass Opacity

Rarely sarcoidosis may present with patchy
ground glass opacity as the predominant
finding (Fig. 12.11), representing the presence
of numerous microscopic granulomas. As

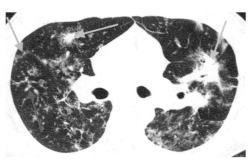

Figure 12.9

Consolidation in sarcoidosis. A combination of
consolidation (*yellow arrows*) in association with
more discrete peribronchovascular (*red arrow*) and
subpleural (*blue arrow*) nodules may be seen in
sarcoidosis. The consolidation represents confluent
granulomatous disease.

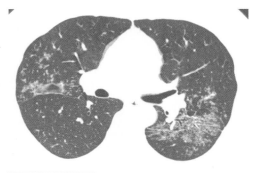

Figure 12.11

Sarcoidosis with ground glass opacity (GGO).
Patchy GGO is present in the left lung, but even
within areas of GGO, small discrete nodules can be
appreciated. GGO as an isolated finding is a rare
manifestation of sarcoidosis.

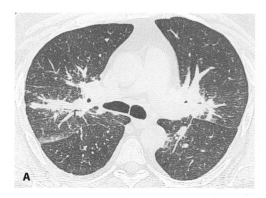

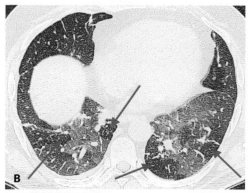

Figure 12.12

Sarcoidosis with air trapping. A. Typical peribronchovascular interstitial thickening is present in the upper lobes in this patient with sarcoidosis. **B.** On a post-expiratory image, patchy areas of air trapping (*arrows*) at the lung bases reflect small airway stenosis or occlusion by granulomas or associated fibrosis.

the lung findings in these cases are not particularly suggestive of sarcoidosis, lymphadenopathy, if present, may be the only clue as to the diagnosis.

Airway Abnormalities

Mosaic perfusion and/or air trapping may be seen in association with obstruction or narrowing of small airways by granulomas (Fig. 12.12). Depending upon the level of bronchial/bronchiolar obstruction, the distribution of these findings may be lobular, segmental, or lobar (Fig. 12.4).

Mosaic perfusion and air trapping are not usually isolated abnormalities in patients with sarcoidosis. At presentation, airway abnormalities are almost always associated with other findings, such as nodules (Fig. 12.12). However, after treatment, the airways disease may persist, even after the nodules resolve.

A combination of air trapping and nodules may be seen with several other diffuse lung diseases such as hypersensitivity pneumonitis, respiratory bronchiolitis, follicular bronchiolitis, and atypical infections. The nodules in these cases differ from sarcoidosis in that they are of ground glass opacity, whereas the nodules in sarcoidosis tend to be dense and well defined. Pneumoconioses and LIP may show perilymphatic nodules and associated mild mosaic perfusion and air trapping. It is unusual for lymphangitic spread of tumor and amyloidosis to produce mosaic perfusion and air trapping.

Fibrosis

Fibrosis occurs in approximately 20% of patients with sarcoidosis and is associated with a poor outcome. The fibrosis is usually upper lobe, central, and peribronchovascular in distribution. Irregular reticulation is common (Fig. 12.13). Fibrotic masses may be seen in some patients (Fig. 12.14). Masses are often associated with traction bronchiectasis, and irregular air bronchograms may be seen within them. Honeycombing may also

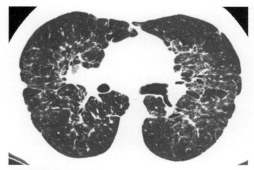

Figure 12.13

Sarcoidosis with fibrosis and irregular reticulation. Irregular reticular opacities predominate in the parahilar and peribronchovascular regions of the upper lobes. There is distortion of the fissures and subpleural areas of fibrosis are also visible.

12

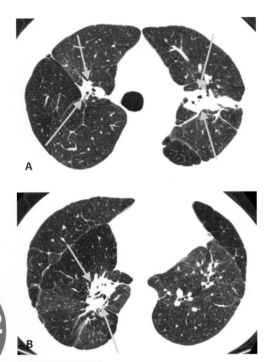

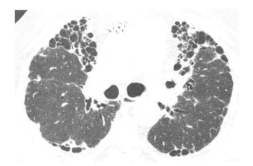

Figure 12.15

Honeycombing in sarcoidosis. Honeycombing may be seen as a manifestation of end-stage sarcoidosis. The distribution differs from idiopathic pulmonary fibrosis by being predominant in the upper lobes and/or having significant involvement of the central lung regions.

Figure 12.14

Sarcoidosis with fibrotic masses. A. Lung fibrosis associated with sarcoidosis typically predominates in the upper lobes and peribronchovascular regions (*arrows*). Masses of fibrous tissue may result. As in this case, there is associated volume loss and architectural distortion, and dilated bronchi (i.e., traction bronchiectasis) may be visible within the masses. **B.** In some patients, similar masses of fibrosis (*arrows*) are seen in the lower lobes.

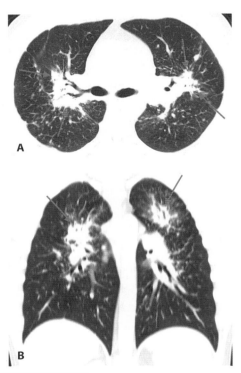

Figure 12.16

Sarcoidosis with findings resembling progressive massive fibrosis. Axial **(A)** and coronal **(B)** images show masses of consolidative fibrosis (*arrows*) and traction bronchiectasis within the central lung regions in a patient with sarcoidosis. These findings resemble progressive massive fibrosis seen in patients with silicosis.

be present (Fig. 12.15), but the overall distribution of fibrosis differs from idiopathic pulmonary fibrosis (IPF). IPF usually presents with a basilar and peripheral distribution of fibrosis.

Confluent areas of fibrosis may be manifested as mass-like areas of consolidation with architectural distortion, usually surrounding central bronchi (Fig. 12.16). This may be termed *progressive massive fibrosis (PMF)*, although PMF is usually used to refer to similar abnormalities occurring in silicosis. Consolidative areas of fibrosis can be

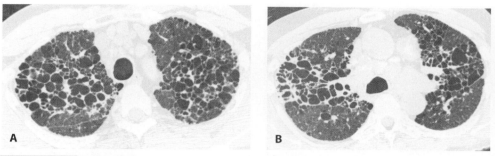

Figure 12.17

End-stage sarcoidosis with traction bronchiectasis and cyst formation. Images through the upper **(A)** and mid **(B)** lungs show extensive parahilar and upper lobe cystic disease may be seen with end-stage sarcoidosis. Differentiating dilated bronchi from cysts or emphysema may be difficult. Mycetoma is common in patients with this manifestation of fibrosis in sarcoidosis.

distinguished from "alveolar sarcoidosis" by the presence of associated traction bronchiectasis and architectural distortion. Given the upper lobe predominance of disease, the hila are often retracted superiorly.

Large cysts may be seen in areas of fibrosis in patients with sarcoidosis. These may represent dilated bronchi (traction bronchiectasis) or areas of emphysema (Fig. 12.17). Traction bronchiectasis is common in end-stage sarcoidosis. Mycetoma is a common complication of cystic sarcoidosis.

The differential diagnosis of sarcoidosis with fibrosis includes other chronic lung diseases that are upper lobe predominant including many pneumoconioses, most specifically silicosis or coal worker's pneumoconiosis, prior tuberculosis or fungal infection, radiation fibrosis, and ankylosing spondylitis. While hypersensitivity pneumonitis is typically mid-lung predominant, an upper lobe distribution of fibrosis is not uncommon and findings may overlap those typical of sarcoidosis. PMF is most commonly seen with sarcoidosis, pneumoconioses, or prior granulomatous infections.

LYMPHADENOPATHY

Hilar and mediastinal lymphadenopathy are common manifestations of sarcoidosis and may be seen as an isolated abnormality or in conjunction with parenchymal lung disease. The lymphadenopathy is typically symmetric in distribution, with involvement of the hilar, paratracheal, aortopulmonary window and/or subcarinal regions (Fig. 12.18). Hilar involvement is most characteristic.

Although the presence of typical lymph node enlargement on CT can be helpful in supporting a diagnosis of sarcoidosis, keep in mind that many patients with HRCT findings diagnostic or strongly suggestive of sarcoidosis have no evidence of lymph node enlargement. The diagnosis can be made on typical lung abnormalities alone.

Lymphadenopathy in sarcoidosis may be hypermetabolic on positron emission tomography with standard uptake values that overlap with malignancy (Fig. 12.19). This distribution of lymphadenopathy in a patient of the appropriate demographic is very suggestive of sarcoidosis. Lymph nodes may be calcified or noncalcified. The morphology of calcification may be diffuse, hazy, and central; may have an eggshell pattern (Fig. 12.20); or may be heterogeneous. Necrosis in lymph nodes is rare.

The differential diagnosis (Table 12.3) includes other causes of symmetrical lymphadenopathy including pneumoconioses, amyloidosis, and Castleman's disease. Metastases are an uncommon cause of symmetrical disease, but

12

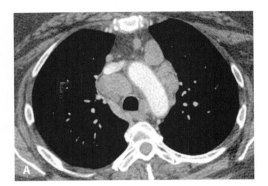

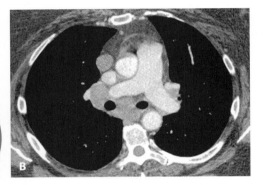

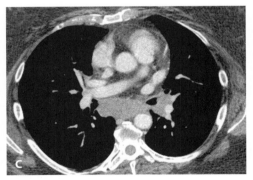

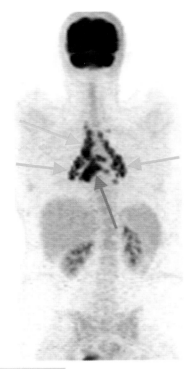

Figure 12.19

Positron emission tomography (PET) in sarcoidosis.
The distribution of lymph node activity on PET
scanning is the same as on CT, with paratracheal
(*yellow arrow*), subcarinal (*red arrow*), and hilar (*blue
arrows*) involvement. The PET avidity of these nodes
may be in the same range as malignancy.

Figure 12.18

Lymphadenopathy in sarcoidosis. A–C.
Symmetric lymphadenopathy is present in the
paratracheal, aortopulmonary, subcarinal, and hilar
regions. The combination of symmetric and hilar
involvement is strongly suggestive of sarcoidosis.
However, lymph node enlargement is not
necessary for the HRCT diagnosis of this disease.

disease, are typically asymmetric. Lymphoma is
often a concern in patients with suspected sarcoidosis; however, the majority of cases of lymphoma are asymmetric.

Table 12.3	Differential diagnosis of lymphadenopathy in sarcoidosis
Commonly symmetric	Pneumoconioses
	Amyloidosis
	Castleman's disease
Rarely symmetric	Metastases
	Lymphoma
	Mycobacterial/fungal infection

this pattern is occasionally seen with gastrointestinal tumors, genitourinary tumors, lung cancer,
breast cancer, and leukemia. Granulomatous
infections, such as mycobacterial and fungal

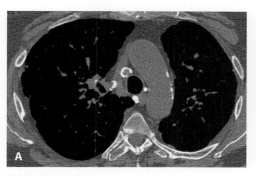 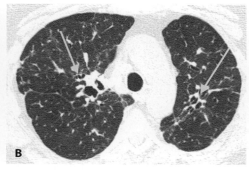

Figure 12.20

Eggshell calcification of mediastinal lymph nodes in sarcoidosis. The nodes of sarcoidosis may be calcified. The pattern of calcification is variable, but may be peripheral/eggshell in distribution, dense, or hazy. In this patient, eggshell calcification **(A)** is associated with parahilar fibrosis and traction bronchiectasis (*arrows*, **B**).

FURTHER READING

Brauner MW, Grenier P, Mompoint D, et al. Pulmonary sarcoidosis: evaluation with high-resolution CT. *Radiology.* 1989;172:467-471.

Brauner MW, Lenoir S, Grenier P, et al. Pulmonary sarcoidosis: CT assessment of lesion reversibility. *Radiology.* 1992;182:349-354.

Criado E, Sánchez M, Ramírez J, et al. Pulmonary sarcoidosis: typical and atypical manifestations at high-resolution CT with pathologic correlation. *Radiographics.* 2010; 30:1567-1586.

Gleeson FV, Traill ZC, Hansell DM. Evidence of expiratory CT scans of small-airway obstruction in sarcoidosis. *AJR Am J Roentgenol.* 1996;166:1052-1054.

Hamper UM, Fishman EK, Khouri NF, et al. Typical and atypical CT manifestations of pulmonary sarcoidosis. *J Comput Assist Tomogr.* 1986;10:928-936.

Hansell DM, Milne DG, Wilsher ML, Wells AU. Pulmonary sarcoidosis: morphologic associations of airflow obstruction at thin-section CT. *Radiology.* 1998;209:697-704.

Lee KS, Kim TS, Han J, et al. Diffuse micronodular lung disease: HRCT and pathologic findings. *J Comput Assist Tomogr.* 1999;23:99-106.

Lenique F, Brauner MW, Grenier P, et al. CT assessment of bronchi in sarcoidosis: endoscopic and pathologic correlations. *Radiology.* 1995;194:419-423.

Lynch DA, Webb WR, Gamsu G, et al. Computed tomography in pulmonary sarcoidosis. *J Comput Assist Tomogr.* 1989;13:405-410.

Miller BH, Rosado-de-Christenson ML, McAdams HP, Fishback NF. Thoracic sarcoidosis: radiologic-pathologic correlation. *Radiographics* 1995;15:421-437.

Müller NL, Kullnig P, Miller RR. The CT findings of pulmonary sarcoidosis: analysis of 25 patients. *AJR Am J Roentgenol.* 1989;152:1179-1182.

Müller NL, Mawson JB, Mathieson JR, et al. Sarcoidosis: correlation of extent of disease at CT with clinical, functional, and radiographic findings. *Radiology.* 1989;171:613-618.

Nakatsu M, Hatabu H, Morkawa K, et al. Large coalescent parenchymal nodules in pulmonary sarcoidosis: "Sarcoid Galaxy" sign. *AJR Am J Roentgenol.* 2002;178:1389-1393.

Nishimura K, Itoh H, Kitaichi M, et al. Pulmonary sarcoidosis: correlation of CT and histopathologic findings. *Radiology.* 1993;189:105-109.

Padley SP, Padhani AR, Nicholson A, Hansell DM. Pulmonary sarcoidosis mimicking cryptogenic fibrosing alveolitis on CT. *Clin Radiol.* 1996;51:807-810.

Remy-Jardin M, Beuscart R, Sault MC, et al. Subpleural micronodules in diffuse infiltrative lung diseases: evaluation with thin-section CT scans. *Radiology.* 1990;177:133-139.

Remy-Jardin M, Giraud F, Remy J, et al. Pulmonary sarcoidosis: role of CT in the evaluation of disease activity and functional impairment and in prognosis assessment. *Radiology.* 1994;191:675-680.

Traill ZC, Maskell GF, Gleeson FV. High-resolution CT findings of pulmonary sarcoidosis. *AJR Am J Roentgenol.* 1997;168:1557-1560.

12

Hypersensitivity Pneumonitis and Eosinophilic Lung Disease

HYPERSENSITIVITY PNEUMONITIS

Hypersensitivity pneumonitis (HP) represents an immune reaction to inhaled organic antigens. The possible sources of these antigens are diverse and include microbes, animals, plant material, and various chemicals.

There are three possible presentations of HP: acute, subacute, and chronic. *Acute HP* is rare and involves a large antigen exposure leading to the rapid onset of cough, dyspnea, and fever. Exposure to moldy hay in farmer's lung is the most typical example of acute HP. *Subacute HP* is common and demonstrates symptoms that are similar to, but less severe than acute HP. Exposures leading to the development of symptoms are more prolonged, extending over weeks to months. *Chronic HP* is also common and involves long-term exposure to low levels of antigen over a period of years.

There are striking differences in the prevalence of HP based upon antigen exposure. For instance, up to 15% of pigeon breeders will develop HP. Of note, however, only 50% of patients with HP will have an identifiable exposure. This is one of the major challenges in the diagnosis of HP as most other inhaled diseases, such as pneumoconioses, have an easily identifiable exposure. Smoking is thought to be relatively protective against the development of HP, but it does not preclude this diagnosis.

HRCT Findings

The HRCT findings of HP vary depending upon the clinical presentation.

Acute HP

The findings of acute HP have not been well studied, as most patients are not imaged in this stage. The HRCT findings are likely similar to subacute HP (discussed below), but may be more extensive (Fig. 13.1) and demonstrate an increased incidence of consolidation.

Subacute HP

The diagnosis of subacute HP is usually based on the presence of a combination or constellation of abnormalities, including ground glass opacity (GGO), centrilobular nodules of GGO, mosaic perfusion or air trapping, and the headcheese sign (Table 13.1).

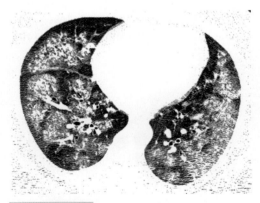

Figure 13.1

Acute hypersensitivity pneumonitis (HP).
Extensive bilateral ground glass opacity is seen in a patient with acute HP secondary to mold exposure. These abnormalities are nonspecific and more severe than that typically present with subacute HP.

Table 13.1	HRCT findings of subacute hypersensitivity pneumonitis

Patchy GGO
Centrilobular nodules of GGO
Mosaic perfusion and air trapping
Headcheese sign (combination of GGO and mosaic perfusion/air trapping)
Mid–lower lung distribution, spares costophrenic angles

GGO, ground glass opacity.

Ground Glass Opacity

GGO in HP is often patchy and bilateral in distribution. It may be seen in isolation, in which case it is a nonspecific finding (Fig. 13.2). Isolated GGO may be seen with a variety of acute diseases (infections, edema, diffuse alveolar damage, and hemorrhage) and chronic diseases (invasive mucinous adenocarcinoma, interstitial pneumonias, organizing pneumonia, eosinophilic pneumonia, lipoid pneumonia, and alveolar proteinosis). When associated with other findings of subacute HP, such as air trapping, the specificity of GGO for a diagnosis of HP increases.

Centrilobular Nodules of GGO

This is a common finding in subacute HP and reflects peribronchiolar inflammation, cellular infiltration, and poorly marginated granulomas. HP is the most common cause of centrilobular GGO nodules in association with chronic symptoms. The nodules are often diffuse or symmetric (Fig. 13.3). In the setting of an identifiable exposure to an organic antigen, centrilobular GGO nodules are considered diagnostic of subacute HP. The differential diagnosis of centrilobular GGO nodules includes respiratory bronchiolitis, follicular bronchiolitis, atypical infections, and vascular diseases, including pulmonary hemorrhage.

Mosaic Perfusion, Air Trapping, and the Headcheese Sign

Mosaic perfusion and air trapping may be seen in association with other abnormalities (Figs. 13.3B and 13.4) or may be seen as an isolated abnormality (Fig. 13.5). Mosaic perfusion appears as one or more focal areas of decreased lung attenuation associated with reduced size of vessels within the lucent region (see Chapter 5). It reflects the presence of bronchiolitis and bronchiolar obstruction occurring as a result of bronchiolar inflammation. It may persist after treatment of HP and following resolution of GGO or nodules. When seen as an isolated abnormality, the differential diagnosis includes asthma and constrictive bronchiolitis.

The combination of patchy mosaic perfusion and GGO has been termed the *headcheese sign*; it is highly suggestive of HP (Fig. 13.6). Both GGO and mosaic perfusion must be present. GGO reflects the cellular infiltration

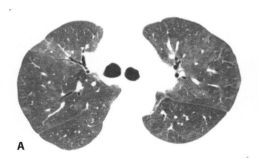
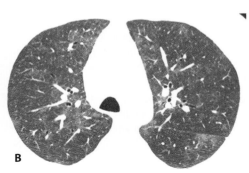

A **B**

Figure 13.2

Subacute hypersensitivity pneumonitis (HP) with ground glass opacity in two patients. A and B. Patchy ground glass opacity is a nonspecific finding that may be seen in a variety of disorders. It may be the only manifestation of subacute HP, but more commonly is associated with other findings such as mosaic perfusion and centrilobular nodules.

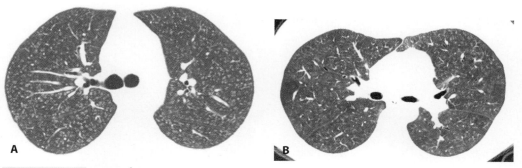

Figure 13.3

Subacute hypersensitivity pneumonitis (HP) with centrilobular ground glass opacity nodules in two patients. A and **B.** HP is the most common cause of diffuse centrilobular nodules of ground glass opacity. In the setting of an appropriate exposure, such as this patient with a chronic mold exposure, the HRCT should be considered diagnostic of that disease. In the absence of an exposure, biopsy is required for diagnosis. In **(B)** note that the centrilobular nodules are associated with areas of low-attenuation mosaic perfusion.

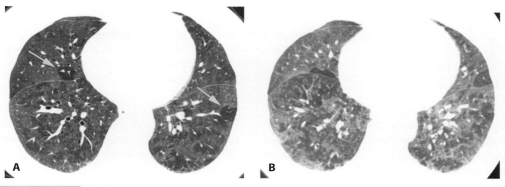

Figure 13.4

Subacute hypersensitivity pneumonitis (HP) with mosaic perfusion and air trapping. A. HRCT in a 66-year-old bird fancier shows patchy and lobular areas of decreased lung attenuation (arrows) representing mosaic perfusion. Ground glass opacity is also likely present. **B.** Air trapping within the regions of mosaic perfusion is seen on a dynamic expiratory scan. Mosaic perfusion and/or air trapping may be seen in combination with other abnormalities or as an isolated finding in patients with HP, either at initial presentation or after treatment. Not uncommonly, these are the only abnormalities that persist after treatment of subacute HP.

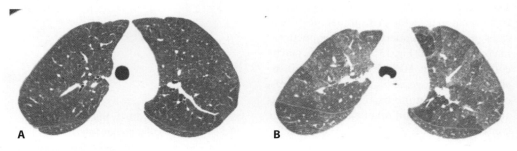

Figure 13.5

Subacute hypersensitivity pneumonitis (HP) with isolated mosaic perfusion and air trapping. A. Other than subtle mosaic perfusion, the inspiratory scan appears nearly normal. **B.** On expiration, air trapping is clearly seen. This appearance may be seen in patients with subacute HP before or after treatment.

13

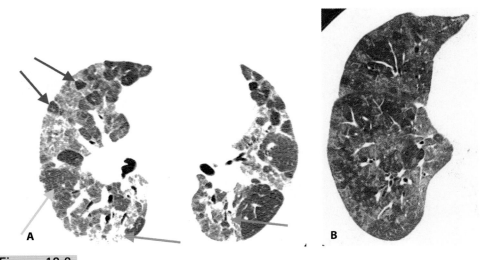

Figure 13.6

Subacute hypersensitivity pneumonitis (HP) with the "headcheese" sign in two patients. A. The combination of lobular mosaic perfusion (*dark blue arrows*), geographic areas of ground glass opacity (*red arrows*), and normal lung (*light blue arrow*) constitutes the headcheese sign and is highly suggestive of HP. **B.** In a different patient with HP, geographic areas of mosaic perfusion and ground glass opacity are well demonstrated.

typical of HP, while the mosaic perfusion reflects bronchiolar obstruction. It is called the headcheese sign because of its resemblance to a sausage of the same name.

The differential diagnosis of the headcheese sign includes desquamative interstitial pneumonia (DIP)/respiratory bronchiolitis, follicular bronchiolitis/lymphoid interstitial pneumonia, and atypical infections. Of note, mosaic perfusion and air trapping may persist after treatment even when other findings have resolved.

Consolidation

The presence of consolidation is rare in HP. However, it may be the predominant feature in cases in which secondary organizing pneumonia is also present (Fig. 13.7). On HRCT, patchy consolidation in HP may be indistinguishable from cryptogenic organizing pneumonia, eosinophilic pneumonia, invasive mucinous adenocarcinoma, and other causes of chronic consolidation.

Distribution of Abnormalities

In patients with HP, abnormalities typically predominate in the mid-lungs, with sparing of the inferior costophrenic angles (Fig. 13.8).

However, an upper lobe distribution is not uncommon. Distribution may help distinguish HP from the interstitial pneumonias (usual interstitial pneumonia [UIP], nonspecific interstitial pneumonia [NSIP], and DIP) that

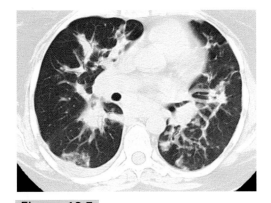

Figure 13.7

Subacute hypersensitivity pneumonitis (HP) with organizing pneumonia. Patchy peribronchovascular consolidation is present in a patient with HP, typical of organizing pneumonia. While organizing pneumonia is commonly seen pathologically in patients with HP, it is only rarely seen as the predominant abnormality on HRCT.

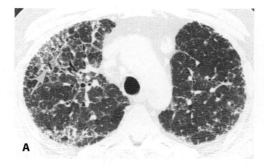

A

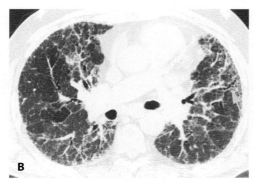

B

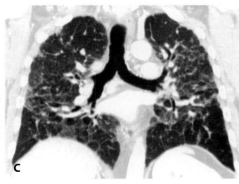

C

Figure 13.8

Chronic hypersensitivity pneumonitis (HP), distribution. A and **B.** In a patient with chronic HP with fibrosis, reticulation and traction bronchiectasis (*yellow arrows*) involve the entire cross section of the lung, both central and subpleural regions. **C.** Coronal reformatted image shows the mid-lung predominance typical of HP.

Table 13.2	HRCT findings of chronic hypersensitivity pneumonitis

HRCT findings
Irregular reticulation
Traction bronchiectasis
Honeycombing
Associated findings of subacute HP (centrilobular nodules, mosaic perfusion, air trapping)
Mid–lower lung distribution, spares costophrenic angles
Diffuse or central distribution in the axial plane

HP, hypersensitivity pneumonitis.

Chronic HP

The cardinal finding of chronic HP is fibrosis. The pattern of fibrosis and associated abnormalities may be used to distinguish HP from other fibrotic lung diseases (Table 13.2). The most common findings of fibrosis seen with HP are traction bronchiectasis and irregular reticulation (Fig. 13.8). Honeycombing may also be present (Fig. 13.9). The distribution of fibrosis is the same as the distribution of abnormalities in subacute HP, often involving the central lung regions and the mid- or upper lungs (Figs. 13.8 and 13.9). This helps distinguish chronic HP from fibrosis in UIP or NSIP.

The combination of lung fibrosis with mosaic perfusion or air trapping, similar to the *headcheese sign*, is highly suggestive of chronic hypersensitivity pneumonitis (Figs. 13.9 and 13.10). The presence of significant mosaic perfusion or air trapping (multiple lobules in three or more lobes) is considered inconsistent with a diagnosis of UIP.

There may be an overlap of the findings of chronic and subacute HP. Fibrosis may be present in association with GGO and/or centrilobular nodules (Fig. 13.11).

EOSINOPHILIC LUNG DISEASES

Eosinophilic lung diseases (Table 13.3) are a heterogeneous group of disorders that are characterized by the presence of a lung abnormality and increased eosinophils in the lung and/or blood. Of note, many noneosinophilic

typically predominate in the lung bases, with involvement of the costophrenic angles. Also, in the axial plane, HP is usually diffuse or central in distribution, whereas the interstitial pneumonias are typically peripheral and subpleural.

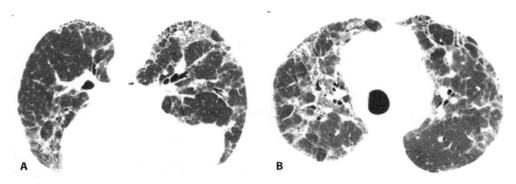

Figure 13.9

Chronic hypersensitivity pneumonitis with honeycombing. A. Honeycombing is visible posteriorly at the lung base. **B.** A scan through the upper lobes shows more extensive fibrosis, involving the entire cross section of the lung. Lobular areas of sparing likely reflect mosaic perfusion. As opposed to idiopathic pulmonary fibrosis, the distribution of fibrosis in this patient shows significant involvement of the central lung and upper lobes.

lung diseases may a show mild increase in eosinophils. For example, asthma may show mild elevations of serum eosinophils and eosinophils on lung biopsy, but it is not a disease whose primary abnormality is eosinophilic infiltration. Peripheral eosinophilia is present in the majority of eosinophilic lung diseases, with the exception of acute eosinophilic pneumonia (AEP).

Eosinophilic lung diseases can be classified by whether their cause is known or unknown (idiopathic). Those with a known cause include parasitic infections, allergic

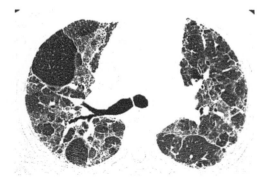

Figure 13.10

Chronic hypersensitivity pneumonitis with fibrosis and mosaic perfusion. Reticulation and traction bronchiectasis involve the upper lobes. Multiple lobular and multilobular lucencies reflect mosaic perfusion.

bronchopulmonary aspergillosis (ABPA), and bronchocentric granulomatosis.

Those with an unknown cause include simple pulmonary eosinophilia, AEP, chronic eosinophilic pneumonia (CEP), hypereosinophilic syndrome, and Churg-Strauss syndrome. The idiopathic diseases may be further subclassified by whether they have an acute or chronic presentation. Acute presentations are seen with simple pulmonary eosinophilia and AEP. Chronic symptoms are seen with CEP and hypereosinophilic syndrome.

Idiopathic Eosinophilic Disorders

Simple Pulmonary Eosinophilia (Loeffler's Syndrome)

Loeffler's syndrome is a rare disease of unknown cause that is characterized by an acute presentation followed by spontaneous regression, usually within 1 month. Patients have mild or absent symptoms in the presence of chest x-ray or CT abnormalities.

The most typical HRCT finding is migratory, nonsegmental consolidation (Fig. 13.12). This is often peripheral and involves the mid- or upper lungs. While new areas of consolidation appear, others resolve, and complete regression within 1 month is typical. GGO, nodules, and bronchial wall thickening may be associated with the consolidation, but are not particularly suggestive of this disease.

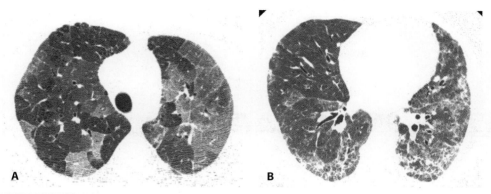

Figure 13.11

Overlap of subacute and chronic hypersensitivity pneumonitis. A. HRCT through the upper lobes shows findings typical of subacute hypersensitivity pneumonitis, with patchy ground glass opacity (GGO) and mosaic perfusion, the headcheese sign. **B.** HRCT through the lung bases shows GGO with extensive reticulation indicative of fibrosis. Hypersensitivity pneumonitis not uncommonly presents with a combination of findings of subacute and chronic disease on the same HRCT.

Table 13.3   Features of eosinophilic disorders

Disease	Features	HRCT findings
Idiopathic eosinophilic disorders		
Simple pulmonary eosinophilia	Acute, spontaneous regression within 1 mo, mild symptoms	Migratory, peripheral upper lung consolidation
Acute eosinophilic pneumonia	Acute, single episode, absence of peripheral eosinophilia, may progress to ARDS	Diffuse GGO and consolidation
CEP	Chronic, most common idiopathic eosinophilic disease, asthma in 50%	Peripheral and peribronchovascular consolidation
Hypereosinophilic syndrome	Multiorgan involvement, nervous systemic and cardiac most common, male in third or fourth decade	Diffuse /consolidation and interlobular septal thickening
Churg-Strauss Syndrome	Involvement of the lungs, central nervous system, and skin	Nonsegmental consolidation or GGO often in a peripheral distribution, and resembling CEP
Known eosinophilic disorders		
Allergic bronchopulmonary aspergillosis	Hypersensitivity reaction to Aspergillus in airways, asthma, or cystic fibrosis history	Upper–mid-lung bronchiectasis (often cystic), other evidence of airways disease
Drugs	Most common drugs: bleomycin, amiodarone, nitrofurantoin, phenytoin, and methotrexate	Resembles idiopathic eosinophilic disorders
Bronchocentric granulomatosis	Idiopathic or due to asthma, immunosuppression, or connective tissue disease	Masses, lobular consolidation, airway impaction
Parasitic infections	Rare in developed countries, travel to endemic regions	Variable: nodules, consolidation, CEP

ARDS, acute respiratory distress syndrome; GGO, ground glass opacity; CEP, chronic eosinophilic pneumonia.

13

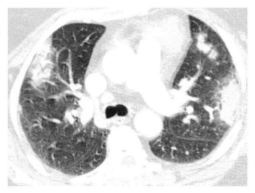

Figure 13.12

Simple pulmonary eosinophilia (Loeffler's syndrome). Peripheral nonsegmental consolidation is seen in the upper lobes bilaterally in a patient presenting with 2 wk of cough. On sequential chest x-rays, this was migratory. This appearance is typical of simple pulmonary eosinophilia; however, correlation with increased serum and lung eosinophils is necessary.

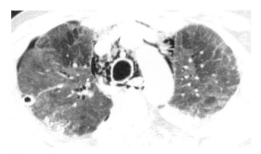

Figure 13.13

Acute eosinophilic pneumonia. Diffuse ground glass opacity is present. This finding is nonspecific, but most often seen with edema, infection, diffuse alveolar damage, and hemorrhage. There was no clinical evidence of any of these diseases, and lung biopsy was performed. Acute eosinophilic pneumonia was proven pathologically. Pneumomediastinum, pneumothorax, and right chest tube are present.

13

Acute Eosinophilic Pneumonia

AEP is characterized by a rapid onset of symptoms, usually less than 1 week prior to presentation. AEP presents with a single episode that does not recur after treatment; however, progression to acute respiratory distress syndrome and death may occur.

As opposed to other eosinophilic lung diseases, AEP often does not show a peripheral eosinophilia, although increased eosinophils on bronchoalveolar lavage is typical. Most cases are idiopathic; however, exposures to cigarette smoking and drugs have been described as associations.

Typical HRCT findings include diffuse or extensive GGO (Fig. 13.13) or consolidation. Pathologically, this corresponds to eosinophilic infiltration and diffuse alveolar damage. Associated findings may include smooth interlobular septal thickening and nodules. These findings are usually indistinguishable from other causes of diffuse lung disease in the acute setting such as pulmonary edema, acute respiratory distress syndrome, atypical infection, and hemorrhage.

Chronic Eosinophilic Pneumonia

CEP is the most common of the idiopathic eosinophilic disorders. Patients present with chronic symptoms, often of several months duration. Asthma is a commonly associated disorder, seen in approximately half the patients. Treatment with steroids often leads to prompt resolution.

Consolidation is the most frequent HRCT finding (Fig. 13.14). Classically, this is peripheral and upper lobe in distribution (Fig. 13.15A–C), but peribronchovascular consolidation is also commonly present. Areas of consolidation are focal, patchy, usually bilateral, and interspersed between areas of normal lung. The *atoll* or *reversed halo sign* may be present (Fig. 13.16). Less typical findings include small nodules, GGO, and reticulation. After treatment, the consolidation may lead to linear areas of atelectasis or scar, which may parallel the pleural surface.

These findings are very similar to those of organizing pneumonia, and in fact, these two entities may be indistinguishable. Pathologically, organizing pneumonia is often seen in association with CEP, and significant overlap between these two entities exists. An upper lobe predominance of abnormalities

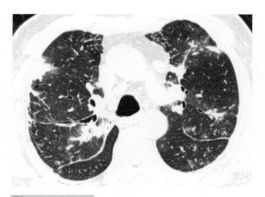

Figure 13.14

Chronic eosinophilic pneumonia (CEP). Patchy, peripheral, nonsegmental consolidation is seen in the upper lobes in this patient with 4 mo of dyspnea and cough. While this finding is nonspecific by itself, the presence of increased eosinophils in the lung or serum in association with these findings is highly suggestive of CEP.

is more typical of CEP (Fig. 13.17), while organizing pneumonia often has a lower lobe predominance, but their distinction is not always possible. Other causes of chronic consolidation that may resemble CEP include sarcoidosis, mucinous adenocarcinoma, lymphoma, and lipoid pneumonia.

Hypereosinophilic Syndrome

Hypereosinophilic syndrome is a systemic disorder that has a course that is prolonged, usually more than 6 months, and is characterized by eosinophilic tissue infiltration of multiple organs. Central nervous systemic and cardiac involvement are most common, but lung disease occurs in approximately 40% of patients. A typical patient is male and aged 20 to 40 years.

HRCT abnormalities are usually a reflection of pulmonary edema from cardiac involvement, rather than pulmonary disease. Findings include diffuse or symmetric GGO (Fig. 13.18) and/or consolidation. Smooth interlobular septal thickening is also a common finding. When eosinophilic infiltration is present, nodules are most characteristic. These tend to be 1 cm or less in diameter, often with an associated halo of GGO.

Churg-Strauss (Eosinophilic Vasculitis) Syndrome

Churg-Strauss syndrome is a disease that has features of both an eosinophilic disorder

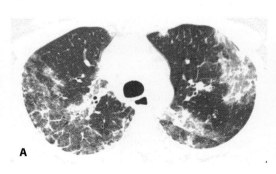

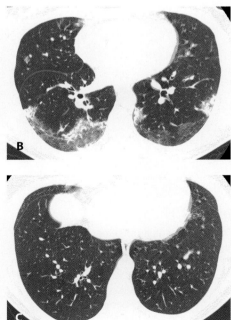

Figure 13.15

Chronic eosinophilic pneumonia. Images through the upper (**A**) mid (**B**) and lower (**C**) lungs show peripheral and upper lobe predominant consolidation and ground glass opacity. These findings are typical of chronic eosinophilic pneumonia.

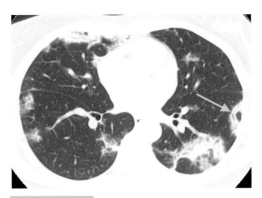

Figure 13.16

Chronic eosinophilic pneumonia (CEP) with the atoll sign. Patchy bilateral, predominantly peripheral consolidation is present. A ring of consolidation surrounding an area of central clearing (*arrow*), the atoll sign, is compatible with organizing pneumonia (OP). In this case, OP is a secondary reaction associated with eosinophilic lung disease. OP and CEP are closely related.

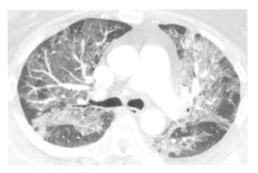

Figure 13.18

Hypereosinophilic syndrome. Diffuse nonspecific ground glass opacity is present in a patient with 8 mo of dyspnea. This finding may be seen in a variety of disorders, but in the setting of hypereosinophilic syndrome, it is either due to eosinophilic infiltration of lung or pulmonary edema from cardiac disease.

13

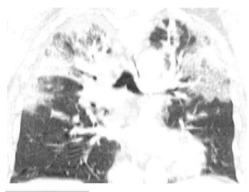

Figure 13.17

Chronic eosinophilic pneumonia (CEP) with upper lobe distribution. Coronal CT shows extensive, peripherally predominant consolidation in a patient with chronic dyspnea. This is a typical appearance and distribution of CEP. Organizing pneumonia, which may closely resemble CEP, usually has a lower lobe predominance.

and vasculitis. It is seen predominantly in patients with a history of asthma or allergy, but often presents in patients who are significantly older than the usual initial onset of asthma. It is a systemic disorder with predominant involvement of the lungs, central nervous system, and skin. Other typical features include eosinophilia, greater than 10% of the white blood cell count, neuropathy, transient or migratory pulmonary opacities, sinus abnormalities, and increased tissue eosinophils.

Typical HRCT findings include nonsegmental consolidation or GGO often in a peripheral distribution, and resembling CEP. These abnormalities may have a lobular distribution (Fig. 13.19); this finding may be a distinguishing feature compared with other eosinophilic lung diseases such as CEP. Other findings include centrilobular nodules, interlobular septal thickening, and bronchial wall thickening.

Eosinophilic Disorders with a Known Etiology

Allergic Bronchopulmonary Aspergillosis

ABPA is a disease predominantly seen in asthmatics or patients with cystic fibrosis (see Chapter 6). The diagnosis is usually clinical and based upon peripheral eosinophilia, increased serum IgE levels, and reactivity to Aspergillus on skin tests in a patient with symptoms unresponsive to traditional asthma treatments. This disease is characterized by a hypersensitivity reaction to Aspergillus that

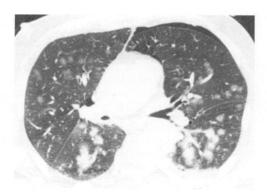

Figure 13.19

Churg-Strauss syndrome. Centrilobular, lobular areas, and nodular areas of consolidation and ground glass opacity are present in a patient with a history of asthma. In a patient with suspected eosinophilic disease, the lobular nature of abnormalities may suggest Churg-Strauss syndrome.

colonizes the airways. The Aspergillus does not invade the lung itself, but induces inflammation within the airway lumen.

The most characteristic HRCT finding of ABPA is bronchiectasis involving the central mid- or upper lungs. The bronchiectasis is usually unilateral or asymmetric, as opposed to the symmetric diseases such as cystic fibrosis. The bronchiectasis may be cylindrical, varicose, or cystic (Fig. 13.20). Bronchial wall thickening and mucoid impaction are usually

associated with the bronchial dilatation. The mucoid impaction may be high in attenuation because Aspergillus accumulates calcium and metal ions.

The combination of bronchiectasis with high-density mucoid impaction is particularly suggestive of this diagnosis. There may be signs of small airways inflammation (centrilobular nodules, tree-in-bud opacities, and bronchiolectasis), but the large airways findings usually predominate.

Drugs

Drug reactions involving the lungs are described in greater detail in Chapter 15. These reactions may be associated with one of several different patterns. Eosinophilic lung disease is a rare manifestation of a drug reaction; it may closely resemble any of the idiopathic eosinophilic disorders. Thus, prior to making the diagnosis of an idiopathic eosinophilic disorder, an examination of drug history is important. The most common drugs to present with this pattern include chemotherapeutic agents such as bleomycin, amiodarone, nitrofurantoin, phenytoin, and methotrexate.

Bronchocentric Granulomatosis

This is a rare disease characterized pathologically by necrotizing granulomatosis inflammation around bronchioles and small bronchi. It is commonly seen in asthmatics and is associated with Aspergillus organisms and thus

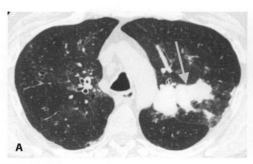
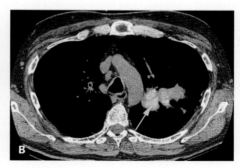

Figure 13.20

Allergic bronchopulmonary aspergillosis. A. Focal bronchiectasis with mucoid impaction (*arrow*) is seen in the left upper lobe. **B.** The mucoid impaction (*arrow*) is of high attenuation. This is highly suggestive of allergic bronchopulmonary aspergillosis.

shares similarities with ABPA. It may be seen in nonasthmatic patients and, in that case, is either idiopathic or associated with disorders such as immunosuppression or connective tissue disease.

The HRCT findings have not been well documented. Described findings include masses, lobular consolidation, and airway impaction.

Parasitic Infections

Parasitic infections are uncommon in the United States, but are often seen in tropical and subtropical regions such as Africa, South America, and southern Asia. Lung abnormalities may be due to direct invasion by parasites or a secondary allergic reaction to infections elsewhere within the body. Peripheral eosinophilia is typically present.

The HRCT findings of parasitic infections are variable and depend upon the offending organism, but the findings are usually nonspecific, and correlation with travel to endemic regions is most important for diagnosis. Nodules are common and often more than 1 cm in size, with irregular borders or adjacent GGO. These may be migratory and are most characteristic of *Ascaris lumbricoides, Clonorchis sinensis, Paragonimus westermani,* and schistosomiasis. Extensive infection with *Strongyloides stercoralis* may result in diffuse ground glass or consolidation as a manifestation of diffuse lung dissemination of the organism. Allergic reactions to the organisms or antigens released during their treatment can result in eosinophilic pneumonia or other reactions described above.

FURTHER READING

Adler BD, Padley SP, Müller NL, et al. Chronic hypersensitivity pneumonitis: high-resolution CT and radiographic features in 16 patients. *Radiology.* 1992;185:91-95.

Arakawa H, Webb WR. Air trapping on expiratory high-resolution CT scans in the absence of inspiratory scan abnormalities: correlation with pulmonary function tests and differential diagnosis. *AJR Am J Roentgenol.* 1998;170:1349-1353.

Bain GA, Flower CD. Pulmonary eosinophilia. *Eur J Radiol.* 1996;23:3-8.

Buschman DL, Waldron JA Jr, King TE Jr. Churg-Strauss pulmonary vasculitis. High-resolution computed tomography scanning and pathologic findings. *Am Rev Respir Dis.* 1990;142:458-461.

Cheon JE, Lee KS, Jung GS, et al. Acute eosinophilic pneumonia: radiographic and CT findings in six patients. *AJR Am J Roentgenol.* 1996;167:1195-1199.

Ebara H, Ikezoe J, Johkoh T, et al. Chronic eosinophilic pneumonia: evolution of chest radiograms and CT features. *J Comput Assist Tomogr.* 1994;18:737-744.

Glazer CS, Rose CS, Lynch DA. Clinical and radiologic manifestations of hypersensitivity pneumonitis. *J Thorac Imaging.* 2002;17:261-272.

Hansell DM, Moskovic E. High-resolution computed tomography in extrinsic allergic alveolitis. *Clin Radiol.* 1991;43:8-12.

Hansell DM, Wells AU, Padley SP, Müller NL. Hypersensitivity pneumonitis: correlation of individual CT patterns with functional abnormalities. *Radiology.* 1996;199:123-128.

Kang EY, Shim JJ, Kim JS, Kim KI. Pulmonary involvement of idiopathic hypereosinophilic syndrome: CT findings in five patients. *J Comput Assist Tomogr.* 1997;21:612-615.

Kim Y, Lee KS, Choi DC, et al. The spectrum of eosinophilic lung disease: radiologic findings. *J Comput Assist Tomogr.* 1997;21:920-930.

King MA, Pope-Harman AL, Allen JN, et al. Acute eosinophilic pneumonia: radiologic and clinical features. *Radiology.* 1997;203:715-719.

Lynch DA, Newell JD, Logan PM, et al. Can CT distinguish hypersensitivity pneumonitis from idiopathic pulmonary fibrosis? *AJR Am J Roentgenol.* 1995;165:807-811.

Remy-Jardin M, Remy J, Wallaert B, Müller NL. Subacute and chronic bird breeder hypersensitivity pneumonitis: sequential evaluation with CT and correlation with lung function tests and bronchoalveolar lavage. *Radiology.* 1993;198:111-118.

Silva CIS, Müller NL, Lynch DA, et al. Chronic hypersensitivity pneumonitis: differentiation from idiopathic pulmonary fibrosis and nonspecific interstitial pneumonia by using thin-section CT. *Radiology.* 2008;246:288-297.

Silver SF, Müller NL, Miller RR, Lefcoe MS. Hypersensitivity pneumonitis: evaluation with CT. *Radiology.* 1989;173:441-445.

Webb WR. Thin-section CT of the secondary pulmonary lobule: anatomy and the image—The 2004 Fleischner lecture. *Radiology.* 2006;239:322-338.

Winn RE, Kollef MH, Meyer JI. Pulmonary involvement in the hypereosinophilic syndrome. *Chest.* 1994; 105:656-660.

Worthy SA, Müller NL, Hansell DM, Flower CD. Churg-Strauss syndrome: the spectrum of pulmonary CT findings in 17 patients. *AJR Am J Roentgenol.* 1998;170:297-300.

13

14

Pulmonary Infections

Infection is a common cause of lung disease in both immunocompromised patients and those with a normal immune status. This chapter focuses on a general approach to suspected infection, the role of HRCT, and typical HRCT findings and provides a discussion of different patterns of infection based upon the type of organism.

ROLE OF HRCT IN INFECTION

HRCT has several uses in patients with suspected infection. These include the detection of abnormalities, differentiating infections from noninfectious lung disease, and determining the most likely organism or organisms to be involved.

Detection of Abnormalities

HRCT is highly sensitive in the detection of pulmonary infections. With the exception of viral infections that only affect the upper airways, the majority of infections show abnormalities easily detected using HRCT. Detection of disease is particularly important in patients with immune deficiencies in which significant pulmonary infection may be present with minimal or absent symptoms or in the presence of a normal chest radiograph.

Differentiating Infectious versus Noninfectious Lung Disease

Understanding the common HRCT findings of infection, and their specificity, is important in

the interpretation of HRCT. It is also important to be aware of noninfectious causes of lung abnormalities that may mimic infection. As infection is common, it is often assumed to be a cause of lung abnormalities in the acute setting, but this is not always the case. Abnormalities such as pulmonary edema, diffuse alveolar damage, and pulmonary hemorrhage may present with symptoms similar to infection. Additionally, certain inflammatory, noninfectious diffuse lung diseases may present with acute symptoms such as hypersensitivity pneumonitis, organizing pneumonia, and acute eosinophilic pneumonia.

Determining the Most Likely Organism(s)

Once infection is determined to be a likely cause of lung abnormalities, the most likely offending organism(s) should be considered. This determination is fundamentally based on the recognition of specific HRCT findings. It is important to keep in mind that there may be significant overlap between HRCT patterns resulting from different infections or more than one organism may be responsible for abnormalities; a differential diagnosis is almost always required in interpreting HRCT in patients with suspected infection.

HRCT is most helpful in distinguishing infections caused by atypical organisms (i.e., viral organisms, atypical bacterial organisms such as Chlamydia and *Mycoplasma pneumoniae*, and *Pneumocystis jiroveci*) from those caused by more common organisms (typical bacteria, mycobacteria, and fungi).

Atypical organisms tend to present with diffuse, symmetric, or extensive bilateral abnormalities. Ground glass opacity is often a significant component of the HRCT findings. Other organisms usually present with unilateral or asymmetric and patchy abnormalities. Consolidation is often a significant finding with these organisms.

For example, a single focal region of consolidation in a patient with HIV infection or AIDS is more likely a common bacterial infection than *P. jiroveci* infection. This has important implications in terms of diagnostic evaluation and treatment.

CLINICAL CONSIDERATIONS

Immune Status
Knowledge of the patient's immune status plays a major role in determining the most likely infectious cause of HRCT abnormalities.

Infections that occur in patients with normal immune status include bacteria (Streptococcus, Chlamydia, Haemophilus, and Mycoplasma), viruses (Influenza and Adenovirus), environmental fungi (coccidioidomycosis, histoplasmosis, blastomycosis), and mycobacterial (tuberculous and nontuberculous) diseases.

Infections in immunocompromised patients vary depending upon the type of immune suppression. For instance, patients with human immunodeficiency virus infection are predisposed to infection by specific organisms, which are rarely seen in immunocompetent hosts, such as Cryptococcus, *P. jiroveci*, and Cytomegalovirus. Neutropenic hosts have a different group of organisms to which they are predisposed, including Candida, Aspergillus, mucormycosis, and *Escherichia coli*.

Bacterial infections are common regardless of a patient's immune status. Also, keep in mind that immunocompromised patients may be infected by more than one organism at a time, resulting in a mix of HRCT manifestations. An immunocompromised patient may also become superinfected with a second organism during treatment of the initial infection.

Geographic Considerations
Certain infections show significant geographic or regional variability based upon environmental differences. For instance, coccidioidomycosis is a relatively common infection in the southwest United States, but is only rarely encountered in the Midwest and eastern states. Histoplasmosis and blastomycosis have other geographic distributions. Parasitic infections are more commonly encountered in underdeveloped or tropical countries.

HRCT FINDINGS OF INFECTION

In a patient with acute symptoms, infection is almost always considered as a cause of HRCT abnormalities. In a patient with chronic symptoms, infection is less likely, although certain infections, such as atypical mycobacterial and fungal organisms, may have a chronic course, as do diseases with a predisposition to chronic infection, such as cystic fibrosis or immune deficiency. The HRCT findings present will determine the likelihood of infection as the etiology.

Ground Glass Opacity and Consolidation
In patients with ground glass opacity or consolidation resulting from infection, the organism most likely responsible depends upon the distribution of abnormalities. When diffuse or symmetric abnormalities are present, atypical organisms (i.e., virus, atypical bacterial organisms such as Chlamydia and *M. pneumoniae*, and *P. jiroveci*) are most likely (Fig. 14.1). Also atypical organisms are most likely to present with ground glass opacity as the predominant abnormality. The ground glass opacities may have a lobular distribution.

When patchy, focal, or asymmetrical abnormalities are present, bacterial, fungal, and mycobacterial infections are the primary considerations. These most commonly present with consolidation as the predominant abnormality.

Ground glass opacity and consolidation are nonspecific findings and in the acute setting may be seen with infection, aspiration,

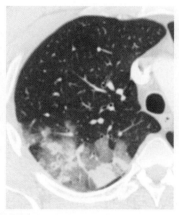

Figure 14.1

Ground glass opacity and consolidation.
Geographic ground glass opacity and consolidation
are seen in a patient with adenoviral infection.

pulmonary edema, diffuse alveolar damage,
and hemorrhage.

Centrilobular Nodules of Soft Tissue Attenuation

In the acute setting, centrilobular nodules of
soft tissue attenuation (Fig. 14.2) are likely due
to infection. Endobronchial spread of bacterial,
mycobacterial, or fungal organisms is the most
common cause. This appearance represents an
early manifestation of bronchopneumonia.

Aspiration is also a consideration when
findings are in dependent lung regions.
Occasionally vascular diseases, such as pulmonary edema or hemorrhage, may present with
centrilobular nodules of soft tissue attenuation. A vascular etiology should be considered
when the abnormalities are diffuse or bilateral
and symmetric. In the chronic setting, chronic
or recurrent infection/aspiration and invasive
mucinous adenocarcinoma are the most common causes of centrilobular nodules of soft tissue attenuation.

Centrilobular Nodules of Ground Glass Opacity

In a patient with acute symptoms, infection
is one of several causes of centrilobular nodules of ground glass opacity (Fig. 14.3). It is
most characteristic of infections that produce
peribronchiolar inflammation without bronchiolar impaction, such as viral and atypical
bacterial infections such as Chlamydia and *M.
pneumoniae*.

The differential diagnosis includes vascular
etiologies such as pulmonary edema and pulmonary hemorrhage, in addition to hypersensitivity
pneumonitis. In the chronic setting, nodules of
this type are unlikely to represent infection and
are most typical of hypersensitivity pneumonitis, respiratory bronchiolitis, follicular bronchiolitis, and pulmonary hypertension.

Tree-in-Bud

Tree-in-bud (TIB) in a patient with acute
symptoms (Fig. 14.4) is highly suggestive of
infection. It is not specific with regard to the
type of infection, but bacterial and mycobacterial infections are most likely. Fungal infections and viral infections are less likely to be
associated with this abnormality. Aspiration
without infection also occasionally produces
TIB with acute symptoms.

14

Figure 14.2

**Centrilobular nodules of soft tissue
attenuation in tuberculosis.** Soft
tissue attenuation centrilobular nodules
are seen in the right lower lobe. This
centrilobular distribution is compatible
with endobronchial spread of infection in
this patient with reactivation tuberculosis.
Note the cavitary lesions.

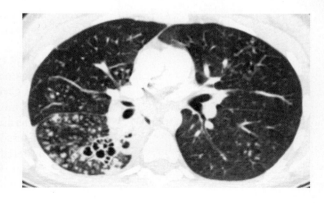

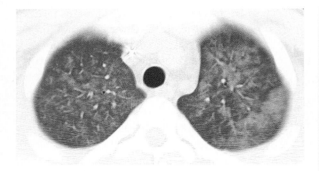

Figure 14.3

Centrilobular nodules of ground glass opacity (GGO) in cytomegalovirus infection. Symmetric, evenly spaced GGO nodules are noted in a centrilobular distribution. Among infections, this appearance is most typical of atypical organisms. Possible noninfectious etiologies in the acute setting include pulmonary edema, diffuse alveolar damage, hemorrhage, and hypersensitivity pneumonitis.

In patients with chronic symptoms, TIB is also commonly due to infection. This may be due to chronic or recurrent acute infections. A common cause of chronic infection with TIB is atypical mycobacteria. Bronchiectasis of any cause, cystic fibrosis, immunodeficiency, primary ciliary dyskinesia, allergic bronchopulmonary aspergillosis, and disorders of the bronchial cartilage may also lead to chronic infection with TIB, but these also show prominent involvement of the large airways.

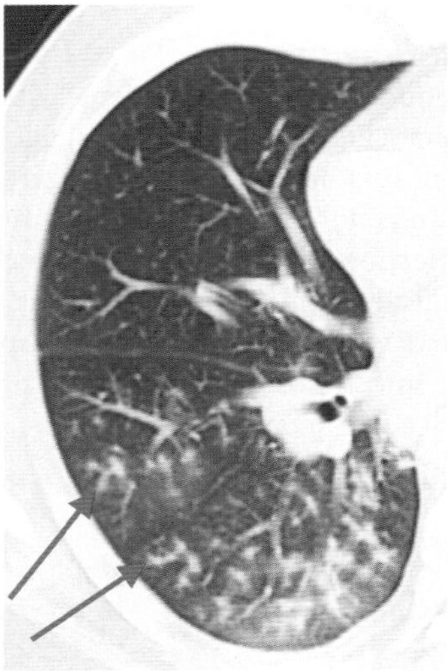

Panbronchiolitis is predominantly a small airways disease that presents with chronic TIB; it is uncommon. In the appropriate clinical setting, noninfectious causes of TIB to consider include invasive mucinous adenocarcinoma, follicular bronchiolitis, talcosis, and intravascular metastases.

Airway Wall Thickening and Impaction

Large airway infection, associated with bronchial wall thickening and sometimes luminal impaction (Fig. 14.5A, B), in a patient with suspected infection is often associated with other abnormalities, such as centrilobular nodules, consolidation, or TIB (see Chapter 6). It is occasionally seen as an isolated finding, in which case atypical organisms (viral, Chlamydia, *M. pneumoniae*) are the most likely etiologies.

Other common etiologies of isolated airway thickening and impaction include asthma and acute or chronic bronchitis. This finding should be distinguished from thickening of the peribronchovascular interstitium that may be seen with pulmonary edema and lymphangitic spread of tumor.

Large Nodules and Cavities

Large nodules (more than 1 cm in diameter) and cavities are commonly due to infection. The most likely infections to produce these patterns include septic embolism (Fig. 14.6), bacterial lung abscess, and fungal and mycobacterial infections. Nocardia and Actinomyces are rare infections that commonly present with large nodules and/or cavities. An air-fluid level

14

Figure 14.4

Tree-in-bud. Branching tubular opacity with associated nodules (*arrows*) is seen in the peripheral regions of the right lower lobe in a patient with bacterial bronchopneumonia. The tree-in-bud sign is highly suggestive of infection and the diagnosis can often be made by sputum analysis.

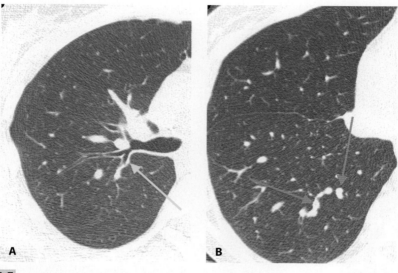

Figure 14.5

Airway inflammation. A and B. Airway wall thickening (*arrow*, **A**) and impaction (*arrows*, **B**) may be the only signs of infection. In isolation, this is most typical of viral infection, such as in this patient with rhinovirus infection.

within a cavitary nodule or mass suggests bacterial infection.

Noninfectious causes of large nodules and cavities include malignancy, vasculitis such as Wegener's granulomatosis, and rare disorders such as tracheobronchial papillomatosis. Clinical history is important in distinguishing

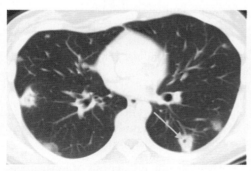

Figure 14.6

Large nodules and cavities. Infection is the most common cause of large nodules and cavities (arrow). The most common infections to produce this pattern include septic emboli, bacterial abscesses, fungal infection, and mycobacterial infection. This patient was diagnosed with septic emboli from infective endocarditis.

infectious versus noninfectious causes of this pattern. The thickness of the cavity wall may also be helpful in making this distinction. A wall thickness less than 5 mm suggests a benign process, whereas a wall thickness greater than 15 mm suggests a malignancy (Fig. 14.7A, B). A wall thickness between 5 and 15 mm is not helpful in predicting the likelihood of a benign versus malignant process.

A Random Pattern of Small Nodules (Miliary Infection)

Random nodules have no particular distribution with respect to the lung structures or the pulmonary lobule (see Chapter 3). They typically show a diffuse and homogeneous distribution with involvement of the subpleural interstitium. Overall, random nodules are diffuse and uniform in distribution. Random nodules are usually of soft tissue attenuation, sharply marginated, and easily visible when only a few millimeters in size.

The differential diagnosis of random nodules primarily includes miliary tuberculosis (TB) or other mycobacteria, miliary fungal infection (e.g., histoplasmosis and coccidioidomycosis), and hematogenous spread of malignancy.

14

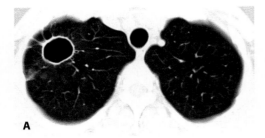

A

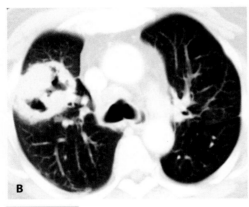

B

Figure 14.7

Cavities, thickness of wall. The thickness of the wall of a cavity helps determine the likelihood of a benign or malignant etiology. A wall thickness <5 mm is likely due to a benign etiology **(A)** such as in this patient with a resolving coccidioidomycosis infection. A wall thickness >15 mm is likely due to a malignant etiology **(B)** such as in this patient with a primary lung squamous cell carcinoma.

BACTERIAL INFECTIONS

Bacterial infections are common and, in general, should be considered the most likely infectious cause of most HRCT abnormalities. They may be hospital or community acquired. The most common hospital-acquired organisms include *Staphylococcus aureus*, *Pseudomonas aeruginosa*, *E. coli*, Acinetobacter, Klebsiella, and *Haemophilus influenzae*. The most common community-acquired organisms include *Streptococcus pneumoniae*, *H. influenzae*, *S. aureus*, and gram-negative organisms. Atypical bacterial infections such as Chlamydia and *M. pneumoniae* are also common bacterial infections acquired in the community, but have unique imaging features. These will be discussed later in conjunction with viral

Table 14.1	HRCT findings of lobar and bronchopneumonia

Lobar pneumonia	Bronchopneumonia
Consolidation, single lobe or multiple lobes, nonsegmental distribution	Consolidation, patchy, asymmetric, segmental distribution
Nodules usually absent	Centrilobular nodules, tree-in-bud
Air bronchograms in regions of consolidation	Airway wall thickening and impaction

organisms and *P. jiroveci*, as these organisms all share many features.

Bacterial infections classically result in one of three patterns: lobar pneumonia, bronchopneumonia (Table 14.1), and atypical pneumonia (discussed later in this chapter). Note that there may be significant overlap between these patterns, particularly between bronchopneumonia and lobar pneumonia.

Lobar Pneumonia

In lobar pneumonia, the infection originates in, and is predominantly centered in, the alveolar spaces. Spread to adjacent alveoli occurs through the pores of Kohn, small interalveolar pores, and the canals of Lambert. Associated spread via the airways is typically absent. The infection is limited by fissures.

This pattern is most typical of Streptococcus, *H. influenzae*, Klebsiella, and *Moraxella catarrhalis*. The HRCT findings (Fig. 14.8) include the following:

1. Consolidation marginated by fissures
2. Prominent air bronchograms
3. Single lobe, or multiple lobes, affected, nonsegmental distribution

The differential diagnosis of lobar pneumonia includes mycobacterial and fungal infections, both of which can produce an isolated region of consolidation. An upper lobe distribution might suggest one of these, but this is not a constant feature.

Bronchopneumonia

The defining feature of this pattern is endobronchial spread of infection. The infection is

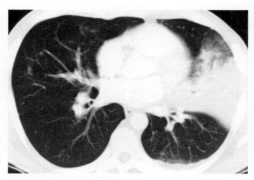

Figure 14.8

Lobar pneumonia. HRCT shows consolidation in the lingula of a patient with *Streptococcus pneumoniae* infection. Note that the consolidation is limited by the major fissure. Only minimal abnormality is seen elsewhere. Nodules and tree-in-bud are not a feature of this pattern. This is typical of infections centered within the alveolar spaces.

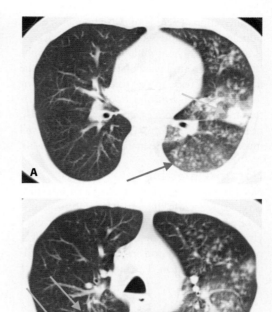

Figure 14.9

Bronchopneumonia. A. Bacterial infections that spread via the airways are characterized by patchy, asymmetric, ill-defined centrilobular nodules of varying sizes (*red arrow*) progressing to areas of confluent consolidation (*yellow arrow*). **B.** Note the segmental distribution of findings in the upper lobes (*arrows*).

centered within airways and is often associated with airway impaction. The process spreads outward from the centrilobular bronchiole, forming a centrilobular nodule, and may continue to spread until the entire pulmonary lobule is involved. Adjacent involved lobules may coalesce to form confluent areas of consolidation. This pattern is typical of *S. aureus*, *P. aeruginosa*, Klebsiella, and *E. coli*. The HRCT findings (Fig. 14.9A, B) of this type of spread include the following:

1. Centrilobular nodules of soft tissue attenuation (various sizes, ill-defined borders)
2. TIB opacities
3. Airway wall thickening, impaction, and dilatation
3. Consolidation
4. Patchy, lobular, or segmental distribution

The differential diagnosis of a bronchopneumonia includes mycobacterial and fungal infections. Mycobacterial disease very commonly demonstrates endobronchial spread. In TB, there is often, but not always, a dominant focus of cavitary pneumonia in the upper lobes. Nontuberculous mycobacterial (NTMB) infection such as Mycobacterium avium-intracellulare (MAI) often demonstrates extensive

inflammation of the airways with little associated consolidation. Except in immunosuppressed patients, fungal diseases do not commonly produce this pattern. Airway-invasive aspergillosis is an example of this type of infection.

RARE BACTERIAL INFECTIONS

Actinomyces Infection

Actinomyces is a normal part of the oral flora that, when aspirated, may produce a pneumonia. Predisposing factors for developing infection include alcoholism, poor dental hygiene, and preexisting lung disease such as emphysema or bronchiectasis. On HRCT, Actinomyces usually presents with nodule(s), mass(es), or consolidation. A nodule or mass may be the earliest

14

manifestation. There is often only one or a few nodules present and widespread nodular disease is not typical. The nodule may show a peripheral rim of ground glass opacity. Over time, the nodule(s) increase in size to produce a mass or focal region of consolidation. The consolidation frequently cavitates, producing low-density, nonenhancing regions. Pleural and chest wall involvement may be seen in advanced infections.

Nocardia Infection

Nocardia is present in soil. Nocardia infection is typically seen in the setting of immunocompromise, such as human immunodeficiency virus infection, organ transplantation, leukemia, lymphoma, and chronic immunosuppressive medication. The radiographic features are similar to Actinomyces infection and include nodule(s), mass(es) (Fig. 14.10A–D), and consolidation. These may be associated with lymphadenopathy.

MYCOBACTERIAL INFECTIONS

Mycobacterial infection is usually classified as tuberculous (i.e., TB) and nontuberculous or atypical mycobacterial infection. While there is overlap in their presentation and HRCT appearances, they often can be differentiated.

Tuberculosis

TB is a very common disease worldwide, but its prevalence in the United States and other developed nations is significantly lower than

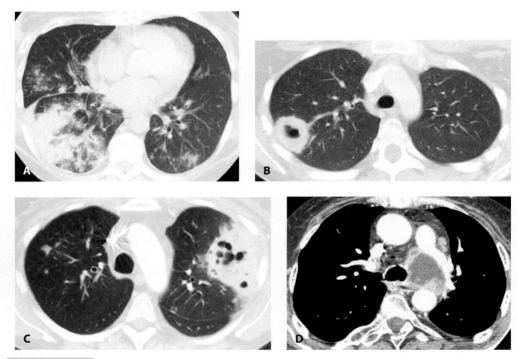

Figure 14.10

Nocardia pneumonia. A. Focal consolidation in the right lower lobe is associated with centrilobular nodules. This is most suggestive of typical bacterial bronchopneumonia, but this patient was eventually diagnosed with nocardia. **B.** A solitary cavitary mass is present in the right upper lobe. This is one possible manifestation of nocardia but is more commonly seen in bacterial, fungal, and mycobacterial infections. **C.** Focal left upper lobe consolidation with cavitation is present. The most common etiologies of this abnormality are mycobacterial or fungal infection, but nocardia may present with this finding. **D.** Necrotic mediastinal lymphadenopathy is present in the aortopulmonary window. This was associated with cavitary consolidation in the left lower lobe (not shown).

Primary	Reactivation	Miliary
Consolidation, upper or lower lung	Consolidation, upper lobes or superior segment of lower lobes	Well-defined nodules
Lymphadenopathy	Cavities	Nodules usually <3 mm
Nonspecific nodule	Centrilobular nodules and/or tree-in-bud opacities	Diffuse, homogeneous
Consolidation + lymphadenopathy most suggestive	Pleural effusions/thickening	Random distribution on HRCT

Table 14.2 HRCT findings of tuberculosis

in third world countries. Within the United States, there is a higher incidence of TB in patients with human immunodeficiency virus infection and other immunocompromised patients than in the general population. It is a major public health problem and thus rapid diagnosis and treatment is important.

Imaging plays an important role in the detection of TB and its differentiation from other diseases. There are several different patterns of infection with TB (Table 14.2), although overlap between the patterns may occur. TB cannot be excluded based solely on imaging, but if HRCT findings do not fit into one of these typical patterns of infection, TB is an unlikely cause of the radiographic abnormalities. Fungal infection may produce identical findings to TB of any pattern.

Primary TB

The infection associated with an initial exposure to TB usually elicits an inflammatory response that sequesters the bacilli and prevents further progression of disease. In many patients, this does not result in a recognizable abnormality on radiographs or CT.

If an abnormality is visible on CT, the most common abnormality is a solitary nodule, representing a granulomatous reaction to the initial focus of infection (Fig. 14.11A, B). Draining lymph node enlargement may or may not be present; enlarged lymph nodes are commonly low in attenuation. Both the nodule and the abnormal lymph nodes may eventually calcify.

Primary TB may also have a more aggressive course, progressing to a symptomatic infection; this is most typical in children

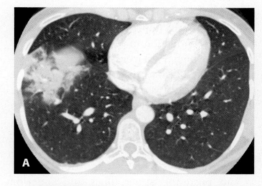
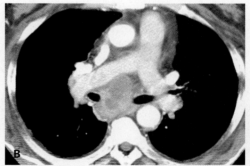

Figure 14.11

Primary tuberculosis in two different patients. A. A nonspecific area of consolidation is seen in the anterior segment of the right lower lobe. This appearance is most commonly a manifestation of community-acquired bacterial pneumonia. This patient was diagnosed with tuberculosis via sputum analysis. **B.** Necrotic lymphadenopathy is visible in the subcarinal space. This finding, in isolation, may also be a manifestation of primary tuberculosis. This patient was diagnosed at bronchoscopy, by Wang needle biopsy.

and immunocompromised patients. This tends to appear on CT as a nonspecific lung consolidation, which may be lobar or patchy, a pulmonary nodule, and/or lymphadenopathy. The combination of lung consolidation and lymphadenopathy is most suggestive, as significant lymphadenopathy is unusual with community-acquired bacterial infection.

Post-Primary (Reactivation or Secondary) TB

At some point after the initial infection, TB may disseminate. When this occurs, the organisms deposit in regions of the body with a high oxygen tension. The highest oxygen tension within the lungs is in the upper lobes because of a relatively high ventilation to perfusion ratio. As TB thrives in a high oxygen environment, the infection is more likely to recur in this region. If it does, it induces a very pronounced inflammatory reaction characterized by necrosis, scarring, and pleural reaction. The typical HRCT findings of reactivation TB include the following:

1. Consolidation in typical locations (apical and posterior upper lobes and superior segments of lower lobes) (Fig. 14.12)
2. Cavities
3. Endobronchial spread (centrilobular nodules of soft tissue attenuation and TIB)
4. Lung scarring (even relatively early in the course of infection)
5. Pleural effusions and/or thickening

Other causes of upper lobe cavitary consolidation include fungal infections (particularly coccidioidomycosis and histoplasmosis) and bacterial infections.

Miliary TB

When hematogenous spread of TB is not limited by an immune response, extensive dissemination of organisms may occur, with diffuse lung involvement. This may occur with primary or secondary infection.

On HRCT, miliary TB results in multiple small nodules having a random distribution (Fig. 14.13). Nodules do not show a predominance in relation to any specific lung structures. Subpleural nodules are present. The nodules tend to be 1 to 2 mm in size, but without treatment they may grow larger. The differential of miliary TB includes hematogenous spread of fungal disease (coccidioidomycosis, histoplasmosis, and blastomycosis) or metastatic disease.

Nontuberculous (Atypical) Mycobacteria

The various organisms included in the category of NTMB produce similar abnormalities on HRCT. Of these, MAI, also known as Mycobacterium avium-intracellulare complex

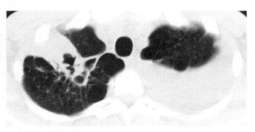

Figure 14.12

Reactivation tuberculosis. Upper lobe cavitary consolidation with architectural distortion is present in a patient with sputum positive for tuberculosis. The location and presence of cavitation favors reactivation tuberculosis, but this appearance could also be seen with fungal and bacterial infection.

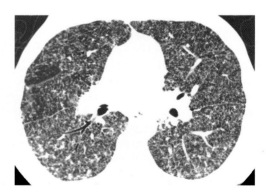

Figure 14.13

Miliary tuberculosis. Diffuse very small discrete nodules are present. They appear evenly distributed. Pleural surfaces, including the fissures, are involved. This indicates a random distribution. The differential diagnosis includes miliary tuberculosis, miliary fungal infection, and hematogenous spread of malignancy.

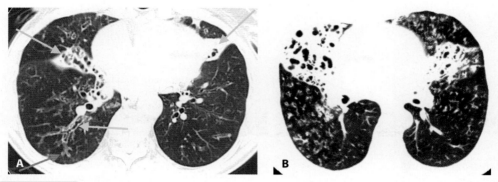

Figure 14.14

Nontuberculous mycobacterial (Mycobacterium avium-intracellulare complex, MAC) infection in two patients. A. Extensive airways inflammation with wall thickening is present in this patient with Mycobacterium avium-intracellulare infection. Varicose bronchiectasis (*yellow arrow*), bronchiolar wall thickening (*red arrow*), and near-complete collapse of the middle lobe and lingula (*blue arrows*) are strongly suggestive of an atypical mycobacterial infection. **B.** In a 67-year-old woman with cough, there is severe bronchiectasis involving the middle lobe and lingual, and numerous centrilobular nodules and examples of tree-in-bud are visible. In a woman of this age, this appearance is strong evidence that MAC infection is present.

(MAC), is the most common. There are several patterns of disease that may affect either immunocompetent or immunocompromised individuals.

The most common HRCT pattern seen with NTMB (Fig. 14.14) occurs in patients with normal immune status, most frequently elderly women (older than 60 years). The predominant feature is airways disease that predominates in the middle lobe and lingula. Bronchiectasis, airway wall thickening, and mucous impaction are typically present. Centrilobular nodules and TIB opacities are also frequently seen.

There may be partial or complete collapse of the middle lobe and lingula in severe cases. In most cases, there is a relative paucity of consolidation present. This combination of HRCT abnormalities in an older woman is highly predictive of MAI (MAC) infection. The differential diagnosis includes recurrent bacterial infections or aspiration.

A second manifestation of NTMB (Fig. 14.15A, B) occurs in immunocompromised patients, often elderly men. This tends to resemble TB with upper lung consolidation, cavitation, and endobronchial spread of infection.

14

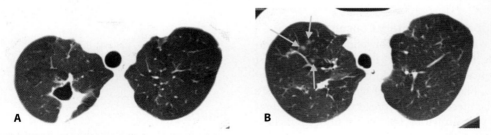

Figure 14.15

Nontuberculous mycobacterial infection. A right upper lobe cavity **(A)** is present in association with a small cluster of centrilobular nodules **(B,** *arrows***)**. This pattern is most suggestive of tuberculosis, but occasionally may be a manifestation of atypical mycobacterial infection.

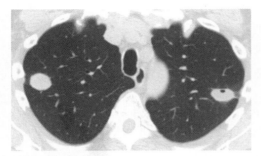

Figure 14.16

Nontuberculous mycobacterial infection.
Discrete, isolated nodules are present bilaterally.
A small area of cavitation is seen in the left-sided
nodule. This pattern is most commonly seen with
fungal infection or septic emboli; however, atypical
mycobacterial infection can occasionally have this
appearance.

Uncommon manifestations of NTMB
include nonspecific lung consolidation resembling bacterial infection and nodules or masses
(Fig. 14.16) resembling fungal infection.

FUNGAL INFECTION

Fungal infection has a wide variety of different
manifestations, and findings show a significant
overlap with those associated with bacterial
and mycobacterial infections. Different fungal
organisms tend to affect immunocompetent
and immunocompromised patients.

HRCT Findings

Several patterns may be present with fungal
infection (Table 14.3).

Upper Lobe Cavitary Consolidation

Cavitary upper lobe consolidation may resemble reactivation TB (Fig. 14.17). It is most
typical of coccidioidomycosis, histoplasmosis, blastomycosis, and chronic aspergillosis.
The mechanism of spread to the upper lungs
is very similar to TB. Typical findings include
consolidation affecting the upper lobes or
superior segments of the lower lobes with cavitation and sometimes endobronchial spread.
Pleural effusion and/or pleural thickening
may also be present. These abnormalities may

Table 14.3	HRCT manifestations of fungal infection
	Upper lobe cavitary consolidation Solitary pulmonary nodule Lymphadenopathy Bronchopneumonia or lobar pneumonia Nodular or mass-like consolidation Random distribution of small nodules

eventually lead to significant upper lung fibrosis and volume loss.

Solitary Pulmonary Nodule and/or Lymphadenopathy

This manifestation of fungal infection resembles primary TB, but is significantly more
common with fungal disease. An isolated pulmonary nodule (Fig. 14.18A–C) is the most
common manifestation. Hilar and mediastinal
lymphadenopathy may be seen in association
with the nodule or as an isolated abnormality.
The nodule typically cavitates and often develops a thin wall over time. These patients are
often asymptomatic, so the primary differential
diagnosis in these cases is malignancy.

Bronchopneumonia or Lobar Pneumonia

Bronchopneumonia associated with fungal disease may be indistinguishable from a typical

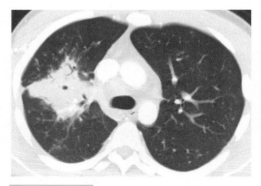

Figure 14.17

Coccidioidomycosis. Right upper lobe cavitary
consolidation is present with scattered nodules
at the periphery of the large mass. Fungal and
mycobacterial infections may show significant
overlap in the HRCT findings.

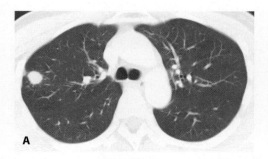

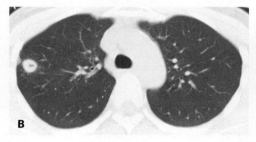

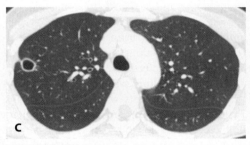

Figure 14.18

Coccidioidomycosis. A. An isolated, soft tissue attenuation pulmonary nodule is seen in the right upper lobe in an asymptomatic patient. This finding is nonspecific, but when it represents infection, either fungal or mycobacterial infections are most likely. **B** and **C.** Over time, this nodule cavitates **(B)** and eventually develops a thin wall **(C).**

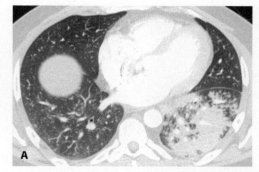

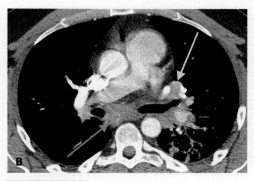

Figure 14.19

Coccidioidomycosis. A and **B.** Focal consolidation is seen in the left lower lobe **(A).** While this finding is nonspecific with regard to the type of infection, there is extensive associated lymphadenopathy **(B)** in the left hilum (*yellow arrow*, **B**) and mediastinum (*red arrow*, **B**). Lymphadenopathy is unusual in uncomplicated bacterial infection and suggests fungal or mycobacterial organisms as an etiology.

Nodular or Mass-Like Areas of Consolidation

Multiple, bilateral nodular or mass-like regions of consolidation (Fig. 14.20) are the most common manifestation of fungal infection in immunocompromised patients. It is characteristic of Aspergillus, mucormycosis, and Candida infections. The abnormalities tend to be scattered bilaterally with large (>1 cm) focal regions of rounded consolidation with ill-defined margins. The lung in between the nodules is relatively unaffected, and endobronchial spread is not a typical manifestation of disease. A halo of ground glass opacity may be seen surrounding nodules, the so-called halo sign. In an

bacterial infection (Fig. 14.19A, B). Patchy unilateral or bilateral, asymmetric segmental consolidation with centrilobular nodules and airway inflammation may resemble bacterial bronchopneumonia. A nonsegmental region of consolidation involving a single lobe may resemble a bacterial lobar pneumonia. This is not a common manifestation of fungal infection and is usually seen with primary infections. As with bacterial infections, an overlap of bronchopneumonia and lobar pneumonia may be present.

14

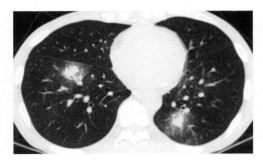

Figure 14.20

Aspergillosis. Focal, nodular areas of consolidation are seen with adjacent ground glass opacity (i.e., the halo sign is present) in a neutropenic patient. In this clinical setting, fungal infection such as angioinvasive aspergillosis is the most likely etiology.

Table 14.4	Features of atypical infections
Organisms	Viral infections
	Atypical bacterial organisms
	(*Mycoplasma pneumoniae*,
	Chlamydia pneumoniae,
	Legionella pneumophila)
	Pneumocystis jiroveci
HRCT findings	Airway wall thickening
	Mild bronchial dilatation
	Centrilobular nodules
	Mosaic/perfusion air trapping
	Symmetric or diffuse ground
	glass opacity and consolidation

immunosuppressed patient with neutropenia, the halo sign suggests angioinvasive aspergillosis infection, but otherwise the halo sign is not specific for any one organism.

In immunocompromised patients, the differential diagnosis includes organizing pneumonia (e.g., from drug reaction or graft vs. host disease), lymphoproliferative disease, and infarcts from pulmonary emboli. Other etiologies that may resemble this pattern include invasive mucinous adenocarcinoma, eosinophilic pneumonia, and sarcoidosis; however, the clinical presentation of these diseases is quite different.

Random Distribution of Small Pulmonary Nodules

A pattern of small nodules with a random distribution may be present with fungal infection. This closely resembles miliary TB. Random nodules may be seen in association with the other patterns described above and represents diffuse hematogenous spread of infection to the lungs. This pattern is most typical of coccidioidomycosis, histoplasmosis, and blastomycosis.

ATYPICAL INFECTIONS

Included in this category are atypical bacterial infections, viral infections, and infection with *P. jiroveci* (Table 14.4). The most common atypical bacterial organisms within this category include *M. pneumoniae*, *Chlamydia pneumoniae*, and *Legionella pneumophila*.

Atypical infections share clinical and radiographic features that distinguish them from typical bacterial infections such as Streptococcus, TB, and fungal infections. Symptoms attributable to the respiratory system tend to be milder than those in patients with other infections. Extrapulmonary symptoms are more frequent and severe, and leukocytosis is often absent. Also, these organisms are often not responsive to antibiotics given to treat typical bacterial organisms.

Atypical infections may be predominantly associated with patchy, diffuse, or centrilobular ground glass opacity (Figs. 14.21 and 14.22). This appearance is most typical of pneumocystis or some viral infections. The presence of ground glass opacity and air-filled cysts (pneumatoceles) in an immunosuppressed patient suggests pneumocystis. Cysts are more likely of *P. jiroveci* infection than other atypical infections (Fig. 14.23).

Atypical infections also may be manifested by findings similar to bronchopneumonia (Fig. 14.24). Initially, these produce inflammation of airway walls and the peribronchiolar interstitium with limited airway impaction. As the infection progresses, areas of bronchiolar impaction, centrilobular nodules, and peribronchiolar consolidation

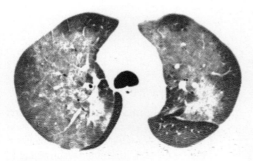

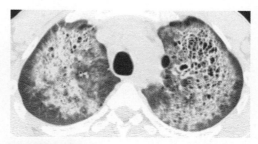

Figure 14.23

***Pneumocystis jiroveci* pneumonia in a patient with HIV.** Symmetric ground glass opacity and consolidation are seen in association with cysts (i.e., pneumatoceles). Pneumatoceles are most commonly seen with *Pneumocystis jiroveci*, viral, and bacterial infections. The distribution and history of human immunodeficiency virus infection favor *Pneumocystis jiroveci* infection.

Figure 14.21

Atypical pneumonia. Extensive bilateral ground glass opacity and consolidation are present. The bilateral distribution and presence of ground glass favor atypical pneumonias such as viral, atypical bacterial, and *Pneumocystis jiroveci*. This patient was diagnosed with adenovirus infection.

may develop. Early, the centrilobular nodules are often of ground glass opacity, but they may evolve and be of soft tissue attenuation. More extensive areas of ground glass opacity and consolidation may appear. Pathologically, these represent areas of diffuse alveolar damage. Associated mosaic perfusion and/or air trapping reflects narrowing of small airways by inflammation.

Typical HRCT findings in patients with this pattern of infection include the following:

1. Airway wall thickening with or without dilatation
2. Centrilobular nodules (ground glass opacity early, soft tissue attenuation late)
3. Mosaic perfusion and/or air trapping
4. Symmetric or diffuse ground glass opacity and consolidation

In patients with an infection, HRCT is most accurate in distinguishing atypical infections from other types. Atypical infections often present with abnormalities that are bilateral and extensive in distribution. Ground glass opacity is more commonly seen with atypical infections, as compared with bacterial, mycobacterial, and fungal infections.

Viral and atypical bacterial infections also may be associated with airway thickening, impaction, centrilobular nodules (Fig. 14.24), and TIB opacities. These abnormalities also tend to be symmetric in distribution. Mosaic perfusion and/or air trapping may also be present, underlying the airway-centric nature of this process. Airways inflammation is not typical of *P. jiroveci* infection.

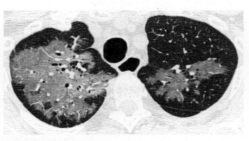

Figure 14.22

Atypical pneumonia. Extensive bilateral ground glass opacity is present in a patient with cytomegalovirus pneumonia. The bilateral distribution and presence of ground glass as a significant abnormality makes atypical infections the most likely infectious etiology.

14

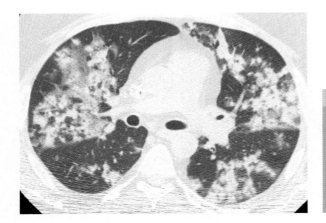

Figure 14.24

Varicella pneumonia. Extensive bilateral soft tissue attenuation nodules and consolidation are present. The nodules have a centrilobular distribution. Soft tissue attenuation nodules may be seen with any type of infection, but the bilateral distribution in this case favors an atypical infection.

FURTHER READING

Brecher CW, Aviram G, Boiselle PM. CT and radiography of bacterial respiratory infections in AIDS patients. *AJR Am J Roentgenol.* 2003;180:1203-1209.

Cattamanchi A, Nahid P, Marras TK, et al. Detailed analysis of the radiographic presentation of *Mycobacterium kansasii* lung disease in patients with HIV infection. *Chest.* 2008;133:875-880.

Elicker BM, Schwartz BS, Liu C, et al. Thoracic CT findings of novel influenza A (H1N1) infection in immunocompromised patients. *Emerg Radiol.* 2010;17:299-307.

Erasmus JJ, McAdams HP, Farrell MA, Patz EF Jr. Pulmonary nontuberculous mycobacterial infection: radiologic manifestations. *Radiographics.* 1999;19:1487-1505.

Franquet T, Müller NL, Gimenez A, et al. Spectrum of pulmonary aspergillosis: histologic, clinical, and radiologic findings. *Radiographics.* 2001;21:825-837.

Gotway MB, Dawn SK, Caoili EM, et al. The radiologic spectrum of pulmonary *Aspergillus* infections. *J Comput Assist Tomogr.* 2002;26:159-173.

Gruden JF, Huang L, Turner J, et al. High-resolution CT in the evaluation of clinically suspected *Pneumocystis carinii* pneumonia in AIDS patients with normal, equivocal, or nonspecific radiographic findings. *AJR Am J Roentgenol.* 1997;169:967-975.

Im JG, Itoh H, Shim YS, et al. Pulmonary tuberculosis: CT findings—early active disease and sequential change with antituberculous therapy. *Radiology.* 1993;186:653-660.

Kim EA, Lee KS, Primack SL, et al. Viral pneumonias in adults: radiologic and pathologic findings. *Radiographics.* 2002;22:S137-S149.

Lee KS, Song KS, Lim TH, Kim PN, Kim IY, Lee BH. Adult-onset pulmonary tuberculosis: findings on chest radiographs and CT scans. *AJR Am J Roentgenol.* 1993;160:753-758.

Leung AN. Pulmonary tuberculosis: the essentials. *Radiology.* 1999;210:307-322.

Leung AN, Brauner MW, Gamsu G, et al. Pulmonary tuberculosis: comparison of CT findings in HIV-seropositive and HIV-seronegative patients. *Radiology.* 1996;198:687-691.

Lieberman D, Porath A, Schlaeffer F, Boldur I. *Legionella* species community-acquired pneumonia. A review of 56 hospitalized adult patients. *Chest.* 1996;109:1243-1249.

Lynch DA, Simone PM, Fox MA, Bucher BL, Heinig MJ. CT features of pulmonary Mycobacterium avium complex infection. *J Comput Assist Tomogr.* 1995;19:353-360.

McAdams HP, Rosado de Christenson ML, Lesar M, Templeton PA, Moran CA. Thoracic mycoses from endemic fungi: radiologic-pathologic correlation. *Radiographics.* 1995;15:255-270.

McAdams HP, Rosado de Christenson ML, Templeton PA, et al. Thoracic mycoses from opportunistic fungi: radiologic-pathologic correlation. *Radiographics.* 1995;15:271-286.

Primack SL, Logan PM, Hartman TE, Lee KS, Müller NL. Pulmonary tuberculosis and Mycobacterium avium-intracellulare: a comparison of CT findings. *Radiology.* 1995;194:413-417.

Reittner P, Muller NL, Heyneman L, et al. *Mycoplasma pneumoniae* pneumonia: radiographic and high-resolution CT features in 28 patients. *AJR Am J Roentgenol.* 2000;174:37-41.

Saurborn DP, Fishman JE, Boiselle PM. The imaging spectrum of pulmonary tuberculosis in AIDS. *J Thorac Imaging.* 2002;17:28-33.

14

15

Complications of Medical Treatment: Drug-Induced Lung Disease and Radiation

DRUG-INDUCED LUNG DISEASE

Drug-induced lung disease is often overlooked or misdiagnosed. The most common categories of drugs that result in lung disease include chemotherapeutic agents, cardiac medications, and antibiotics.

Drug-induced diffuse lung disease may be associated with a number of possible appearances on HRCT (Table 15.1). These appearances reflect the typical manifestations of different patterns of lung injury reviewed in other parts of this book and include many of the interstitial pneumonias reviewed in Chapter 9.

The most common patterns of lung injury associated with drug toxicity include pulmonary edema and pulmonary hemorrhage, diffuse alveolar damage (DAD), organizing pneumonia (OP), nonspecific interstitial pneumonia (NSIP), usual interstitial pneumonia (UIP), and eosinophilic pneumonia. Less common patterns of drug toxicity include hypersensitivity pneumonitis (HP), a sarcoid-like reaction, constrictive bronchiolitis, pulmonary vasculitis and pulmonary hypertension, desquamative interstitial pneumonia, and lymphoid interstitial pneumonia.

There are no HRCT findings that specifically suggest drug toxicity. Drug reactions must be considered in the differential diagnosis of the various patterns described above. A high degree of suspicion and correlation with medication history is necessary to make a confident diagnosis. The patterns of lung disease related to drugs are reviewed below.

Pulmonary Edema

Hydrostatic pulmonary edema may result from drugs that affect the heart or systemic vasculature. An example is cocaine. HRCT findings are typical of any cause of hydrostatic edema (Fig. 15.1). Pleural effusion may be present.

Increased permeability pulmonary edema also may occur with drug treatment. Onset is usually sudden. HRCT findings are typical of pulmonary edema, including interlobular septal thickening, ground glass opacity, and to a lesser extent consolidation. This occurrence is typical of interleukin-2, but many other drugs are capable of causing increased permeability pulmonary edema. These include aspirin, nitrofurantoin, heroin, and cytotoxic agents such as methotrexate, cyclophosphamide, and carmustine. Unlike hydrostatic edema, pleural effusion is typically absent. Prompt resolution may occur with appropriate treatment.

Pulmonary Hemorrhage

Drug-related diffuse pulmonary hemorrhage is uncommon. Typical causes include anticoagulants, cyclophosphamide, and penicillamine. Hemoptysis may or may not be present. HRCT findings are typical of pulmonary hemorrhage, with bilateral patchy ground glass opacity or consolidation. Pleural effusion is typically absent.

Diffuse Alveolar Damage

DAD, the histologic pattern associated with acute respiratory distress syndrome (ARDS), is a common manifestation of drug toxicity.

15

Table 15.1 — Patterns of drug-induced lung disease and the most common offending agents

Pattern	Drugs
Pulmonary edema	Aspirin, nitrofurantoin, heroin, methotrexate, cyclophosphamide, carmustine, interleukin-2
Pulmonary hemorrhage	Anticoagulants, cyclophosphamide, penicillamine
Diffuse alveolar damage	Carmustine, busulfan, cyclophosphamide, bleomycin, amiodarone, methotrexate, aspirin, narcotics, cocaine
Organizing pneumonia	Carmustine, bleomycin, doxorubicin, cyclophosphamide, amiodarone, nitrofurantoin, cephalosporins, tetracycline, amphotericin B, gold salts, phenytoin, sulfasalazine, cocaine
Nonspecific interstitial pneumonia	Bleomycin, busulfan, cyclophosphamide, methotrexate, amiodarone, nitrofurantoin, hydrochlorothiazide, statins, phenytoin, gold
Usual interstitial pneumonia	Cyclophosphamide, chlorambucil, nitrofurantoin, pindolol
Eosinophilic pneumonia	Bleomycin, amiodarone, nitrofurantoin, antidepressants, beta-blockers, hydrochlorothiazide, nonsteroidal anti-inflammatory drugs, phenytoin, sulfasalazine, cocaine
Hypersensitivity pneumonitis	Methotrexate, cyclophosphamide, mesalamine, fluoxetine, amitriptyline, paclitaxel
Sarcoid-like reaction	Interferon
Vasculitis and pulmonary hypertension	Fenfluramine, busulfan, methylphenidate, and methadone
Constrictive bronchiolitis	Penicillamine and sulfasalazine

DAD is characterized by edema, intra-alveolar hyaline membranes, and acute interstitial inflammation, followed by fibroblast proliferation, and progressive fibrosis with collagen deposition.

Not all patients with DAD meet the clinical criteria for ARDS (see Chapter 8); this is particularly true in the setting of drug toxicity.

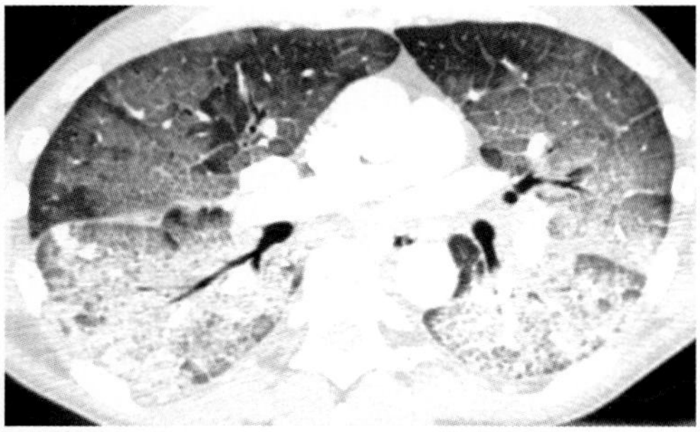

15

Figure 15.1

Pulmonary edema with cocaine use. Diffuse ground glass opacity and smooth interlobular septal thickening is present, representing the *crazy paving* pattern. This patient had an acute onset of pulmonary edema after the inhalational use of cocaine.

The most common drugs associated with this pattern include carmustine, busulfan, cyclophosphamide, bleomycin, amiodarone, methotrexate, aspirin, narcotics, and cocaine.

HRCT findings are identical to those of DAD from other causes. Diffuse ground glass opacity and consolidation are present (Fig. 15.2). Early, this may have a peripheral distribution, but the abnormalities quickly become diffuse. If early treatment is instituted, complete resolution of findings may be seen; otherwise patients may progress to ARDS. Eventually fibrosis may develop, often peripherally, and is anterior in distribution.

Organizing Pneumonia

OP is a common pattern associated with drug toxicity. Conversely, drug toxicity is one of the most common causes of OP. This pattern is most commonly associated with carmustine, bleomycin, doxorubicin, cyclophosphamide, amiodarone, nitrofurantoin, cephalosporins, tetracycline, amphotericin B, gold salts, phenytoin, sulfasalazine, and cocaine.

The predominant HRCT findings are the same as in other causes of OP, including bilateral patchy, nodular, or mass-like areas of

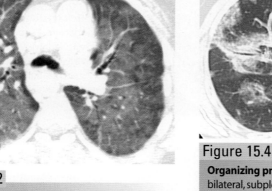

Figure 15.2

Diffuse alveolar damage due to carmustine treatment. Diffuse ground glass opacity is present in a patient being treated with carmustine for lymphoma. Pathologically, this corresponded to diffuse alveolar damage. This finding resolved after steroid treatment.

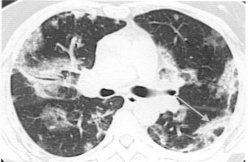

Figure 15.4

Organizing pneumonia with amiodarone. Patchy, bilateral, subpleural and peribronchovascular consolidation and ground glass opacity are present without evidence of fibrosis. Note the presence of the *atoll sign* in the left lower lobe (*arrow*). These findings are compatible with organizing pneumonia.

peribronchovascular and subpleural consolidation (Fig. 15.3). The *atoll sign or reversed halo sign*, a peripheral rim of consolidation surrounding a central area of ground glass opacity (Fig. 15.4), is highly specific for OP. The findings of drug-related OP are indistinguishable from those of cryptogenic organizing pneumonia.

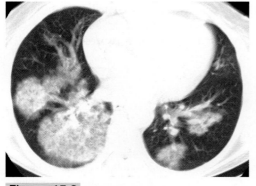

Figure 15.3

Organizing pneumonia with crack cocaine use. Patchy, bilateral, mass-like areas of consolidation are seen in a patient presenting with subacute symptoms after the recurrent usage of crack cocaine.

Nonspecific Interstitial Pneumonia

The most common cause of NSIP is connective tissue disease. Next on the list of likely causes is drug toxicity.

The most common drugs to cause this pattern include bleomycin, busulfan, cyclophosphamide, methotrexate, amiodarone, nitrofurantoin, hydrochlorothiazide, statins, phenytoin, and gold.

NSIP secondary to drugs may be cellular, fibrotic, or a combination of both. HRCT may be helpful in making this distinction; differentiation of cellular and fibrotic NSIP has significant implications for treatment, as cellular NSIP is most likely to respond to treatment and has a better prognosis.

Typical HRCT findings of NSIP include ground glass opacity and/or irregular reticulation with a subpleural and basilar distribution (Fig. 15.5). A peripheral distribution of abnormalities with sparing of the immediate subpleural lung is particularly suggestive of NSIP. The presence of ground glass opacity, with or without reticulation, suggests cellular NSIP. Reticulation associated with traction bronchiectasis suggests the fibrotic subtype of NSIP. Honeycombing is typically absent or minimal in extent, but when present indicates fibrotic NSIP.

15

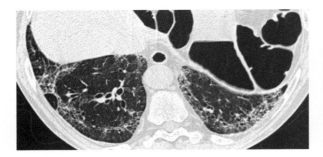

Figure 15.5

Nonspecific interstitial pneumonia with amiodarone. Peripheral and basilar irregular reticulation and mild traction bronchiectasis are seen. There is subpleural sparing. After cessation of the drug and treatment with steroids, the majority of these abnormalities resolved.

Usual Interstitial Pneumonia

A UIP pattern may be seen as a manifestation of drug treatment, closely resembling idiopathic pulmonary fibrosis. The most common drugs to present in this manner include cyclophosphamide, chlorambucil, nitrofurantoin, and pindolol. HRCT findings include fibrosis, characterized by reticulation, traction bronchiectasis, and honeycombing, with subpleural and basilar predominance (Fig. 15.6).

Eosinophilic Pneumonia

A common cause of eosinophilic lung disease is drug toxicity. Patients with an eosinophilic reaction show a combination of lung abnormalities on imaging and increased serum or tissue eosinophils. This pattern is most closely associated with bleomycin, amiodarone, nitrofurantoin, antidepressants, beta-blockers, hydrochlorothiazide, nonsteroidal anti-inflammatory drugs, phenytoin, sulfasalazine, and cocaine.

HRCT findings resemble those seen in the idiopathic eosinophilic disorders, particularly chronic eosinophilic pneumonia (see Chapter 13). Peripheral, upper lobe predominant consolidation is most characteristic, although not commonly seen. Patchy bilateral nodular or mass-like consolidation is a more frequent finding and may closely resemble OP. Eosinophilic pneumonia often shows an upper lobe predominance, while OP often shows a lower lobe predominance.

Hypersensitivity Pneumonitis

HP is an uncommon pattern associated with drug toxicity but may be seen with methotrexate, cyclophosphamide, mesalamine, fluoxetine, amitriptyline, and paclitaxel.

HRCT findings are similar to those present with inhalational causes of HP, including ground glass opacity, centrilobular nodules, and mosaic perfusion or air trapping (see Chapter 13). If fibrosis is present (Fig. 15.7),

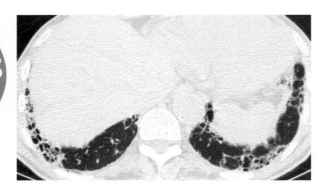

Figure 15.6

Usual interstitial pneumonia with bleomycin. Subpleural and basilar fibrosis is present with significant honeycombing. This finding developed during treatment for breast cancer with bleomycin. This appearance is indistinguishable from other causes of usual interstitial pneumonia, such as idiopathic pulmonary fibrosis.

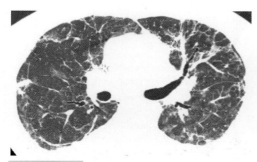

Figure 15.7

Hypersensitivity pneumonitis with infliximab. Patchy, bilateral irregular reticulation is seen in both peripheral and central locations. This finding by itself is nonspecific with regard to pattern, but suggests fibrosis. Pathology showed a hypersensitivity reaction.

it usually presents with irregular reticulation and traction bronchiectasis with a patchy distribution.

Sarcoid-Like Reaction

Sarcoidosis is an idiopathic disease, but rarely, a similar reaction may be seen with drug toxicity. This pattern is most commonly associated with interferon treatment. HRCT findings are identical to those typical of sarcoidosis (see Chapter 12), including nodules with a perilymphatic distribution (Fig. 15.8).

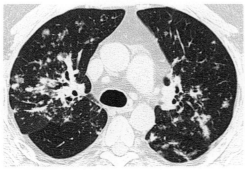

Figure 15.8

Sarcoid-like reaction with interferon. Nodules are noted with a peribronchovascular and subpleural predominance. This perilymphatic distribution is most commonly due to sarcoidosis. These CT abnormalities developed while this patient was on interferon for hepatitis infection.

Fibrosis is not common with drug-induced sarcoidosis.

Pulmonary Vasculitis and Pulmonary Hypertension

The use of various drugs may result in acute or chronic abnormalities of small pulmonary vessels, with histologic abnormalities including pulmonary vasculitis, plexogenic arteriopathy, pulmonary capillary hemangiomatosis, and pulmonary veno-occlusive disease. The most common offending medications include fenfluramine, busulfan, methylphenidate, and methadone.

The HRCT appearances of these vary with the specific abnormalities present. Pulmonary vasculitis may result in an appearance similar to that of pulmonary edema or pulmonary hemorrhage, with patchy or diffuse consolidation or ground glass opacity. Plexogenic arteriopathy shows findings of pulmonary hypertension, with enlargement of central pulmonary arteries. Pulmonary veno-occlusive disease and pulmonary capillary hemangiomatosis mimic hydrostatic pulmonary edema, but with normal heart size.

Constrictive Bronchiolitis

The least common lung reaction to drugs is constrictive bronchiolitis, a finding primarily described in association with penicillamine therapy for rheumatoid arthritis. However, the role of penicillamine is controversial, as constrictive bronchiolitis can be seen in patients with rheumatoid arthritis who have not been treated with this drug. Constrictive bronchiolitis has also been seen in patients treated with sulfasalazine.

Abnormalities seen on HRCT consist of bronchial wall thickening and a pattern of mosaic perfusion, similar to that seen with other causes of constrictive bronchiolitis (Fig. 15.9); air trapping on expiratory scans is typically present.

RADIATION

Radiation treatment of thoracic malignancies may induce lung inflammation and eventually lead to lung fibrosis. The pattern

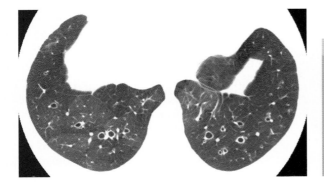

Figure 15.9

Constrictive bronchiolitis with penicillamine treatment. Extensive mosaic perfusion is present and associated with bronchiectasis. Pathology confirmed constrictive bronchiolitis. This patient was on penicillamine treatment for rheumatoid arthritis. Both medications and connective tissue disease are causes of this pattern.

of radiation-induced lung injury depends primarily upon the location (Table 15.2) and dose of radiation given. Lung injury due to radiation is most commonly seen with the treatment of breast cancer, lung cancer, lymphoma, esophageal cancer, and neck malignancies.

Radiation injury is divided into two stages: radiation pneumonitis and radiation fibrosis. *Radiation pneumonitis* occurs early, typically less than 6 months after treatment, and is primarily characterized by DAD that is localized to the region of treatment. Over time, *radiation fibrosis* may develop in the same lung regions.

HRCT findings are usually limited to areas of lung that are included in the radiation field. Breast radiation is localized to the anterior subpleural lung just deep to the treated breast (Fig. 15.10). Axillary and supraclavicular radiation manifests with findings in the lung apex on the treated side (Fig. 15.11). Radiation for

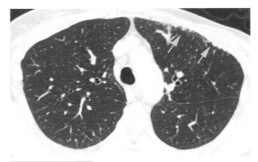

Figure 15.10

Radiation fibrosis after treatment of breast cancer. Isolated irregular reticulation is seen in the subpleural region of the left upper lobe (*yellow arrows*). Note volume loss as evidenced by displacement of the major fissure anteriorly (*red arrow*) and superiorly. This is a typical location for fibrosis due to tangential breast radiation.

Table 15.2	Typical locations of radiation-induced lung injury
Location	**Tumor**
Anterior, subpleural lung	Breast cancer, radiation to primary tumor
Unilateral lung apex	Breast cancer, axillary radiation
Bilateral lung apices	Neck malignancy
Paramediastinal	Lymphoma or esophageal cancer

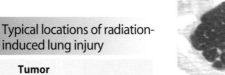

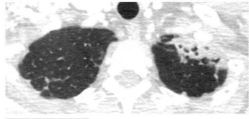

Figure 15.11

Radiation fibrosis after treatment of breast cancer. Irregular reticulation and traction bronchiectasis are seen at the left lung apex. When asymmetric, this location is typical of radiation to the axillary or supraclavicular regions.

15

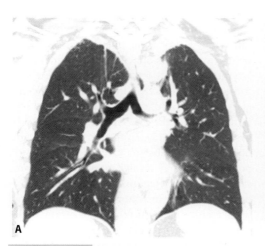
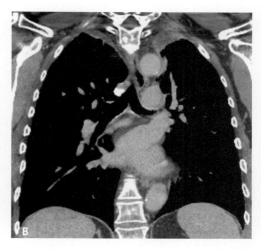

Figure 15.12

Radiation fibrosis in head and neck cancer. Lung **(A)** and mediastinal **(B)** windows from a coronal reformatted CT scan show biapical consolidation, reticulation, and architectural distortion. This is a classic location for fibrosis from radiation treatment of a head and neck malignancy.

cancer of the neck shows findings in both lung apices (Fig. 15.12). Mediastinal radiation for lymphoma or esophageal cancer shows abnormalities in the medial lungs, directly adjacent to the mediastinum (Fig. 15.13). Radiation for lung cancer shows abnormalities that surround the radiated tumor (Fig. 15.14). These changes should not be confused with enlargement of the tumor itself.

Newer radiation techniques, such as CyberKnife therapy, limit the affects on lung uninvolved by tumor. When radiation pneumonitis or fibrosis is seen in this setting, it commonly presents with abnormalities directly adjacent to the treated tumor.

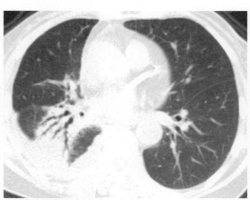

Figure 15.14

Radiation fibrosis in lung cancer. This patient with lung cancer was treated with radiation therapy rather than surgery because of his advanced age. After treatment, fibrosis with traction bronchiectasis, consolidation, and architectural distortion are seen predominantly in the right lower lobe, in the region of the tumor.

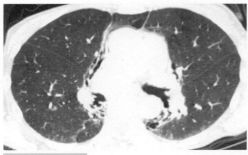

Figure 15.13

Radiation fibrosis in lymphoma. Traction bronchiectasis, reticulation, and architectural distortion are seen in a paramediastinal location bilaterally. This patient had a remote history of mediastinal radiation for lymphoma.

15

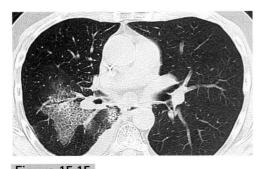

Figure 15.15

Radiation pneumonitis with crazy paving.
A combination of ground glass opacity and
reticulation is noted in the right lower lobe, in the
same region as a treated lung cancer. Note the
relative lack of architectural distortion or significant
signs of fibrosis.

The HRCT findings that are present
depend upon the acuity of radiation-induced
lung injury. Radiation pneumonitis presents
with ground glass opacity or consolidation in
a typical distribution, usually associated with
some volume loss. A combination of ground
glass opacity and smooth interlobular septal thickening, the *crazy paving* sign, may be
present (Fig. 15.15). In the early stages, signs
of fibrosis are absent. Over time, radiation
pneumonitis may resolve or evolve into fibrosis (Fig. 15.16). Regions of radiation fibrosis
decrease further in volume and are associated
with architectural distortion, traction bronchiectasis, and irregular reticulation. Regions
of fibrosis may show straight edges, reflecting
the location of the radiated field.

In a small percentage of cases, radiation
treatment may induce a more generalized
lung reaction, with abnormalities visible
on HRCT outside the area of treatment.
Abnormalities usually represent OP or eosinophilic pneumonia. These tend to present
with similar findings. Patchy consolidation is
the most common HRCT finding (Fig. 15.17).
The consolidation is typically nodular or
mass-like and often has a peribronchovascular
and subpleural distribution.

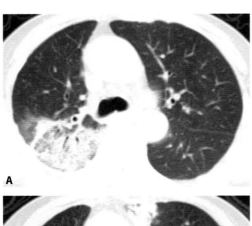

A

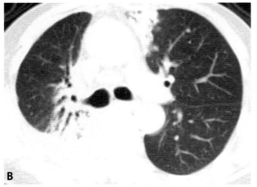

B

15

Figure 15.16

Radiation pneumonitis progressing to fibrosis.
A. Weeks after radiation treatment for lung cancer,
focal ground glass opacity and consolidation
are seen in the right upper lobe. **B.** Months later,
traction bronchiectasis, architectural distortion, and
volume loss indicate the development of fibrosis.

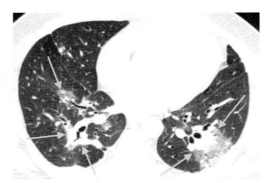

Figure 15.17

**Radiation treatment with organizing
pneumonia.** Patchy bilateral areas of
peribronchovascular consolidation and ground
glass opacity (*arrows*) are seen in a patient with
organizing pneumonia occurring after stereotactic
body radiotherapy for colon cancer metastases.

FURTHER READING

Aquino SL, Webb WR, Golden J. Bronchiolitis obliterans associated with rheumatoid arthritis: findings on HRCT and dynamic expiratory CT. *J Comput Assist Tomogr.* 1994;18:555-558.

Aronchick JM, Gefter WB. Drug-induced pulmonary disorders. *Semin Roentgenol.* 1995;30:18-34.

Bellamy EA, Husband JE, Blaquiere RM, Law MR. Bleomycin-related lung damage: CT evidence. *Radiology.* 1985;156:155-158.

Bush DA, Dunbar RD, Bonnet R, et al. Pulmonary injury from proton and conventional radiotherapy as revealed by CT. *AJR Am J Roentgenol.* 1999;172:735-739.

Cooper JAD, White DA, Matthay RA. Drug induced pulmonary disease, part 1: cytotoxic drugs. *Am Rev Respir Dis.* 1986;133:321-340.

Cooper JAD, White DA, Matthay RA. Drug induced pulmonary disease, part 2: noncytotoxic drugs. *Am Rev Respir Dis.* 1986;133:488-503.

Davis SD, Yankelevitz DF, Henschke CI. Radiation effects on the lung: clinical features, pathology, and imaging findings. *AJR Am J Roentgenol.* 1992;159:1157-1164.

Gotway MB, Marder SR, Hanks DK, et al. Thoracic complications of illicit drug use: an organ system approach. *Radiographics.* 2002;22:119-135.

Kuhlman JE. The role of chest computed tomography in the diagnosis of drug-related reactions. *J Thorac Imaging.* 1991;6:52-61.

Kuhlman JE, Teigen C, Ren H, et al. Amiodarone pulmonary toxicity: CT findings in symptomatic patients. *Radiology.* 1990;177:121-125.

Logan PM. Thoracic manifestations of external beam radiotherapy. *AJR Am J Roentgenol.* 1998;171:569-577.

Padley SPG, Adler B, Hansell DM, Müller NL. High-resolution computed tomography of drug-induced lung disease. *Clin Radiol.* 1992;46:232-236.

Pietra GG. Pathologic mechanisms of drug-induced lung disorders. *J Thorac Imaging.* 1991;6:1-7.

Rosenow EC, Myers JL, Swensen SJ, Pisani RJ. Drug-induced pulmonary disease: an update. *Chest.* 1992; 102:239-250.

Rossi SE, Erasmus JJ, McAdams HP, et al. Pulmonary drug toxicity: radiologic and pathologic manifestations. *Radiographics.* 2000;20:1245-1259.

15

16

Pneumoconioses

The incidence of pneumoconioses is decreasing in relation to other diffuse lung diseases, because of a greater emphasis on prevention in high-risk occupations. Because they often have HRCT findings that resemble other diseases, such as sarcoidosis or idiopathic pulmonary fibrosis (IPF), a clinical history of exposure is vital in suggesting the correct diagnosis of pneumoconiosis.

GENERAL APPROACH TO DIAGNOSIS

Most patients with a pneumoconiosis have an identifiable long-term exposure to a known offending agent. However, without knowledge of the exposure history, HRCT findings are commonly mistaken for another disease.

The most common HRCT abnormalities of pneumoconioses include nodules, fibrosis, and lymphadenopathy. Nodules may be perilymphatic or centrilobular in distribution. Fibrosis may appear on HRCT as honeycombing, irregular reticulation, traction bronchiectasis, and consolidation with architectural distortion, so-called progressive massive fibrosis (PMF).

Pneumoconioses have characteristic patterns on HRCT. Each of these patterns is associated with one or more possible inhaled dusts. The archetype of each of these patterns is discussed below, with a review of other dusts that may also be associated with a similar appearance.

PNEUMOCONIOSES PATTERNS ON HRCT

Silicosis and a "Silicosis Pattern"

Silicosis (Table 16.1) is caused by chronic inhalation of silicon dioxide and is associated with professions such as glass manufacturing, sandblasting, mining, stone cutting, and quarrying. Silicosis results from inhalation of dust and subsequent drainage via the lymphatics. It is primarily characterized by nodules, lymphadenopathy, and fibrosis. Silicosis associated with chronic exposure is usually classified as either *simple silicosis* or *complicated silicosis*.

Table 16.1	Features of silicosis and a "silicosis pattern"
HRCT findings	Perilymphatic nodules, posterior/upper lung distribution, bilateral and symmetrical
	Fibrosis, upper/central lung distribution
	Progressive massive fibrosis
	Lymphadenopathy and/or calcification
Other pneumoconioses with similar findings	Coal worker's pneumoconiosis
	Talcosis
	Berylliosis
Complications	Tuberculosis
	Primary bronchogenic carcinoma

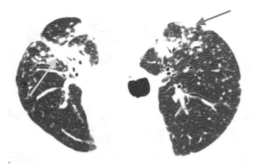

Figure 16.1

Perilymphatic nodules in silicosis. Prone HRCT shows nodules clustered in relation to the peribronchovascular (*yellow arrow*) and subpleural interstitium (*red arrow*). This appearance is indistinguishable from sarcoidosis.

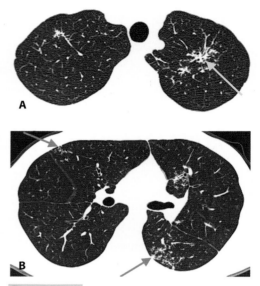

Figure 16.2

Perilymphatic nodules in silicosis. HRCT through the lung apices **(A)** and mid-lungs **(B)** shows patchy, clustered nodules. The nodules are predominantly located within the peribronchovascular (*yellow arrow*, **A**) and subpleural interstitium (*red arrow*, **B**).

A third form of silicosis, *acute silicosis (silicoproteinosis)*, is less frequently seen.

HRCT Findings

Simple silicosis is characterized by scattered nodules (Fig. 16.1). These predominate in the posterior upper lungs and demonstrate a perilymphatic distribution, affecting the centrilobular regions, peribronchovascular interstitium, interlobular septa, and subpleural interstitium (Fig. 16.2). As opposed to other causes of perilymphatic nodules, a predominance of centrilobular nodules (Fig. 16.3) may

be present. Lung involvement is usually bilateral and symmetrical. The nodules are usually of soft tissue attenuation, are well defined, and may calcify.

Hilar and mediastinal lymphadenopathy may also be present (Fig. 16.4). Similar to

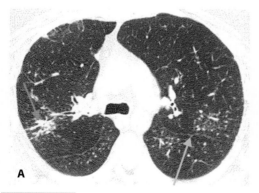

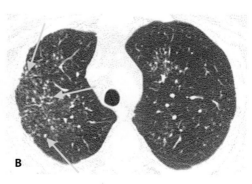

Figure 16.3

Perilymphatic nodules in silicosis. A. A perilymphatic distribution of nodules is present, with nodules seen in the peribronchovascular (*red arrow*) and subpleural regions (*blue arrow*). **B.** A number of centrilobular nodules (region delineated by *yellow arrows*) are present, reflecting the inhaled nature of the disease.

16

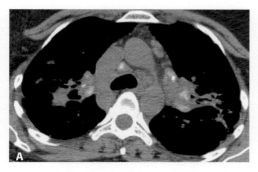

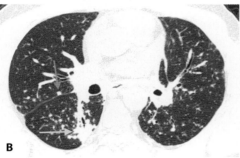

Figure 16.4

Lymphadenopathy in silicosis. Symmetric mediastinal and hilar lymphadenopathy with calcification is present **(A)** indistinguishable from that seen in sarcoidosis. Lung window **(B)** shows peribronchovascular (*yellow arrow*) and subpleural nodules (*red arrow*).

sarcoidosis, the distribution of adenopathy is usually symmetric. Calcification of nodes may be present and may be diffuse or have a so called eggshell pattern, involving the periphery of the node.

Some patients with chronic exposure develop progressive fibrosis, termed *complicated silicosis*. Fibrosis may be seen in association with perilymphatic nodules (Fig. 16.5) or as an isolated abnormality. Fibrosis is manifested by irregular reticulation and traction bronchiectasis with an upper lobe and peribronchovascular distribution. Confluent areas of fibrosis may produce consolidation with architectural distortion and traction bronchiectasis (Fig. 16.6). This is termed *PMF*. Pneumoconioses progress to PMF more commonly than sarcoidosis.

Acute exposure to large amounts of silica dust can result in a clinical syndrome and HRCT appearance that is markedly different from classic silicosis. In these cases, the exposure results in alveolar filling that closely resembles pulmonary alveolar proteinosis (PAP), both pathologically and on HRCT. This is termed *acute silicosis* or *silicoproteinosis*. The HRCT manifestations include extensive or diffuse bilateral ground glass opacity and consolidation. The combination of ground glass opacity and interlobular septal thickening in the same lung regions (i.e., crazy paving) is typical and indistinguishable from other causes of PAP (Fig. 16.7). Centrilobular nodules may also be seen, reflecting the inhaled nature of this disease.

Differential Diagnosis of a Silicosis Pattern

Other pneumoconioses that may show HRCT abnormalities similar to those of silicosis include coal worker's pneumoconiosis (CWP), talcosis, and berylliosis (Fig. 16.8). Rare pneumoconioses that may demonstrate a pattern similar to that of silicosis include those associated with rare earth and cerium.

Figure 16.5

Silicosis with perilymphatic nodules and fibrosis. HRCT through the upper lobes shows fibrosis with architectural distortion, volume loss, and traction bronchiectasis. Nodules are also present. Note the clustered peribronchovascular (*yellow arrow*), subpleural (*red arrow*), and centrilobular (*blue arrow*) nodules.

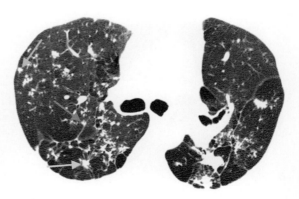

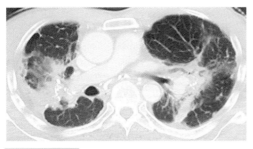

Figure 16.6

Progressive massive fibrosis, silicosis. Large mass-like conglomerates of central fibrosis are present, associated with architectural distortion and bronchiectasis. This appearance is most characteristic of silicosis, but can be seen with other pneumoconioses and sarcoidosis.

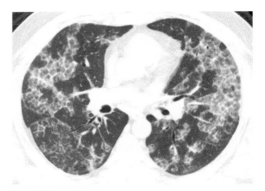

Figure 16.7

Silicoproteinosis. After an acute exposure to large amounts of silica dust, this patient presented with dyspnea and cough. HRCT showed a combination of ground glass opacity and interlobular septal thickening in the same lung regions. This "crazy paving" pattern is identical to that seen with alveolar proteinosis.

Exposure history is more important than HRCT findings in differentiating these causes of lung abnormalities.

Coal Worker's Pneumoconiosis

CWP exposure occurs in patients with an appropriate mining history. The nodules of CWP may be more ill-defined than those of silicosis, and calcification tends to be less common and central in location. Eggshell calcification is unusual in CWP. Fibrosis is less severe with CWP than with complicated silicosis, but conglomerate masses may be seen.

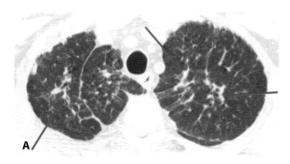

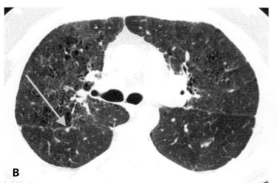

Figure 16.8

Fibrosis in berylliosis. Upper lobe predominant irregular reticulation is present in a central, peribronchovascular distribution (*arrows*, **A**). Minimal nodularity is present, predominantly in the subpleural interstitium (*arrow*, **B**).

16

Talcosis

Talcosis is acquired through high-risk occupations such as the production of textiles, paper, and rubber. Talc is commonly mixed with other dusts such as silica and asbestos, thus a mix of different patterns may be present. Inhaled talcosis, which resembles silicosis, should be distinguished from the intravenous injection of talc, which has a distinct appearance and is discussed in Chapter 7.

Berylliosis

Berylliosis is acquired in the aerospace and ceramic industries in addition to nuclear weapons production. Berylliosis is radiographically and pathologically identical to sarcoidosis (Fig. 16.8). The distinction between these two diseases may be made using a lymphocyte proliferation test that examines the sensitivity of plasma lymphocytes for beryllium.

Complications of Silicosis

Patients with silicosis and other pneumoconioses have an increased risk of developing tuberculosis. The diagnosis of tuberculosis may be challenging because both diseases may produce nodules, consolidation, and fibrosis. The presence of cavitation with a mass of PMF should raise the possibility of tuberculosis (Fig. 16.9), although occasionally, silicosis by itself may result in necrosis of fibrotic masses.

Primary bronchogenic carcinoma has an increased incidence in patients with silicosis. It may be difficult to differentiate areas of PMF from malignancy. Positron emission

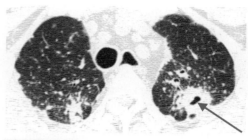

Figure 16.9

Silicosis with cavitation. Cavitation (*arrow*) in a patient with a known silicosis should raise the possibility of infection, particularly tuberculosis, to which these patients are predisposed. Rarely cavitation can be seen in uncomplicated pneumoconioses without evidence of infection. Note typical nodules with a perilymphatic distribution.

tomography or magnetic resonance imaging may be helpful in making this distinction.

Asbestosis and an "Asbestosis Pattern"

Asbestos (Table 16.2) exposure occurs in occupations such as mining, shipbuilding, construction, textiles manufacturing, manufacture of brake linings, and exposure to insulation materials containing asbestos. This exposure may result in various abnormalities, including pleural disease, interstitial lung disease, and malignancy.

HRCT Findings

The earliest manifestation of asbestos exposure may be a pleural effusion. This may be unilateral or bilateral. Effusions are commonly exudative

Table 16.2	Features of asbestosis and an "asbestosis pattern"
HRCT findings	Honeycombing with a usual interstitial pneumonia pattern Other signs of fibrosis (irregular reticulation, traction bronchiectasis) Subpleural and basilar distribution 90% associated with typical pleural disease (plaques, calcification)
Other pneumoconioses with similar findings	Mixed dust pneumoconiosis containing asbestos Lung disease indistinguishable from other causes of usual interstitial pneumonia (idiopathic pulmonary fibrosis, connective tissue disease, drug toxicity)
Complications	Bronchogenic carcinoma Mesothelioma

16

and thus pleural thickening, enhancement, and loculation may be associated. Effusions resolve spontaneously.

Pleural plaques are a characteristic feature of asbestos exposure, occurring after a latent period of many years. Plaques represent focal areas of pleural thickening that are variable in size, but often 1 to 2 cm in diameter. The edges of plaques are often elevated, as opposed to the tapered thickening that occurs at the edges of other benign causes of pleural thickening. Plaques commonly calcify, but even when they are not calcified, they are often high in attenuation because of the mineral they contain. Diffuse pleural thickening is an uncommon finding in patients with asbestos exposure, but may be seen.

Asbestosis is the interstitial lung disease associated with asbestos exposure. It is predominantly fibrotic. A peripheral and basilar distribution of fibrosis is typical (Fig. 16.10), while other pneumoconioses are usually upper lobe predominant.

HRCT abnormalities common in asbestosis result in a usual interstitial pneumonia (UIP) pattern (see Chapter 9). These include irregular reticulation, traction bronchiectasis, and honeycombing occurring in the peripheral, posterior, and subpleural lung, typically the lower lobes. The costophrenic angles are usually involved. An absence of ground glass opacity, nodules, and mosaic perfusion/air trapping is characteristic. Rarely, small ill-defined centrilobular nodules are seen in the peripheral lung (Fig. 16.11); these tend to be

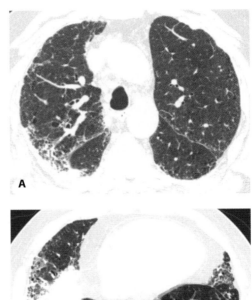

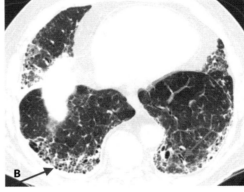

Figure 16.10

Asbestosis. A and **B.** Peripheral and basilar predominant fibrosis is present, with mild honeycombing **(B,** *blue arrow***)**, irregular reticulation, and traction bronchiectasis **(B,** *red arrow***)**. This pattern is indistinguishable in most cases from idiopathic pulmonary fibrosis.

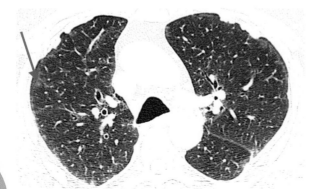

Figure 16.11

Asbestosis. Peripheral ground glass is seen in a patient with early, biopsy-proven, asbestosis. Note ground glass opacity centrilobular nodules *(arrow)* in the peripheral lung. Centrilobular arteries are seen to be associated with some of these nodules.

seen in early disease and reflect the presence of peribronchiolar fibrosis.

Differential Diagnosis of an Asbestosis Pattern

The HRCT pattern of lung disease present with asbestosis is nearly indistinguishable from other causes of UIP. As approximately 90% of patients with asbestosis demonstrate pleural plaques on CT, this may be a helpful distinguishing feature (Fig. 16.12). Otherwise, exposure history is most helpful in making the distinction between asbestosis and the other causes of UIP, such as IPF.

Small centrilobular nodules in the peripheral lung have been described as a differentiating feature of asbestosis, but these are only

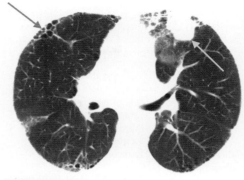

Figure 16.13

Malignancy in asbestosis. Peripheral honeycombing (*red arrow*) is present in a patient with asbestosis complicated by a lung cancer (*yellow arrow*).

seen rarely. Longitudinal evaluation of the progression of lung disease may also be helpful in distinguishing asbestosis from IPF. IPF often shows progression of lung abnormalities over a period of several years, but asbestosis may show long-term stability.

Complications

Of the pneumoconioses, asbestosis is associated with the highest risk of malignancy (Fig. 16.13). Because of the lung distortion associated with fibrosis, malignancies often have an atypical appearance; they may be ill-defined or may mimic consolidation.

Also, *rounded atelectasis* may complicate the diagnosis of bronchogenic carcinoma in patients with asbestos exposure. Rounded atelectasis is common in asbestos exposure because of pleural thickening. It is seen in the peripheral lung, is associated and in contact with adjacent pleural thickening, and is associated with volume loss.

Asbestos exposure also places a patient at risk for mesothelioma. It may be difficult to distinguish mesothelioma from the benign pleural abnormalities associated with asbestos exposure. Features to suggest malignant pleural disease include pleural thickening >1 cm, significant mediastinal pleural involvement, concentric pleural thickening, and development of a pleural effusion.

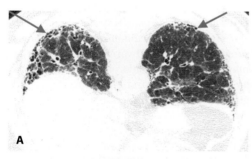

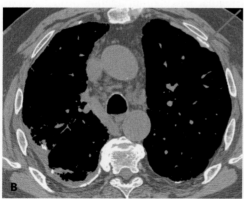

Figure 16.12

Asbestosis. A. Prone HRCT shows a typical pattern of usual interstitial pneumonia (UIP) with peripheral areas of honeycombing (*arrows*). **B.** The lung fibrosis is associated with pleural plaques, some of which are calcified (*arrow*). This combination indicates asbestosis as the likely cause of the UIP pattern.

16

Table 16.3	Features of siderosis and a "siderosis pattern"
HRCT findings	Centrilobular nodules of ground glass opacity Ground glass opacity Mild mosaic perfusion/air trapping Fibrosis is rare except with a mixed dust exposure
Other dusts with similar findings	Baritosis Stannosis Hard metal pneumoconiosis
Complications	Rare Primary bronchogenic carcinoma (mixed dust exposures)

Siderosis and a "Siderosis Pattern"

Siderosis (Table 16.3) is caused by inhalation of iron oxide, most commonly due to exposure during welding. Iron oxide is a material that, in general, does not elicit a significant granulomatous or inflammatory reaction. When inhaled, the dust is deposited around the small airways, but there is minimal associated immune reaction or fibrosis. Mixed dusts, particularly a combination of iron oxide and silica, may be inhaled. Mixed dusts may result in a mixed pattern.

HRCT Findings

Typical HRCT findings resemble subacute hypersensitivity pneumonitis and include centrilobular nodules of ground glass opacity (Fig. 16.14) or more generalized patchy ground glass opacity. Associated mosaic and perfusion air trapping may be present, but these tend to be mild in severity.

These abnormalities rarely progress to fibrosis. This primarily occurs in patients with a mixed dust exposure, including silica. In these cases, traction bronchiectasis, irregular reticulation, and PMF may be present. Cases in which fibrosis is present may closely resemble an interstitial pneumonia, particularly non-specific interstitial pneumonia or UIP.

Differential Diagnosis

Other rare pneumoconioses may closely resemble siderosis. These include *baritosis* (exposure to barium sulfate) and *stannosis* (exposure to tin oxide).

Hard metal pneumonconiosis, an alloy of tungsten, cobalt, and various other materials, may also resemble siderosis with centrilobular nodules of ground glass opacity, ground glass opacity, and mosaic perfusion/air trapping (Fig. 16.15). Hard metal pneumoconiosis more commonly progresses to fibrosis in patients with chronic exposure and may show irregular reticulation, traction bronchiectasis, and honeycombing.

The subacute type of hypersensitivity pneumonitis closely resembles siderosis and

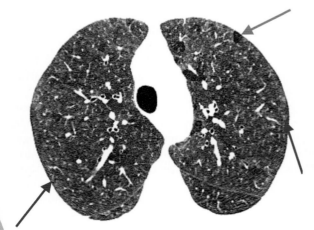

Figure 16.14

Siderosis. Centrilobular ground glass nodules (*blue arrows*), ground glass opacity, and minimal mosaic perfusion (*red arrow*) are typical manifestations of siderosis and other pneumoconioses that do not elicit a prominent fibrotic reaction.

16

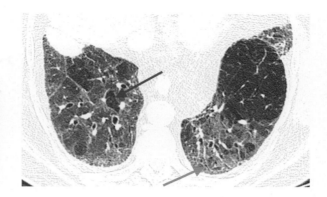

Figure 16.15

Hard metal pneumoconiosis. Patchy ground glass opacity is present at the lung bases and associated with patchy mosaic perfusion (*blue arrow*). There is also mild fibrosis in the posterior peripheral lung regions with irregular reticulation and traction bronchiectasis (*red arrow*).

its mimics. There are likely no accurate distinguishing HRCT features, and exposure history is paramount in differentiating these two entities. The air trapping in siderosis tends not to be as severe as in certain patients with hypersensitivity pneumonitis. Other causes of chronic centrilobular nodules of ground glass opacity include respiratory bronchiolitis and follicular bronchiolitis.

Complications

Complications from siderosis are rare, unless silica is also present, in which case malignancy can occur. Given its greater association with fibrosis, hard metal pneumonconiosis is more commonly complicated by bronchogenic carcinoma.

FURTHER READING

Aberle DR, Balmes JR. Computed tomography of asbestos-related pulmonary parenchymal and pleural diseases. *Clin Chest Med*. 1991;12:115-131.

Akira M. Uncommon pneumoconioses: CT and pathologic findings. *Radiology*. 1995;197:403-409.

Akira M. High-resolution CT in the evaluation of occupational and environmental disease. *Radiol Clin North Am*. 2002;40:43-59.

Akira M, Kozuka T, Yamamoto S, et al. Inhalational talc pneumoconiosis: radiographic and CT findings in 14 patients. *AJR Am J Roentgenol*. 2007;188:326-333.

Akira M, Yamamoto S, Yokoyama K, et al. Asbestosis: high-resolution CT-pathologic correlation. *Radiology*. 1990; 176:389-394.

Akira M, Yokoyama K, Yamamoto S, et al. Early asbestos: evaluation with high-resolution CT. *Radiology*. 1991;178:409-416.

Alper F, Akgun M, Onbas O, Araz O. CT findings in silicosis due to denim sandblasting. *Eur Radiol*. 2008;18: 2739-2744.

Antao VC, Pinheiro GA, Terra-Filho M, et al. High-resolution CT in silicosis: correlation with radiographic findings and functional impairment. *J Comput Assist Tomogr*. 2005;29:350-356.

Chong S, Lee KS, Chung MJ, et al. Pneumoconiosis: comparison of imaging and pathologic findings. *Radiographics*. 2006;26:59-77.

Copley SJ, Wells AU, Sivakumaran P, et al. Asbestosis and idiopathic pulmonary fibrosis: comparison of thin-section CT features. *Radiology*. 2003;229: 731-736.

Henry DA. International Labor Office Classification System in the age of imaging: relevant or redundant. *J Thorac Imaging*. 2002;17:179-188.

Kim KI, Kim CW, Lee MK, et al. Imaging of occupational lung disease. *Radiographics*. 2001;21:1371-1391.

Marchiori E, Souza CA, Barbassa TG, et al. Silicoproteinosis: high-resolution CT findings in 13 patients. *AJR Am J Roentgenol*. 2007;189:1402-1406.

Newman LS, Buschman DL, Newell JD, Lynch DL. Beryllium disease: assessment with CT. *Radiology*. 1994;190:835-840.

Remy-Jardin M, Degreef JM, Beuscart R, et al. Coal worker's pneumoconiosis: CT assessment in exposed workers and correlation with radiographic findings. *Radiology*. 1990;177:363-371.

Savranlar A, Altin R, Mahmutyazicioglu K, et al. Comparison of chest radiography and high-resolution computed tomography findings in early and low-grade coal worker's pneumoconiosis. *Eur J Radiol*. 2004;51:175-180.

Sette A, Neder JA, Nery LE, et al. Thin-section CT abnormalities and pulmonary gas exchange impairment in workers exposed to asbestos. *Radiology*. 2004;232:66-74.

Shida H, Chiyotani K, Honma K, et al. Radiologic and pathologic characteristics of mixed dust pneumoconiosis. *Radiographics*. 1996;16:483-498.

Silva CI, Müller NL, Neder JA, et al. Asbestos-related disease: progression of parenchymal abnormalities on high-resolution CT. *J Thorac Imaging*. 2008;23:251-257.

Ward S, Heyneman LE, Reittner P, et al. Talcosis associated with IV abuse of oral medications: CT findings. *AJR Am J Roentgenol*. 2000;174:789-793.

16

Neoplastic and Lymphoproliferative Diseases

Pulmonary neoplasm and lymphoproliferative disorders may present with diffuse lung abnormalities. The goal of this chapter is to discuss the various patterns of diffuse pulmonary neoplasm and lymphoproliferative disease and when these entities should be considered in the differential diagnosis.

PULMONARY MALIGNANCIES: MECHANISM OF SPREAD

Neoplasms may result in diffuse lung abnormalities by several different mechanisms (Table 17.1). These result in different appearances on HRCT.

Hematogenous Spread

Hematogenous spread of tumor to small pulmonary arteries is the most common mechanism by which malignancy results in diffuse lung involvement. The primary HRCT manifestation of hematogenous spread is randomly distributed pulmonary nodules (see Chapter 3) (Fig. 17.1).

Nodules involve the entire lung and have a diffuse and uniform distribution with involvement of pleural surfaces. The nodules may be lower lobe predominant because there is usually greater blood flow to this location. Nodules are usually of soft tissue attenuation and may range in size from a few millimeters in size, when first recognized, to many centimeters. The nodules tend to be similar in size.

The differential diagnosis includes other causes of random nodules, including miliary tuberculosis and miliary fungal infection.

Clinical history may be helpful in distinguishing infections from neoplasm. The size of nodules may be helpful when the clinical presentation is unclear. Large nodules are more likely to represent metastases than infection. Miliary infections uncommonly produce nodules larger than 5 mm.

Intravascular Metastases

In occasional patients, tumor embolism to pulmonary arteries results in intravascular metastases, tumor deposits that grow within the lumen of the artery. These may be seen with various neoplasms, but are most common with very vascular primary tumors (e.g., sarcomas) and tumors that result in invasion of large veins (e.g., hepatoma and renal cell carcinoma).

Intravascular metastases result in focally dilated, nodular, beaded, or lobulated pulmonary artery branches (Fig. 17.2). Intravascular filling defects may be visible if contrast agent is injected. This appearance may mimic pulmonary embolism, but smooth luminal filling defects, resembling thrombotic pulmonary emboli, are rare as an isolated finding.

Lymphangitic Spread

Pulmonary lymphatics predominate in the parahilar peribronchovascular interstitium, centrilobular regions, interlobular septa, and subpleural interstitium. Tumors that spread via the lymphatics may demonstrate abnormalities associated with these structures, particularly the interlobular septa and peribronchovascular interstitium (Fig. 17.3).

Table 17.1	Mechanisms of spread of pulmonary malignancies
Type of spread	**HRCT finding(s)**
Hematogenous spread	Random distribution of nodules
Intravascular metastases	Dilated, nodular, unopacified pulmonary arterial branches
Lymphangitic spread	Smooth or nodular thickening of the interlobular septa or peribronchovascular interstitium
Endobronchial spread	Centrilobular nodules

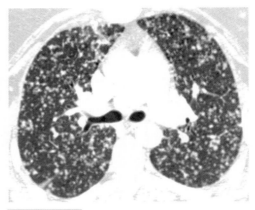

Figure 17.1

Hematogenous metastases. HRCT in a patient with metastatic medullary thyroid carcinoma shows diffuse nodules, less than 1 cm in diameter, with a random distribution. The random distribution reflects hematogenous spread of tumor to the lungs.

Thickening of these structures may be smooth or nodular.

The most common tumors to produce this pattern include lymphoma and cancers of the lung, breast, thyroid gland, stomach, pancreas, prostate, and head and neck. In many cases, lymphangitic spread occurs as a result of hematogenous dissemination to small vessels, with tumor invasion of the interstitium. Thus an overlap between the appearance of hematogenous spread and lymphangitic spread may be seen in some patients.

Interlobular septal thickening is the result of direct invasion of the pulmonary lymphatics and interstitium by a lung metastasis or primary tumor. Peribronchovascular interstitial thickening is most commonly seen in patients with mediastinal metastases that spread peripherally via lymphatics.

The differential diagnosis of nodular interlobular septal and peribronchovascular interstitial thickening includes other causes of perilymphatic disease including sarcoidosis, pneumoconioses, amyloidosis, and lymphoid interstitial pneumonia (LIP). When smooth thickening of these structures is present, the

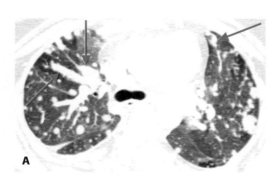

A

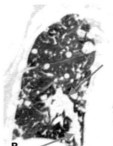

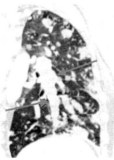

B

Figure 17.2

Intravascular metastases in chondrosarcoma. A. Dilated tubular, branching pulmonary arteries (*arrows*) are visible in the central and peripheral lung. These represent pulmonary arterial branches whose lumens are filled with tumor. Multiple nodular metastases are also visible. **B.** Coronal reformatted image shows the irregularly dilated arteries supplying the lower lobes (*arrows*). This reflects the presence of extensive intravascular tumor emboli (*arrows*).

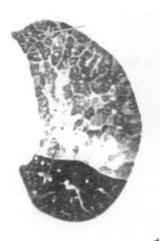

Figure 17.3

Lymphangitic metastases. Focal smooth interlobular septal thickening is noted in the left upper lobe in a patient with lung cancer. Note the polygonal lobules outlined by the thickened septa. Centrilobular arteries are visible in their centers (*yellow arrow*). Central peribronchovascular interstitial thickening is also present (*red arrow*).

primary differential consideration is pulmonary edema.

Endobronchial Spread

Endobronchial spread of tumor is rare with extrathoracic malignancies. It is more commonly seen with primary bronchogenic carcinomas, particularly invasive mucinous adenocarcinoma or squamous cell carcinoma. Endobronchial spread of tumor may closely resemble bronchopneumonia with airway impaction and centrilobular nodules. Consolidation or ground glass opacity may be due to atelectasis or post-obstructive pneumonitis (Fig. 17.4A, B). The most common extrathoracic primaries to show endobronchial spread include melanoma, breast, renal, pancreatic, and colon cancers. Tracheobronchial papillomatosis is associated with infection by the human papilloma virus. Papillomas involving the larynx may spread via the airways to involve the trachea, bronchi, and lung parenchyma. Squamous cell carcinoma may result. HRCT may show cysts, nodules, cavitary nodules, and endobronchial lesions (Fig. 17.4C). Papillomas may be seen within cysts.

INVASIVE MUCINOUS PULMONARY ADENOCARCINOMA

Invasive mucinous adenocarcinoma (formerly diffuse bronchioloalveolar carcinoma or BAC) is a subtype of pulmonary adenocarcinoma, characterized by endobronchial spread and diffuse or multifocal lung involvement. The nonmucinous subtype of adenocarcinoma is much less likely to result in this type of dissemination; it more frequently appears as a solitary nodule, often of ground glass opacity.

The HRCT findings of invasive mucinous adenocarcinoma often resemble lobar pneumonia or bronchopneumonia. Consolidation and ground glass are the most frequent abnormalities; these abnormalities often result from filling of alveoli by mucin or fluid secreted by the tumor. The tumor itself is characterized by *lepidic growth*, or growth along alveolar walls, without filling or replacement of the alveolar spaces.

Abnormalities may be focal, patchy, or diffuse (Fig. 17.5). The distribution may be unilateral, bilateral, asymmetric, or symmetric. When intravenous contrast is administered, the vessels with areas of consolidation may appear dense compared with the low-density consolidation. This is called the *CT angiogram sign* and is common with invasive mucinous adenocarcinomas. However, this sign may be seen in many causes of consolidation and not specific for this diagnosis.

Centrilobular nodules may also be present, reflecting endobronchial spread of tumor (Fig. 17.6). Similar to bronchopneumonia, the nodules are often heterogeneous in size, with variable spread into the alveoli surrounding the centrilobular bronchiole. Nodules are most commonly of soft tissue attenuation, but ground glass opacity nodules may also be seen.

Interlobular septal thickening may be present and is typically seen in areas of ground glass opacity. This combination is termed *crazy paving*, and while classically associated with pulmonary alveolar proteinosis, it may be seen with a variety of other acute and chronic lung diseases.

The differential diagnosis of invasive mucinous adenocarcinoma includes infections with endobronchial spread. However, the clinical presentations of these two entities are quite different; pneumonia presents with acute

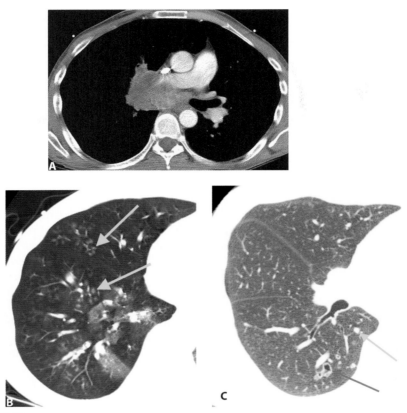

Figure 17.4

Endobronchial spread of tumor in two patients. A and B. A large central squamous cell carcinoma causes obstruction of the bronchus intermedius. **B.** In the same patient as **(A)**, patchy centrilobular nodules are present in the right middle and lower lobes distal to this obstruction (*arrows*). These could represent post-obstructive bronchial impaction or tumor. Pathologically, there was endobronchial spread of tumor in these regions. **C.** In a patient with tracheobronchial papillomatosis, HRCT shows nodules (*yellow arrow*) and a thick-walled cavitary nodule or cyst (*red arrow*).

symptoms and mucinous adenocarcinoma presents with chronic symptoms, usually of greater than 3 months duration. Invasive mucinous adenocarcinoma may be associated with *bronchorrhea*, the production of liters of watery sputum each day.

In patients presenting with chronic symptoms, the differential diagnosis of invasive mucinous adenocarcinoma includes other causes of chronic consolidation and ground glass opacity, such as organizing pneumonia, chronic eosinophilic pneumonia, sarcoidosis, lymphoma, lipoid pneumonia, and alveolar proteinosis. Centrilobular nodules are rare

with these diseases and relatively common with invasive mucinous adenocarcinoma, although organizing pneumonia and sarcoidosis may rarely have associated centrilobular nodules as a prominent finding. When centrilobular nodules are absent, the various causes of chronic consolidation may be difficult to distinguish from one another.

KAPOSI'S SARCOMA

Kaposi's sarcoma (KS) is a malignancy originally described in elderly men of Mediterranean descent, but is most frequently seen in patients

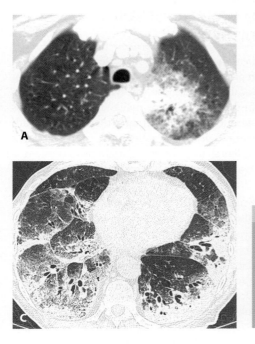

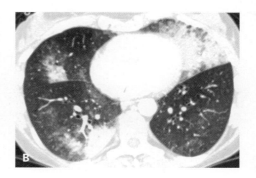

Figure 17.5

Invasive mucinous adenocarcinoma (IMA) in two patients. IMA may present with consolidation or ground glass opacity (GGO) that is focal **(A),** patchy, or bilateral **(B)**. In another patient **(C),** IMA appears extensive and diffuse. These appearances may resemble a variety of other diseases, and IMA should always be considered in the setting of chronic consolidation and GGO.

with human immunodeficiency virus (HIV) infection. Pulmonary involvement is seen in up to 50% of HIV patients with KS, but its incidence has significantly declined after the development of highly active antiretroviral therapy.

The earliest HRCT manifestation of KS is thickening of the peribronchovascular interstitium (Fig. 17.7). A later and more suggestive feature of KS is large (more than 1 cm), irregular, flame-shaped nodules (Fig. 17.8). These typically have a peribroncho-vascular distribution. Other findings include interlobular septal thickening, pleural effu-sions, and mediastinal lymphadenopathy.

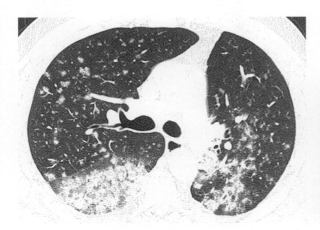

Figure 17.6

Invasive mucinous adenocarcinoma with centrilobular nodules. Patchy, bilateral centrilobular nodules are present, most of which are of soft tissue attenuation. This reflects endobronchial spread of tumor. A more confluent region of lobular consolidation is seen in the right lower lobe reflecting extensive tumor spread.

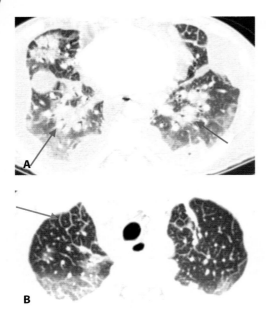

Figure 17.7

Kaposi's sarcoma. A. Extensive peribronchovascular soft tissue thickening (*arrows*) is noted in the lower lobes, reflecting interstitial spread of tumor. **B.** In the upper lobes, interlobular septal thickening (*arrow*) is seen. This could be due to tumor infiltration or lymphatic obstruction.

LYMPHOMA AND LYMPHOPROLIFERATIVE DISORDERS

Lymphoproliferative disorders of the lung represent a spectrum of diseases from benign localized collection of lymphocytes to diffuse proliferation of malignant cells. There is significant overlap among these entities both pathologically and radiographically. These disorders share a common origin from bronchus-associated lymphoid tissue.

Focal Lymphoid Hyperplasia

Also known as pseudolymphoma, focal lymphoid hyperplasia represents a localized collection of non-neoplastic lymphocytes and other immune cells. This rare disorder usually presents with a solitary nodule or focal area of consolidation. Occasionally, multiple nodules or areas of consolidation may be seen (Fig. 17.9).

When presenting as a solitary nodule, focal lymphoid hyperplasia is indistinguishable from primary bronchogenic carcinoma, metastasis, granulomas, hamartomas, or other causes of solitary nodules. When presenting as a focal area of consolidation, the differential often includes adenocarcinoma and other causes of chronic consolidation.

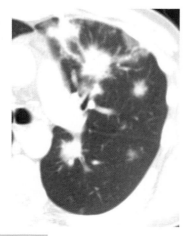

Figure 17.8

Kaposi's sarcoma. Nodules of varying sizes are noted in the left lung. These are peribronchovascular and subpleural in distribution, and their irregular borders result in a characteristic flame shape.

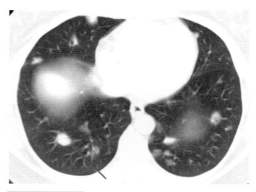

Figure 17.9

Focal lymphoid hyperplasia. Multiple nodules are seen bilaterally, some of which are solid and some of which are of ground glass opacity. Note an air bronchogram in one of the right lower lobe nodules (*arrow*). Lymphoid hyperplasia was confirmed on surgical pathology.

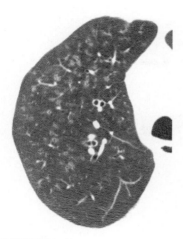

Figure 17.10

Follicular bronchiolitis. Centrilobular nodules of ground glass opacity are seen in this patient with follicular bronchiolitis. The centrilobular distribution of nodules reflects the pathologic correlate of lymphoid follicles around the small airways.

LIP and Follicular Bronchiolitis

LIP and follicular bronchiolitis (FB) are benign lymphoproliferative disorders characterized pathologically by lymphoid follicles predominantly within the interstitium, in the case of LIP, or around the small airways, in the case of FB. They show significant clinical, pathologic, and radiographic overlap and are thought to represent a spectrum of the same disease. They were originally thought to represent a premalignant condition, with some patients progressing to lymphoma, but these cases were likely misclassified, and currently LIP and FB are thought to represent non-neoplastic processes.

LIP and FB are frequently associated with either immunocompromised states or connective tissue disease. The most common diseases to lead to these patterns include HIV infection, common variable immunodeficiency, and Sjögren's syndrome. A history of an associated disease is vital in making this diagnosis, as LIP and FB are rare entities and show features that overlap with other, more common, disorders.

The most typical HRCT finding in FB is centrilobular nodules of ground glass opacity (Fig. 17.10). These nodules are indistinguishable from the nodules seen in hypersensitivity pneumonitis, respiratory bronchiolitis, and atypical infections. Rarely, FB presents with tree-in-bud opacities resembling infection. Mild mosaic perfusion and/or air trapping may be present (Fig. 17.11), but this is rarely as severe as that seen in hypersensitivity pneumonitis.

The findings of LIP are more variable. Ground glass opacity and/or consolidation may be present and is often bilateral and patchy in nature (Fig. 17.12). These are both nonspecific findings. Pulmonary nodules may also be seen. In distinction to FB, these are usually well defined and have a perilymphatic distribution (Fig. 17.13) resembling sarcoidosis, lymphangitic spread of malignancy, silicosis, or amyloidosis. Cysts may be seen in association with any of these abnormalities (Fig. 17.14) or may be an isolated finding. Sjögren's syndrome and collagen vascular disease, in particular, may present with cysts as the only abnormality (Fig. 17.15).

The manifestations of LIP and FB (Table 17.2) reflect a spectrum of abnormalities in this disease; an overlap of findings may be present (Fig. 17.16). For instance, there may be centrilobular nodules with more diffuse patchy ground glass opacity. Regardless, this diagnosis is not usually considered unless there is an appropriate clinical history.

Secondary Pulmonary Lymphoma

Most cases of lymphoma with lung involvement are secondary. In other words, the lymphoma is diffuse or predominantly extrathoracic, and lung involvement is a component of that disease. The cardinal finding of lymphoma is lymphadenopathy.

Lung involvement, while uncommon, is well described and may resemble a variety of focal and diffuse lung diseases. Involvement of the lung is much more common with recurrent lymphoma. This is particularly true in patients with Hodgkin's disease, which only rarely shows lung involvement at initial presentation.

The most common finding of pulmonary involvement by lymphoma is nodules that are often larger than 1 cm in size (Fig. 17.17)

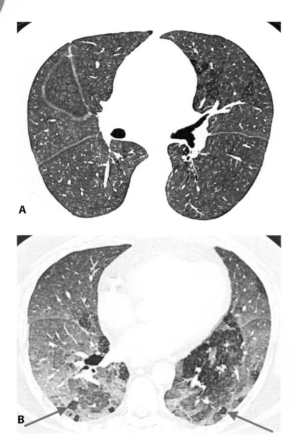

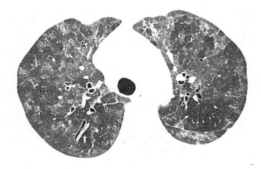

Figure 17.11

Follicular bronchiolitis. A combination of centrilobular nodules of ground glass opacity (**A**) and air trapping (*red arrows* in **B**) is present in a patient with connective tissue disease. Note the sparing of the subpleural lung by the nodules in **A**.

Figure 17.12

Lymphoid interstitial pneumonia (LIP). Nonspecific patchy bilateral ground glass opacity is present in a patient with connective tissue disease (CTD). In the presence of chronic symptoms, the differential diagnosis of this pattern in a patient with CTD is limited and includes LIP and an atypical distribution of nonspecific interstitial pneumonia. This represented LIP.

and typically ill-defined (Fig. 17.18). Nodules less than 1 cm may also be seen, but a pattern resembling miliary spread of disease is rare. Consolidation is also a relatively common pattern (Fig. 17.18). The consolidation may or may not appear mass-like. Air bronchograms may be present within nodules or masses.

In the setting of known lymphoma, the primary differential diagnosis of consolidation includes infections (particularly fungal infection) and drug reaction presenting with an organizing pneumonia pattern.

Primary Pulmonary Lymphoma

Primary pulmonary lymphoma, in which lung involvement is the principle manifestation of disease, is rare. Several criteria must be met for a case to qualify as primary pulmonary lymphoma: no history of lymphoma, lack of mediastinal lymphadenopathy on chest radiographs,

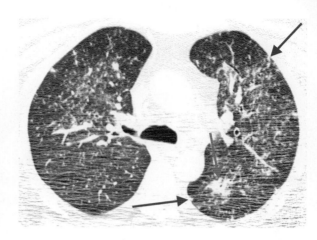

Figure 17.13

Lymphoid interstitial pneumonia. Tiny nodules are present in a patient with human immunodeficiency virus infection and chronic, progressive symptoms. The perilymphatic distribution of these nodules is evidenced by their patchy nature and the presence of subpleural (*blue arrows*) and peribronchovascular (*red arrow*) nodules.

and absent extrathoracic disease initially and for 3 months after presentation. Low-grade tumors are significantly more common than high-grade tumors, thus slow growth is most characteristic of primary lymphoma.

The HRCT findings include single or multiple nodules, masses, and regions of consolidation (Fig. 17.19). Multifocal disease is more common than a solitary abnormality. When nodules are present, they tend to be larger (>2 cm) than benign causes of pulmonary nodules

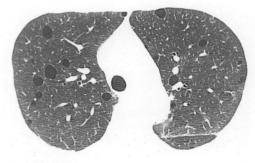

Figure 17.15

Lymphoid interstitial pneumonia. Cysts are usually seen as an isolated finding. This is a common manifestation of lymphoid interstitial pneumonia in the setting of Sjögren's syndrome.

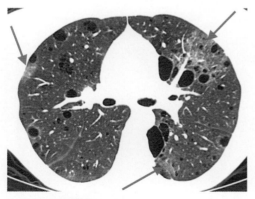

Figure 17.14

Lymphoid interstitial pneumonia (LIP). A combination of cysts and patchy ground glass opacity (arrows) is present in a patient with Sjögren's syndrome. While the ground glass opacity is nonspecific, its association with cysts in a patient with connective tissue disease is strongly suggestive of LIP.

Table 17.2	HRCT findings of lymphoid interstitial pneumonia and follicular bronchiolitis
Follicular bronchiolitis	Centrilobular nodules of ground glass opacity Mild mosaic perfusion and air trapping
Lymphoid interstitial pneumonia	Patchy bilateral ground glass opacity and consolidation Perilymphatic nodules Cysts

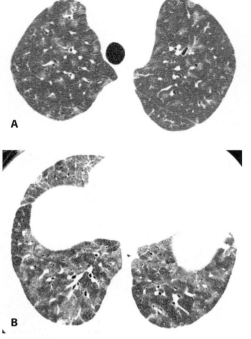

A

B

Figure 17.16

Follicular bronchiolitis/lymphoid interstitial pneumonia. As these two entities are considered a spectrum of the same disease, an overlap of HRCT findings may be present. This patient with common variable immunodeficiency shows a combination of centrilobular nodules of ground glass attenuation in the upper lobes (**A**) and more generalized ground glass opacity in the lower lobes (**B**).

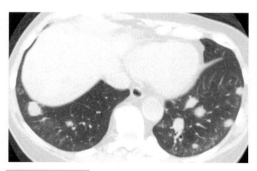

Figure 17.17

Lymphoma with nodules. Scattered, bilateral mass-like regions of nodular consolidation are present in a patient with recurrent lymphoma after treatment. This is a typical appearance of lymphoma involving the lungs.

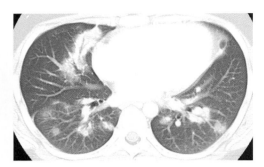

Figure 17.18

Lymphoma with ill-defined nodules and consolidation. Ill-defined nodules and patchy mass-like consolidations with air bronchograms are present in a patient with previously treated lymphoma. This appearance is most typical of recurrent secondary lymphoma.

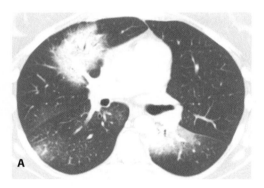

A

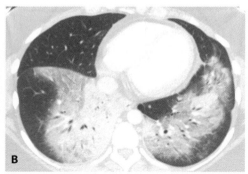

B

Figure 17.19

Primary pulmonary lymphoma. A and B. Patchy bilateral consolidation and ground glass opacity, stable for nearly 2 years, are present. Biopsy showed low-grade B-cell lymphoma. Chronic consolidation as a manifestation of lymphoma is most commonly seen with recurrent disease, but may occasionally be the presenting abnormality.

such as hamartomas or granulomas. Air bronchograms within nodules or consolidation are common. Abnormalities are often peribronchovascular in distribution.

Slow growth over months to years is most typical of primary pulmonary lymphoma. Because of this slow growth, the differential diagnosis of primary pulmonary lymphoma includes slowly growing tumors such as well-differentiated adenocarcinoma and carcinoid tumors, in addition to chronic causes of consolidation such as invasive mucinous adenocarcinoma and lipoid pneumonia.

Lymphomatoid Granulomatosis

The exact nature of lymphomatoid granulomatosis is not clear, but it is likely that the vast majority of cases represent malignant lymphoma. It is unique because of its strong angiocentric nature, sharing features with vasculitis. The lungs are involved in nearly all cases, but the disease may be systemic with additional organs involved, including the skin, nervous system, and other organs.

HRCT shows nodules that are variable in size, but may be quite large (Fig. 17.20). These nodules often have a peribronchovascular distribution and cavitation is common. Reticular opacities associated with these nodules may also be present.

Post-Transplant Lymphoproliferative Disorders

Post-transplant lymphoproliferative disorders (PTLD) may occur with solid organ or bone marrow transplantation. PTLD represents a spectrum of disease from benign proliferation of non-neoplastic lymphocytes to malignant lymphoma. Development of PTLD is closely correlated with Epstein-Barr viral infection. In general, the likelihood of developing PTLD is associated with the severity of immunosuppression, but this may be impacted by chronic antiviral therapy. Presentation within 1 year of transplantation is most typical.

The HRCT findings of PTLD resemble primary or secondary pulmonary lymphoma. Single or multiple pulmonary nodules, masses, or areas of consolidation may be present. These are often associated with mediastinal and/or hilar lymphadenopathy (Fig. 17.21). In transplant patients, the differential diagnosis predominantly includes infections,

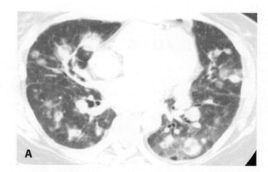

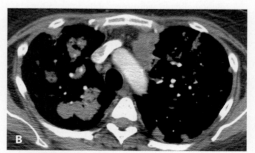

Figure 17.21

Post-transplant lymphoproliferative disorder. Multiple nodules and masses are seen bilaterally **(A)** in this patient with a history of renal transplantation. **B.** These findings are associated with mediastinal lymphadenopathy.

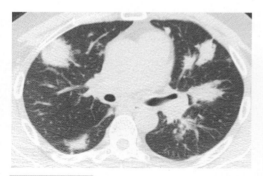

Figure 17.20

Lymphomatoid granulomatosis. Large, irregular nodules are seen bilaterally in a patient with lymphomatoid granulomatosis. This is a typical manifestation of this rare disease, but there are many other more common causes in the setting of chronic symptoms, including tumor, organizing pneumonia, eosinophilic pneumonia, and sarcoidosis.

particularly fungal infection. Organizing pneumonia from drugs or graft versus host disease may also closely resemble PTLD.

LEUKEMIA

Lung abnormalities in patients with leukemia are not uncommon, but many are due to non-neoplastic diseases such as pneumonia, drug reaction, edema, or hemorrhage. Leukemic infiltration occurs in approximately 15% of patients with significant HRCT abnormalities.

On HRCT, leukemic lung infiltration often shows lymphatic dissemination. Thus, thickening of the interlobular septa and peribronchovascular interstitium are common. Small nodules may also be present and are typically perilymphatic or random in distribution. The presence of centrilobular nodules favors a non-neoplastic cause, such as pneumonia. Ground glass opacity and consolidation are uncommon findings of leukemic infiltration and more likely represent pneumonia, diffuse alveolar damage, edema, or hemorrhage.

FURTHER READING

Akira M, Atagi S, Kawahara M, Iuchi K, Johkoh T. High-resolution CT findings of diffuse bronchioloalveolar carcinoma in 38 patients. *AJR Am J Roentgenol*. 1999;173:1623-1629.

Aquino S. Imaging of metastatic disease to the thorax. *Radiol Clin North Am*. 2005;43:481-495.

Bae YA, Lee KS. Cross-sectional evaluation of thoracic lymphoma. *Radiol Clin North Am*. 2008;46:253-264.

Bragg DG, Chor PJ, Murray KA, Kjeldsberg CR. Lymphoproliferative disorders of the lung: histopathology, clinical manifestations, and imaging features. *AJR Am J Roentgenol*. 1994;163:273-281.

Carignan S, Staples CA, Müller NL. Intrathoracic lymphoproliferative disorders in the immunocompromised patient: CT findings. *Radiology*. 1995;197:53-58.

Collins J, Müller NL, Leung AN, et al. EpsteinBarr virus–associated lymphoproliferative disease of the lung: CT and histologic findings. *Radiology*. 1998;208:749-759.

Do KH, Lee JS, Seo JB, et al. Pulmonary parenchymal involvement of low-grade lymphoproliferative disorders. *J Comput Assist Tomogr*. 2005;29:825-830.

Dodd G, LedesmaMedina J, Baron RL, Fuhrman CR. Posttransplant lymphoproliferative disorder: intrathoracic manifestations. *Radiology*. 1992;184:65-69.

Eisner MD, Kaplan LD, Herndier B, Stulbarg MS. The pulmonary manifestations of AIDS related non Hodgkin's lymphoma. *Chest*. 1996;110:729-736.

Gibson M, Hansell DM. Lymphocytic disorders of the chest: pathology and imaging. *Clin Radiol*. 1998;53:469-480.

Gruden JF, Huang L, Webb WR, et al. AIDS-related Kaposi sarcoma of the lung: radiographic findings and staging system with bronchoscopic correlation. *Radiology*. 1995;195:545-552.

Hartman TE, Primack SL, Müller NL, Staples CA. Diagnosis of thoracic complications in AIDS: accuracy of CT. *AJR Am J Roentgenol*. 1994;162:547-553.

Heyneman LE, Johkoh T, Ward S, et al. Pulmonary leukemic infiltrates: high resolution CT findings in 10 patients. *AJR Am J Roentgenol*. 2000;174:517-521.

Howling SJ, Hansell DM, Wells AU, et al. Follicular bronchiolitis: thin-section CT and histologic findings. *Radiology*. 1999;212:637-642.

Johkoh T, Ikezoe J, Tomiyama N, et al. CT findings in lymphangitic carcinomatosis of the lung: correlation with histologic findings and pulmonary function tests. *AJR Am J Roentgenol*. 1992;158:1217-1222.

Johkoh T, Müller NL, Pickford HA, et al. Lymphocytic interstitial pneumonia: thin section CT findings in 22 patients. *Radiology*. 1999;212:567-572.

Knisely BL, Mastey LA, Mergo PJ, et al. Pulmonary mucosa-associated lymphoid tissue lymphoma: CT and pathologic findings. *AJR Am J Roentgenol*. 1999;172:1321-1326.

Lee DK, Im JG, Lee KS, et al. Bcell lymphoma of bronchus-associated lymphoid tissue (BALT): CT features in 10 patients. *J Comput Assist Tomogr*. 2000;24:30-34.

Lee KS, Kim Y, Primack SL. Imaging of pulmonary lymphomas. *AJR Am J Roentgenol*. 1997;168:339-345.

Lee WK, Duddalwar VA, Rouse HC, Lau EW, Bekhit E, Hennessy OF. Extranodal lymphoma in the thorax: cross-sectional imaging findings. *Clin Radiol*. 2009;64:542-549.

Lynch DA, Travis WD, Muller NL, et al. Idiopathic interstitial pneumonias: CT features. *Radiology*. 2005;236:10-21.

Munk PL, Müller NL, Miller RR, Ostrow DN. Pulmonary lymphangitic carcinomatosis: CT and pathologic findings. *Radiology*. 1988;166:705-709.

Naidich DP, Tarras M, Garay SM, et al. Kaposi sarcoma: CT radiographic correlation. *Chest*. 1989;96:723-728.

Okada F, Ando Y, Kondo Y, Matsumoto S, Maeda T, Mori H. Thoracic CT findings of adult T-cell leukemia or lymphoma. *AJR Am J Roentgenol*. 2004;182:761-767.

Rappaport DC, Chamberlain DW, Shepherd FA, Hutcheon MA. Lymphoproliferative disorders after lung transplantation: imaging features. *Radiology*. 1998;206:519-524.

Silva CI, Flint JD, Levy RD, Müller NL. Diffuse lung cysts in lymphoid interstitial pneumonia: high-resolution CT and pathologic findings. *J Thorac Imaging*. 2006;21:241-244.

Stein MG, Mayo J, Müller N, et al. Pulmonary lymphangitic spread of carcinoma: appearance on CT scans. *Radiology*. 1987;162:371-375.

Travis WD, Brambilla E, Noguchi M, et al. International Association for the Study of Lung Cancer/American Thoracic Society/European Respiratory Society International Multidisciplinary Classification of Lung Adenocarcinoma. *J Thorac Oncol*. 2011;6:244-285.

Travis WD, Garg K, Franklin WA, et al. Evolving concepts in the pathology and computed tomography imaging of lung adenocarcinoma and bronchioloalveolar carcinoma. *J Clin Oncol*. 2005;23:3279-3287.

18

Rare Diseases

PULMONARY ALVEOLAR PROTEINOSIS

Pulmonary alveolar proteinosis (PAP) is a rare disorder characterized pathologically by the accumulation of lipoprotein within alveoli.

There are three different forms of the disease. *Congenital PAP* results from mutations in genes encoding surfactant B or C or granulocyte–macrophage colony-stimulating factor (GM-CSF). *Secondary PAP* occurs in association with a wide variety of disorders, including acute silicosis (silicoproteinosis), infections, and hematologic and lymphatic malignancy. *Idiopathic PAP* accounts for nearly 90% of cases. It is an autoimmune disease in which antibodies to GM-CSF interfere with the degradation or clearance of surfactant.

Men with PAP outnumber women. Patients range in age from a few months to more than 70 years, with two-thirds of patients being between 30 and 50 years old. Symptoms are usually mild and of insidious onset. They include cough, fever, and mild dyspnea. About 30% of patients are asymptomatic.

HRCT abnormalities are typically diffuse, bilateral, and often symmetric (Table 18.1). The characteristic HRCT abnormality consists of geographic regions of ground glass opacity and smooth interlobular septal thickening in the same lung regions. This is termed the *crazy paving* pattern (Figs. 18.1 and 18.2). Consolidation or ill-defined nodules may also be present, but are not particularly common. The differential diagnosis of the *crazy paving* pattern in patients

with chronic symptoms is long and includes interstitial pneumonias, organizing pneumonia, eosinophilic pneumonia, hypersensitivity pneumonitis, lipoid pneumonia, and invasive mucinous adenocarcinoma.

HRCT may be used to monitor treatment (Fig. 18.2). Large volume bronchoalveolar lavage is used for treatment in an attempt to clear the proteinaceous material from the alveolar spaces. HRCT can help target appropriate regions of lung for bronchoalveolar lavage and to confirm successful treatment. With lavage, ground glass opacities improve or resolve. Septal thickening may sometimes persist (Fig. 18.2B).

LIPOID PNEUMONIA

Lipoid pneumonia reflects the accumulation of fats within the lung parenchyma. It may be endogenous or exogenous. Endogenous lipoid pneumonia is characterized by lipid-laden macrophages within consolidated lung distal to an obstructed airway. HRCT findings are those of a post-obstructive pneumonia.

Exogenous lipoid pneumonia is caused by the aspiration of fatty materials such as mineral oil. As a large amount of lipid needs to be aspirated over a long period of time, patients usually present with chronic symptomatology. Also, CT abnormalities may be incidentally discovered in asymptomatic patients.

The HRCT findings of exogenous lipoid pneumonia include ground glass opacity or consolidation that is patchy, focal, or mass-like

Table 18.1	HRCT findings of pulmonary alveolar proteinosis

Three forms: congenital, secondary, idiopathic (90% of cases)
Diffuse and bilateral
Patchy and geographic regions of GGO and crazy paving
Consolidation less common
GGO decreases with bronchoalveolar lavage

GGO, ground glass opacity.

(Table 18.2). A combination of ground glass opacity and interlobular septal thickening, the *crazy paving* pattern, is not uncommon. Soft tissue windows may show low-attenuation regions within areas of consolidation, with Hounsfield unit measurements consistent with fat (Fig. 18.3). Masses or regions of consolidation may be round or irregular in shape.

Findings are often most severe in the dependent lung regions, reflecting the typical distribution of aspiration. Associated fibrosis may be present, although this is usually not a significant component of disease.

AMYLOIDOSIS

Amyloidosis reflects the accumulation of an extracellular protein in multiple organs. The most commonly involved organs include the kidneys, heart, nervous system, and liver.

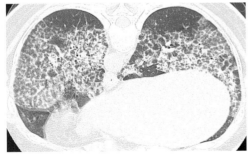

Figure 18.1

Pulmonary alveolar proteinosis. Prone HRCT shows a combination of ground glass opacity and interlobular septal thickening in the same lung regions, the *crazy paving* sign. In a patient with chronic symptoms, alveolar proteinosis is one of several diagnoses that can produce this pattern.

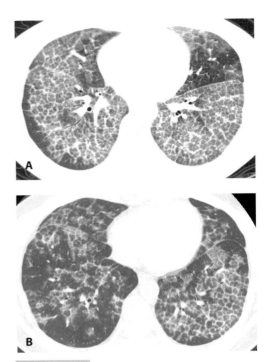

Figure 18.2

Pulmonary alveolar proteinosis, before and after treatment. A. Typical findings of alveolar proteinosis with crazy paving are present on pretreatment HRCT. **B.** After several treatments with large volume bronchoalveolar lavage, there has been significant improvement in the ground glass opacity and septal thickening.

There are two types of amyloid that may be deposited in the lungs, amyloid light chain and amyloid A chain. The former is responsible for the majority of patients with symptomatic lung involvement; it may be idiopathic or associated with myeloma or lymphoma. *A chain amyloidosis* is associated with rheumatoid arthritis, inflammatory bowel disease, chronic

Table 18.2	HRCT findings of lipoid pneumonia

Aspiration of fatty materials (exogenous lipoid pneumonia)
Patchy and dependent
Ground glass opacity or consolidation
Low-attenuation consolidation

18

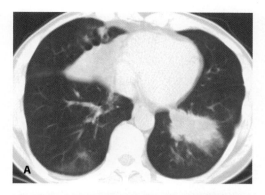

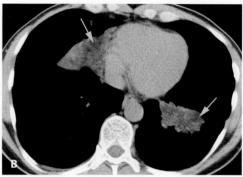

Figure 18.3

Lipoid pneumonia. A. Lung windows show focal regions of consolidation at both lung bases in a patient with chronic symptoms. This finding is nonspecific. **B.** The presence of low-attenuation fat (*arrows*) within regions of consolidation on the mediastinal windows strongly suggests the diagnosis of lipoid pneumonia.

Table 18.3 | HRCT findings of amyloidosis

Focal parenchymal amyloidosis

Single or multiple lung nodules, sometimes calcified

Diffuse parenchymal amyloidosis

Small nodules with a perilymphatic distribution, septal thickening
Consolidation, ground glass opacity, calcification, fibrosis

Tracheobronchial amyloidosis

Diffuse or focal thickening tracheal and bronchial walls
Calcification common

inflammatory disorders (e.g., osteomyelitis), and chronic pulmonary infections (e.g., tuberculosis) and rarely leads to symptoms.

Amyloidosis may involve the lung parenchyma or airways (Table 18.3). Lung parenchymal involvement may be focal or diffuse. Lymphadenopathy may be associated with any of the above patterns of amyloid or as an isolated abnormality. Calcification is often present in mediastinal or hilar lymph nodes.

Focal Parenchymal Amyloidosis

Focal parenchymal amyloidosis presents with a single or multiple discrete lung nodules or masses (Fig. 18.4). These may be calcified. They are difficult to differentiate from other causes of nodules such as primary bronchogenic

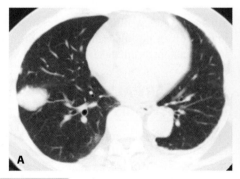
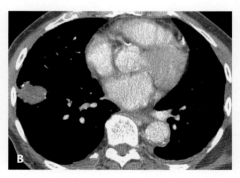

Figure 18.4

Amyloidosis, focal parenchymal. A. A nonspecific nodule is seen in the right lower lobe. **B.** On a soft tissue window, focal areas of calcification are visible within the nodule. Biopsy confirmed amyloidosis in this patient with rheumatoid arthritis.

carcinoma, metastases, granulomatous disease, or hamartoma. Associated airway wall thickening may be present in patients with focal parenchymal amyloid.

Diffuse Parenchymal Amyloidosis

Diffuse parenchymal amyloidosis typically presents with diffuse small (<1.5 cm) nodules. These are often calcified and may have a perilymphatic distribution (Fig. 18.5). Other causes of diffuse, small, calcified lung nodules include sarcoidosis, pneumoconioses such as silicosis, granulomatous infections such as tuberculosis, metastatic calcification, and alveolar microlithiasis. Less characteristic findings include diffuse lung infiltration with consolidation, ground glass opacity, interlobular septal thickening or intralobular interstitial thickening, extensive lung calcification, and fibrosis.

Tracheobronchial Amyloidosis

Involvement of the airways is characterized by diffuse or nodular thickening of the walls of the trachea and/or central bronchi (Fig. 18.6). Calcification may be present. The differential diagnosis of extensive tracheal or central bronchial wall thickening includes relapsing polychondritis, sarcoidosis, Wegener's granulomatosis, inflammatory bowel disease, and infections such as Aspergillosis.

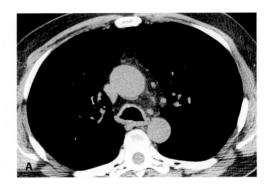
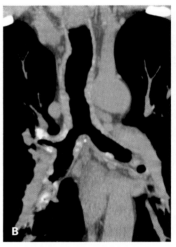

Figure 18.6

Amyloidosis, tracheobronchial. Axial **(A)** and coronal reformatted **(B)** images are shown in a patient with diffuse tracheal wall thickening and calcification from amyloidosis. There is also involvement of the central bronchi.

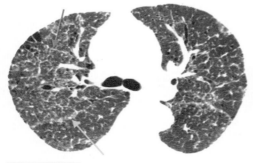

Figure 18.5

Amyloidosis, diffuse parenchymal. HRCT through the upper lobes demonstrates nodules with a perilymphatic distribution. The nodules are clustered along fissures (*yellow arrow*) and in interlobular septa (*red arrow*). Sarcoidosis is the most common cause of this pattern, but this patient was diagnosed with amyloidosis on surgical biopsy.

Tracheobronchopathia osteochondroplastica may result in nodular tracheal and bronchial wall thickening with calcification.

PULMONARY ALVEOLAR MICROLITHIASIS

Pulmonary alveolar microlithiasis (PAM) is a rare idiopathic disorder that pathologically is characterized by the accumulation of small calcified microliths within the alveolar spaces. It may be acquired or familial. Patients typically have no or mild symptoms in the setting of significant lung abnormalities.

The characteristic HRCT finding is that of very small, pinhead-sized, discrete, calcified nodules. These nodules may be perilymphatic or centrilobular in distribution and are most severe in the posterior and inferior lungs. Ground glass opacity and reticulation may be seen, but are not specifically suggestive of PAM. The differential diagnosis includes diffuse parenchymal amyloidosis and metastatic calcification. Granulomatous diseases and pneumoconioses associated with calcification produce nodules larger than those seen in PAM.

ERDHEIM-CHESTER DISEASE

This rare systemic disorder is characterized by infiltration of various organs by non–Langerhans cell histiocytosis (LCH). The bones are most commonly affected, but involvement of the central nervous system, heart, kidneys, and lymphatic system may also be present. Pulmonary involvement is uncommon, but if present has a poor prognosis. Erdheim-Chester disease classically presents in middle-aged men with chronic dyspnea or cough.

The HRCT findings in Erdheim-Chester have a lymphatic distribution. Smooth interlobular septal and fissural thickening resembling pulmonary edema or lymphangitic carcinomatosis are most characteristic. Small nodules may be present in a centrilobular or perilymphatic distribution (Fig. 18.7). Other lung findings such as ground glass opacity may be present but are not particularly characteristic. Hilar, mediastinal, and axillary lymphadenopathy are commonly present. As Erdheim-Chester disease is rare, a combination of HRCT findings and characteristic bone lesions is most suggestive.

LYMPHANGIOLEIOMYOMATOSIS

Lymphangioleiomyomatosis (LAM) is a rare disorder characterized by abnormal smooth muscle proliferation involving the lymphatics, airways, and vessels. It may be sporadic or associated with tuberous sclerosis. The sporadic form is seen almost exclusively in women of childbearing age. The clinical presentation is quite variable. Patients may present with chronic dyspnea or spontaneous pneumothorax.

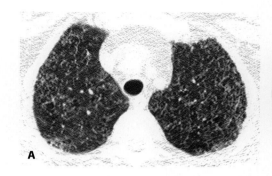

A

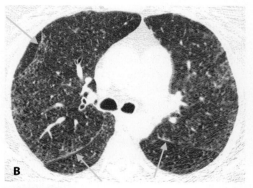

B

Figure 18.7

Erdheim-Chester disease. A. Tiny nodules are present in a patchy and upper lung distribution. The predominance of subpleural nodules (arrows) **(B)** suggests a perilymphatic distribution. This is one manifestation of Erdheim-Chester disease.

Occasionally, lung cysts are discovered as an incidental finding. Pulmonary hypertension is not uncommonly associated with LAM, but is less common than with pulmonary LCH.

The principal HRCT finding is the presence of lung cysts (Table 18.4). Cysts tend to be round and thin walled and show uniform

Table 18.4	HRCT findings of lymphangioleiomyomatosis

Women of childbearing age, sometimes associated with tuberous sclerosis
Round, thin-walled cysts
Diffuse distribution, lung bases equally involved
Low-attenuation consolidation
Nodules rare
Pleural effusion in some
Associated with renal angiomyolipoma

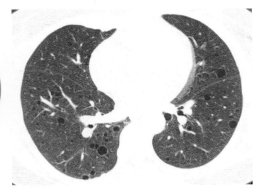

Figure 18.8

Lymphangioleiomyomatosis (LAM). A relatively mild case of LAM in a middle-aged woman is depicted, showing scattered round cysts. This was an incidental finding on a CT performed to evaluate possible malignancy.

involvement of the lung from apex to base. A few scattered cysts may be present (Fig. 18.8) or there may be near-complete replacement of the lung (Fig. 18.9). Associated nodules are rare. Pleural effusions are common and are due to lymphatic obstruction. Patients with tuberous sclerosis and some patients with isolated LAM may show associated abnormalities such as renal angiomyolipomas (Fig. 18.10).

Both LAM and LCH (see Chapter 11) may show extensive cystic lung disease. Demographics are important in distinguishing these diseases as LAM is seen in females of childbearing age (it is very rare in men), whereas LCH is usually associated with cigarette smoking. Nodules are common with LCH and rare

with LAM. The cysts of LCH tend to be irregular and lobulated in contrast to the round cysts of LAM. Pleural effusions in association with cystic lung disease suggest LAM. Other causes of cystic lung disease, such as lymphoid interstitial pneumonia, usually show fewer cysts.

BIRT-HOGG-DUBÉ SYNDROME

Birt-Hogg-Dubé syndrome is an inherited disorder characterized by a combination of skin lesions, renal tumors, and lung cysts. Occasionally, lung cysts are the only manifestation, although the other manifestations may develop later in the course of the disease. It often presents initially with pneumothorax, when a cyst perforates into the pleural space.

The primary HRCT manifestation of Birt-Hogg-Dubé syndrome is lung cysts (Fig. 18.11). These are thin walled and variable in size. The cysts are most numerous in the subpleural and medial lung bases. They are often directly adjacent to the pulmonary veins and arteries. This distribution of cysts may be specifically suggestive of Birt-Hogg-Dubé syndrome, although it is also seen in lymphocytic interstitial pneumonia (LIP). The cysts tend to be less numerous than those seen in LAM and LCH. Other causes of lung cysts include LIP, pneumatoceles from prior infection, and neurofibromatosis.

FAMILIAL PULMONARY FIBROSIS

Some patients with pulmonary fibrosis, resembling idiopathic pulmonary fibrosis, fibrotic sarcoidosis, or fibrotic hypersensitivity

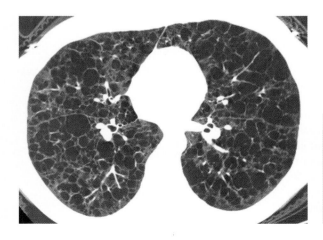

Figure 18.9

Lymphangioleiomyomatosis (LAM). An advanced case of LAM is shown, with extensive replacement of the lung parenchyma by thin-walled cysts. This woman patient presented with dyspnea and pulmonary hypertension.

18

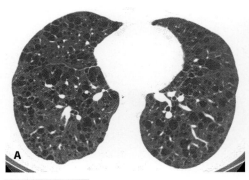
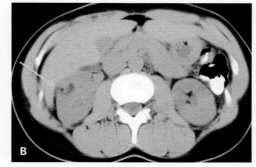

Figure 18.10

Tuberous sclerosis. HRCT and pathologic findings of cystic lung disease in tuberous sclerosis are identical to those of isolated lymphangioleiomyomatosis. **A.** HRCT shows a diffuse distribution of thin-walled, round cysts. **B.** CT through the abdomen shows a fat-containing renal mass (*arrow*) compatible with an angiomyolipoma.

pneumonitis, have a familial history of similar abnormalities. Such patients are considered to have *familial pulmonary fibrosis*. Pathologically, patients with familial fibrosis often have a pattern of usual interstitial pneumonia (similar to idiopathic pulmonary fibrosis), but findings compatible with hypersensitivity pneumonitis or sarcoidosis are also possible. A genetic cause has been identified in a subset of patients with disorders such as surfactant protein C or telomerase mutations, but the majority of cases of familial pulmonary fibrosis are idiopathic.

HRCT findings often show typical features of fibrosis, but the distribution of these is variable and may be atypical (Fig. 18.12). A family history is necessary to make the diagnosis. There may be variable HRCT patterns within the same family.

Hermansky-Pudlak Syndrome

Hermansky-Pudlak syndrome is an inherited disorder characterized by albinism, platelet dysfunction, and pulmonary fibrosis. Renal and intestinal abnormalities may also be present, but pulmonary disease is the most common cause of mortality. This disorder is seen with a particularly high prevalence in Puerto Rico.

There are no HRCT findings that specifically suggests Hermansky-Pudlak syndrome, thus diagnosis is usually made clinically. Fibrosis is the most common finding and manifests as irregular reticulation and traction bronchiectasis (Fig. 18.13). It has a variable distribution, but is often peripheral. HRCT performed early in the progression of the disease shows ground glass opacity and mild reticulation.

Figure 18.11

Birt-Hogg-Dubé syndrome. Scattered cysts are seen in a patient presenting with bilateral pneumothoraces. Some of the cysts are directly adjacent to pulmonary veins in the lower lobes (*arrow*), a finding that may be suggestive of this syndrome.

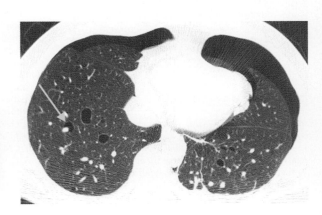

18

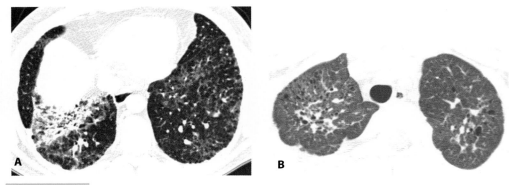

A

B

Figure 18.12

Familial pulmonary fibrosis. Two patients in the same family with familial pulmonary fibrosis are shown (**A** and **B**). On biopsy, the histologic pattern was that of usual interstitial pneumonia. **A.** One patient shows patchy basilar predominant ground glass opacity and mild traction bronchiectasis in the lung base. **B.** The other patient shows upper lobe and centrally predominant reticulation, traction bronchiectasis, and cysts. HRCT findings are often atypical in patients with familial pulmonary fibrosis.

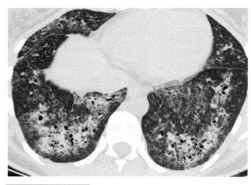

Figure 18.13

Hermansky-Pudlak syndrome. HRCT shows peripheral and basilar predominant irregular reticulation, traction bronchiectasis, and consolidation. The presence of subpleural sparing would be suggestive of nonspecific interstitial pneumonia, but the demographics and other associated abnormalities in this patient were compatible with Hermansky-Pudlak syndrome.

FURTHER READING

Aberle DR, Hansell DM, Brown K, Tashkin DP. Lymphangiomyomatosis: CT, chest radiographic, and functional correlations. *Radiology*. 1990;176:381-387.

Agarwal PP, Gross BH, Holloway BJ, et al. Thoracic CT findings in Birt-Hogg-Dube syndrome. *AJR Am J Roentgenol*. 2011;196:349-352.

Aylwin ACB, Gishen P, Copley SJ. Imaging appearance of thoracic amyloidosis. *J Thorac Imaging*. 2005;20:41-46.

Ayuso MC, Gilabert R, Bombi JA, Salvador A. CT appearance of localized pulmonary amyloidosis. *J Comput Assist Tomogr*. 1987;11:197-199.

Brun AL, Touitou-Gottenberg D, Haroche J, et al. Erdheim-Chester disease: CT findings of thoracic involvement. *Eur Radiol*. 2010;20:2579-2587.

Cluzel P, Grenier P, Bernadac P, et al. Pulmonary alveolar microlithiasis: CT findings. *J Comput Assist Tomogr*. 1991;15:938-942.

Deniz O, Ors F, Tozkoparan E, et al. High resolution computed tomographic features of pulmonary alveolar microlithiasis. *Eur J Radiol*. 2005;55:452-460.

Franquet T, Giménez A, Bordes R, et al. The crazy-paving pattern in exogenous lipoid pneumonia: CT-pathologic correlation. *AJR Am J Roentgenol*. 1998;170:315-317.

Georgiades CS, Neyman EG, Barish MA, et al. Amyloidosis: review and CT manifestations. *Radiographics*. 2004;24:405-416.

Graham CM, Stern EJ, Finkbeiner WE, Webb WR. High-resolution CT appearance of diffuse alveolar septal amyloidosis. *AJR Am J Roentgenol*. 1992;158:265-267.

Helbich TH, Wojnarovsky C, Wunderbaldinger P, et al. Pulmonary alveolar microlithiasis in children: radiographic and high-resolution CT findings. *AJR Am J Roentgenol*. 1997;168:63-65.

Johkoh T, Itoh H, Müller NL, et al. Crazy-paving appearance at thin-section CT: spectrum of disease and pathologic findings. *Radiology*. 1999;211:155-160.

Kirchner J, Stein A, Viel K, et al. Pulmonary lymphangioleiomyomatosis: high-resolution CT findings. *Eur Radiol*. 1999;9:49-54.

Korn MA, Schurawitzki H, Klepetko W, Burghuber OC. Pulmonary alveolar microlithiasis: findings on high-resolution CT. *AJR Am J Roentgenol*. 1992;158:981-982.

Lee KN, Levin DL, Webb WR, et al. Pulmonary alveolar proteinosis: high-resolution CT, chest radiographic, and functional correlations. *Chest.* 1997; 111:989-995.

Lee KS, Müller NL, Hale V, et al. Lipoid pneumonia: CT findings. *J Comput Assist Tomogr.* 1995;19:48-51.

Lenoir S, Grenier P, Brauner MW, et al. Pulmonary lymphangiomyomatosis and tuberous sclerosis: comparison of radiographic and thin-section CT findings. *Radiology.* 1990;175:329-334.

Müller NL, Chiles C, Kullnig P. Pulmonary lymphangiomyomatosis: correlation of CT with radiographic and functional findings. *Radiology.* 1990;175:335-339.

Pickford HA, Swensen SJ, Utz JP. Thoracic cross-sectional imaging of amyloidosis. *AJR Am J Roentgenol.* 1997;168: 351-355.

Templeton PA, McLoud TC, Müller NL, et al. Pulmonary lymphangioleiomyomatosis: CT and pathologic findings. *J Comput Assist Tomogr.* 1989;13:54-57.

18

Index

Index

Note: Locators followed by 'f' and 't' refer to figures and tables respectively.